The Immune Response and its Suppression

Antibiotica et Chemotherapia

Vol. 15

Redactor: A. De Weck, Bern

Collaboratores

Beck, D., Zürich – Gsell, O., Basel – Knothe, H., Frankfurt
Rauenbusch, E., Wuppertal-Elberfeld – Siegenthaler, W., Zürich
Scholtan, W., Leverkusen – Struller, Th., Basel – Weidmann, P., Zürich

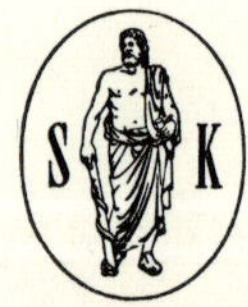

BASEL (Switzerland)   S. KARGER   NEW YORK

An International Symposium held at the Forschungsinstitut Davos
March 1968

The Immune Response and its Suppression

Edited by E. SORKIN, Davos

With 148 figures and 64 tables

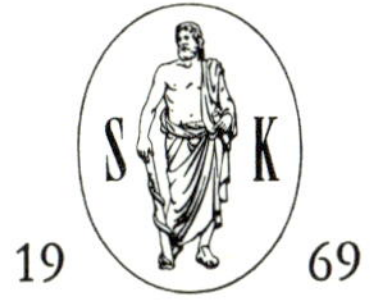

19 69

BASEL (Switzerland)   S. KARGER   NEW YORK

Antibiotica et Chemotherapia

Vol. 1: X + 378 p., 113 fig., 1 plc., 1954. sFr. 52.—.

Vol. 2: VI + 300 p., 21 fig., 1955. sFr. 40.—.

Vol. 3: VIII + 398 p., 45 fig., 1956. sFr. 56.—.

Vol. 4: VIII + 392 p., 49 fig., 1957. sFr. 64.—.

Vol. 5: VI + 337 p., 12 fig., 1958. sFr. 60.—.

Vol. 6: VIII + 530 p., 23 fig., 60 tab., 1959. sFr. 83.—.

Vol. 7: Corticosteroide und Infektion. Teil 1. X + 374 p., 52 fig., 1960. sFr. 64.—.

Vol. 8: 1st International Symposium on Anti-infectious and Antimitotic Chemothera-py/1. Internationales Symposium über antiinfektiöse und antimitotische Chemo-therapie/1er Symposium international de chimiothérapie anti-infectieuse et anti-mitotique, Genève 1959. Hgb. von/edited by/dirigé par H.P. KÜMMERLE (Tü-bingen). P. RENTCHNICK (Genève) und A. SENN (Bern). XII + 430 p., 150 fig., 1960. sFr. 70.—.

Vol. 9: IV + 192 p., 32 fig., 25 tab., 1961. sFr. 40.—.

Vol. 10: VIII + 434 p., 36 fig., 24 tab., 1962. sFr. 75.50.

Vol. 11: 2nd International Symposium of Chemotherapy / 2. Internationales Symposium für Chemotherapie / 2e Symposium international de chimiothérapie, Naples 1961. Part I: New Antibiotics – Neue Antibiotica – Nouveaux antibiotiques. Side Effects of Modern Chemotherapy – Nebenwirkungen der modernen Chemo-therapeutica – Effects secondaires des chimiothérapies modernes. XXII + 354 p., 54 fig., 85 tab., 1963. sFr. 78.—.

Vol. 12: Pharmakokinetik und Arzneimitteldosierung / Pharmacokinetics and Drug Dosage. Kolloquium im Forschungsinstitut Borstel 1962. Hgb. von / edited by: ENNO FREERKSEN (Borstel), unter Mitarbeit von / with the collaboration of L. DETTLI (Basel), E. KRÜGER-THIEMER (Borstel), E. NELSON (Buffalo, N.Y.). XVI + 455 p., 161 fig., 46 tab., 1964. sFr. 70.—.

Vol. 13: VIII + 316 p., 25 fig., 20 tab., 1965. sFr. 74.—.

Vol. 14: VIII + 280 p., 75 fig., 41 tab., 1968. sFr. 69.—.

S. Karger AG, Arnold-Böcklin-Strasse 25, 4000 Basel 11 (Switzerland)

Contents

Contents

Foreword

The aim of this book is to bring together in one volume various aspects of "The immune response and its suppression". This timely issue was discussed at an International Symposium held at the Forschungsinstitut, Davos, Switzerland from March 25 to 28, 1968. Although the freshness of the discussions and the friendly spirit prevailing at the meeting cannot be brought forth in this volume, we feel certain that it will serve the useful purpose of bringing together, perhaps for first time, most aspects of the young and increasingly important field of immunosuppression. It is even hoped that it may help to shape future work on immunosuppression. Outstanding immunologists have set down their thoughts here and presented their work on the immune response and how to interfere with it. It is first of all these active participants whom I wish to thank. Dr. J. H. HUMPHREY F.R.S. and Dr. M. LANDY gave me most valuable advice in the preparatory stages of this meeting.

The generous financial aid of the Swiss Chemical Companies Ciba AG, J. R. Geigy AG, F. Hoffmann-La Roche, Sandoz AG and G. Wander AG is gratefully acknowledged. Without their willing help and the one by Dr. R. M. KUNZ (F. Hoffmann-La Roche), this Symposium would not have taken place. The Landschaft Davos and the Kanton Graubünden also made some financial contributions.

Finally I would like to thank my former secretary, Miss Grethe Simonsen, for her patient and excellent help in organizing the Symposium.

E. SORKIN, Davos

Antibiotica et Chemotherapia, vol. 15, pp. 1–6 (Karger, Basel/New York 1969)

General Introduction

J. H. HUMPHREY

National Institute for Medical Research, London

The opening contribution to a symposium on "The Immune Response and its Suppression" should ideally set out a complete scheme outlining the events from the introduction of antigen and its interaction with immunologically competent cells to the production of antibody or of specifically sensitized cells, indicating at each stage how or where the process might be interfered with or switched off. Since subsequent contributors will be discussing different aspects of this sequence of events, presentation of such a scheme would come much better after than before their formal discussion; the main part of my contribution will, in fact, concern the fate of antigen and its relevance to antibody responses. However, Dr. SORKIN requested that I make a few brief and general remarks about the stages at which interference with immunological responses may occur, and I will do so—largely to confirm that I agree with his choice of subjects and speakers for this symposium!

The picture which I have at the moment (though it is liable to change!) is as follows: Immunologically competent cells are lymphocytes. They originate from stem cells (arising in the bone marrow certainly—elsewhere not proved) and acquire their capacity to exhibit immunological responsiveness as a result of some complex process which requires the presence of a thymus [MILLER and OSOBA, 1967]. Part of this process appears to involve a humoral influence by the thymus epithelium (perhaps a hormone required to confer on thymocytes the property of becoming long lived lymphocytes), and part may be a process of rapid multiplication within the thymus during which "diversity" (i.e. responsiveness to many different antigenic determinants) is generated in the dividing cell populations. Most of the thymus lymphocytes die in the thymus, but some escape into the circulation whence they enter lymphoid tissues and generate the lymphocytes which populate the "thymus dependent" areas of lymphoid tissue [PARROTT, DE SOUSA and EAST, 1966], and circulate via lymphatic ducts to the blood and back to the lymphoid tissue via postcapillary venules as described by GOWANS and KNIGHT [1964]. I am not sure that the traffic from blood to lymphoid tissues via the postcapillary venules is wholly in one direction. GOWANS never claimed that it was so, and others [SAINTE-MARIE, SIN and CHAN, 1967] have provided evidence suggesting a traffic in the reverse direction. Once such lymphocytes have left the thymus they are able to live an independent existence, and to divide and multiply (possibly only when stimulated by specific antigens) in these "thymus dependent" areas. It is in the "thymus dependent" areas of lymphoid tissues that the multiplication of the "sensitized" lymphocytes which engage in cell mediated immunity responses primarily and predominantly takes place [OORT and TURK, 1965]. Whether these cells are stimulated by antigen arriving in the lymphoid tissue, or whether they are stimulated by contact with the antigen at some surface peripherally and then "home" to the draining node via the lymphatic vessels is an open question. What seems certain is that after stimulation has occurred differentiation to "blast" forms and multiplication precedes the appearance of new "sensitized" lymphocytes.

The immunologically competent cells which interact with immunogens so as to go on to form antibody are also lymphocytes—perhaps originally the same population as can engage in cell mediated specific immunity[1]. However, they have become in some way different—perhaps because they have different surface properties and tend to populate and multiply in anatomically different parts of the lymphoid system, and to undergo their cycle of post-thymic free existence in a physiologically different environment. In birds there is good evidence that a separate influence (hormonal or environmental?) exerted by the Bursa of Fabricius is necessary for the development of immunologically competent cells with these different properties. COOPER, GABRIELSEN and GOOD [1967] have made out a persuasive

---

[1] There is increasing evidence that antibody producing cells are derived from the bone marrow without undergoing proliferation in the thymus, although cooperation between marrow-derived and thymus-derived cells is necessary for the antibody response to some, and perhaps to most immunogens [e.g. MITCHELL, G.B. and MILLER, J.F.A.P.; Nature 216: 659–663 (1967)].

case, based on an analysis of congenital immunological deficiency diseases, that a similar developmental influence acts in man and other mammals. They postulate that there are some tissues functionally equivalent to the avian Bursa, and suggest that these lie along the intestinal tract, but the evidence for this is no more than suggestive [Cooper, Perey, McKneally, Gabrielsen, Sutherland and Good, 1966]. Certainly it seems that if the thymus influence is lacking at some early critical stage, even though cells may be able to produce immunoglobulins (under the influence of the bursa or its equivalent) they nevertheless fail to make effective antibody against known determinants—i.e. diversity of response is somehow lacking.

It is not clear to me where and how in lymphoid tissues *in vivo* immunologically competent cells are stimulated by antigen so as to go on to form antibody. In response to a primary stimulus antibody-producing cells are first seen in the medulla of lymph nodes and in the red pulp (or at the border of the red and white pulp) of the spleen, in close proximity to the sinus-lining macrophages which have engulfed antigen. At first sight this suggests that this is where the primary stimulation has occurred. However, when introduction of an immunogen leads to antibody formation this is commonly, though not always accompanied by the rapid enlargement of primary follicles to form germinal centres and/or the enlargement of existing germinal centres in lymph nodes and spleen. As will be mentioned later the earliest antibody forming cells are not found in these germinal centres, although in the presence of "natural" or acquired antibody antigens very soon become trapped on the reticular cells in them. What then are the germinal centres doing? As was shown by the Symposium on "Germinal Centers in Immune Responses" organized by Prof. H. Cottier [1966] we do not really know. The germinal centres contain lymphocytes and rapidly dividing "blast" cells, many of which die there. The origin of the "blast" cells may be lymphocytes which entered from the marginal sinus or from the blood (though rather few appear to enter this way [Parrott, 1966]. The surviving progeny of the "blast" cells appear to provide the lymphocytes in the mantle zone around the centre. What happens to them after this is uncertain. Perhaps they leave and enter the blood via postcapillary venules [in the opposite direction to the circulating lymphocytes studied by Gowans and Knight], or perhaps some migrate into the medulla directly. It is a matter of controversy whether the germinal centre blast cells themselves contain immunoglobulin; however, it is not uncommon in a very active germinal centre to see the blast cells apparently "erupting" through the mantle zone along the tract of a blood vessel and forming a continuous sequence from blast cells which contain no detectable immunoglobulin to cells in the medulla which are typical immunoglobulin-containing plasma cells [BALFOUR and HUMPHREY, 1966]. I shall return to the subject of germinal centres later, and leave it at the moment that they seem to be important in antibody responses, but that we do not really know how they function.

I shall also discuss later the importance of uptake of antigen by macrophages for antibody formation. At this stage I wish only to state that the stimulation of immunologically competent cells to become antibody producers involves differentiation (including the development of the appropriate protein synthesizing mechanisms), usually followed by cell division. The stage of differentiation includes a "lag" period of about 24 h [see review in DUTTON and MISHELL, 1967]. Although there is evidence that antibody production can occur without cell proliferation [STERZL, 1967; BUSSARD and LURIE, 1967] significant antibody responses are usually accompanied by multiplication of antibody forming cells through several cycles of mitotic division. This aspect has been reviewed often [e. g. SERCARZ and COONS, 1962; STERZL, 1967].

"Memory" cells or primed cells—i. e. cells specifically responsive to the same antigenic stimulus—also arise in the course of the cell multiplication which accompanies stimulation of cell mediated immunity and antibody production. Such cells probably do not differ fundamentally from the immunologically competent lymphocytes which are first stimulated by the initial contact with the immunogen, but there are many more of them, and they are likely to have been selected (as a result of selective multiplication of those best fitted to interact with antigen in the first place and of subsequent further selection by competition for antigen with antibody—when this is produced) so that they are able to interact more avidly and specifically with individual determinants on the immunogen. Such cells can then leave the site of origin via the efferent lymphatic vessels and populate other lymphoid tissues [HALL, 1967]. I do not know what decides that a memory cell shall be formed rather than one which goes on to become an antibody secreting plasma cell; the use of small amounts of the immunogen, and perhaps its uptake by macrophages may be important (see STERZL later in this symposium), but for the present purpose it only matters that cell multiplication is involved.

This general outline is superficial, both because of limitations of space and of grasp on my part, but it may help to pin-point some of the steps at which interference with the immune response may occur. These would be by:

a) Preventing the development of stem cells into immunologically competent cells (e.g. by early thymectomy $\pm$ bursectomy; adult thymectomy, and irradiation $\pm$ bursectomy).

b) Destroying immunologically competent cells or inactivating them (e.g. by altering their surface) so that they can no longer interact with antigen (e.g. by antilymphocytic serum or x-rays).

c) Preventing effective contact between antigen and immunologically competent cells—e.g. by concealing the antigenic determinant sites by coating with antibody.

d) When presentation of antigen via macrophages is an important or obligatory step, preventing the function of macrophages e.g. by ingestion of irrelevant materials (blockade, overloading), or by preventing the "processing" of antigen (possibly by x-irradiation or corticosteroid hormones).

e) Interfering during the inductive or lag phase with the intracellular reorganization which follows stimulation of immunologically competent cells by antigen (e.g. by antimetabolites).

f) Preventing multiplication and differentiation of stimulated cells, so as to interfere with the generation of effector cells as well as of memory cells (e.g. by x-irradiation, radiomimetic agents, antimetabolites).

g) Interfering with protein synthetic mechanisms involved in immunoglobulin synthesis (e.g. by amino acid analogues, puromycin etc).

h) Specific paralysis—i.e. the induction of specific immunological unresponsiveness—will be discussed by others, and I mention it here only for completeness. It is an alternative response by immunologically competent cells to successful stimulation and both may occur at the same time. Specific paralysis includes both low zone paralysis and high zone paralysis. Their mechanisms may be quite different, insofar that the one may abort the immune response by killing or inactivating the competent cells before they function at all, and the other may encourage them to premature senescence or suicidal proliferation. It is sufficient to note here that a measure which makes an immunogen less effective in stimulating an immune response is liable to make it more effective in causing immune paralysis.

References

BALFOUR, B.M. and HUMPHREY, J.H.: Localization of labeled antigen in germinal centres and its relationship to the immune response. In: Germinal centres in immune responses. pp. 80–85 (Springer-Verlag, Berlin 1966).

BUSSARD, A.E. and LURIE, M.: Primary antibody response *in vitro* in peritoneal cells. J. exp. Med. *125:* 873–892 (1967).

COOPER, M.D.; GABRIELSEN, A.E. and GOOD, R.A.: Role of the thymus and other central lymphoid tissues in immunological disease. Ann. Rev. Med. *18:* 113–138 (1967).

COOPER, M.D.; PEREY, D.Y.; McKNEALLY, M.F.; GABRIELSEN, A.E.; SUTHERLAND, D.E. and GOOD, R.A.: A mammalian equivalent of the avian bursa of Fabricius. Lancet *i:* 1388–1391 (1966).

COTTIER, H.; ODARTCHENKO, N.; SCHINDLER, R. and CONGDON, C.C. (Eds.): Germinal centres in immune responses (Springer-Verlag, Berlin 1966).

DUTTON, R.W. and MISHELL, R.I.: Proliferation and differentiation in the immune response. In: Symposium on cytoplasmic and environmental influence on nuclear behaviour. Soc. Gen. Physiol. (N.J. Prentice-Hall Inc., 1967).

GOWANS, J.L. and KNIGHT, J.E.: The route of recirculation of lymphocytes in the rat. Proc. roy. Soc. (Lond.) B *159:* 257–282 (1964).

HALL, J.G.: Studies of the cells in the afferent and efferent lymph of lymph nodes draining the site of skin homografts. J. exp. Med. *125:* 737–754 (1967).

MILLER, J.F.A.P. and OSOBA, D.: Current concepts of the immunological function of the thymus. Physiol. Rev. *47:* 437–519 (1967).

OORT, J. and TURK, J.K.: A histological and autoradiographic study of lymph nodes during the development of contact sensitivity in the guinea-pig. Brit. J. exp. Path. *46:* 147–154 (1965).

PARROTT, D.M.V.: The integrity of the germinal center: An investigation of the differential localization of labeled cells in lymphoid organs. In: Germinal centers in immune responses (Ed. H. COTTIER), pp. 168–175 (Springer-Verlag, Berlin 1966).

PARROTT, D.M.V.; DE SOUSA, M.A.B. and EAST, J.: Thymus-dependent areas in the lymphoid organs of neonatally thymectomized mice. J. exp. Med. *123:* 191–203 (1966).

SAINTE-MARIE, G.; SIN, Y.M. and CHAN, C.: The diapedises of lymphocytes through post-capillary venules of rat lymph nodes. Rev. Canad. Biol. *26:* 141–151 (1967).

SERCARZ, E. and COONS, A.H.: The exhaustion of specific antibody producing capacity during a secondary response. In: Mechanisms of immunological tolerance. pp. 73–83, Czech. Acad. Sci. Prague (1962).

ŠTERZL, J.: Factors determining the differentiation pathways of immunocompetent cells. Cold Spring Harbor Symp. on quant. Biology *32:* 493–506 (1967).

Author's address: Dr. J.H. HUMPHREY, National Institute for Medical Research, Mill Hill, *London, N.W. 7* (England).

Antibiotica et Chemotherapia, vol. 15, pp. 7–23 (Karger, Basel/New York 1969)

The Fate of Antigen
and its Relationship to the Immune Response
The Complexity of Antigens

J. H. HUMPHREY

National Institute for Medical Research, London

Before discussing in detail what can be learned by studying the fate of antigens about the nature of their interaction with immunologically competent cells I wish to make two points. The first is that substances used experimentally as antigens or immunogens differ enormously in respect of size, shape, antigenic complexity, chemical nature, electric charge, stability to extracellular and intracellular enzymes, rates of disappearance from body fluids and of catabolism, and many other properties. This seems so obvious that it would not require stating, but for the fact that to lump together anything from a synthetic polypeptide to an erythrocyte under the general term "antigen" is liable to lead to generalizations which are unwarrantable unless it is realized that only the highest common factor of the behaviour of all immunogens is being studied. These strictures will need to be applied to my own contribution!

The second point is that antibodies against immunogens possessing a tertiary or even quaternary structures have been found, when tested suitably, to include antibodies specific for determinants whose conformation depends upon these structures [e.g. CRUMPTON, 1967; SELIGMANN and MIHAESCO, 1967; RAJEWSKI, ROTTLÄNDER, PELTRE and MÜLLER, 1967; HENNEY, STANWORTH and GELL, 1965]. This implies that the immunogen at the time when it initiates stimulation of suitable immunologically competent cells can do so in an undegraded and undistorted form. Since the immunogen may be a large molecule or even a complex of large molecules, this limits the number of ways or sites in which effective interaction with the immunologically competent cells can occur, and argues, I think rather strongly, that this interaction takes place at a surface. The most probable surface would be the exterior of the immunologically competent cell, bearing a "receptor" of the kind which Mitchison will talk about later, although it could conceivably be an internal surface. However, if the immunogen is also on the surface of another cell—e.g. of a macrophage or of a reticulum cell—then the argument for an external surface is strengthened.

Factors Determining Phagocytosis

Antigens, whether particulate or soluble, introduced into the body fluids end up sooner or later in phagocytic cells. On the whole the larger they are, and the less they are in true solution, the more rapidly they are ingested by macrophages and the shorter their survival in the circulation. It is not evident why this should be so. For example, erythrocytes may circulate for many days in homologous animals, and even in a closely related species, until antibodies are formed against them. Yet the same erythrocytes are often rapidly removed and ingested by macrophages (either fixed in the reticuloendothelial system or free) in an unrelated species. This is commonly and perhaps rightly attributed to the presence of cross-reacting "natural" antibodies or opsonins in the unrelated species. However, large molecules such as haemocyanins have short half lives in the circulation, of a few hours only, in rabbits and mice and are rapidly taken up by fixed macrophages of the RES, without any detectable opsonins being present. This rapid disappearance can hardly be a question simply of size and charge, since α_2-macroglobulin, which is not dissimilar from the smaller haemocyanins in these respects, has in man at least a long half life [11–17 days; Kluthe, Hagemann and Kleine, 1967]. Some other immunogens such as salmonella flagellin in polymerized or in the smaller monomeric form, have half lives of a few hours, even in tolerant rats [Mitchell and Nossal, 1966, p. 215]. Various synthetic polypeptides composed either of D- or the L-amino acids, with differing charges, have all been found to be cleared very rapidly from the blood stream and taken up by macrophages—the L-forms, though not the D-forms, being promptly broken down [Gill, Papermaster and Mowbray, 1965; Janeway and Humphrey, 1968]. A variety of serum albumins of comparable size, however, have relatively long half lives (depending upon the species and the extent of loss via the intestine) and are ingested by macrophages very much more slowly. Nevertheless, when the same serum albumins are denatured by heating, sufficiently to diminish their solubility at the isoelectric point, they also are rapidly ingested by medullar macrophages [Lang and Ada, 1967b] although their antigenicity is not much altered. Boyden [1966] has reviewed evidence for the occurrence of natural opsonins which may or may not be cross reacting antibodies reactive with many immunogens, and these may certainly be important in causing rapid phagocytosis by macrophages. There is indeed good evidence, mentioned below, that such natural opsonins are responsible for the rapid localization of some good immunogens, such as flagella, on the reticular macrophages in germinal centres of normal animals. However, rapid uptake of antigens and other materials by *medullary* macrophages is not so obviously correlated with the presence of detectable amounts of "natural" opsonins, and I think that we must confess to being ignorant of what properties ultimately determine whether any potential immunogen will be rapidly and extensively ingested by medullary macrophages. Since its immunogenicity will be greatly influenced by its fate, this reveals an important gap in our knowledge.

The Localization of Antigens

In order to study the fate of antigens in relation to the immune response it is necessary to be able to detect and localize their presence in very small quantities. Immunofluorescence is too insensitive a method. Although some proteins, such as peroxidase [Leduc, Avrameas and Bouteille, 1968] or ferritin [Wellensiek and Coons, 1964] can be detected and localized in cells in minute amounts by electron microscopic techniques, the only general method is to use antigens extrinsically labelled with a radioactive isotope at very high specific activities, and of the isotopes available ^{125}Iodine is the most suitable. A justification for supposing that the presence of this label reflects the presence of undegraded or only partly degraded antigen has been given by Humphrey, Askonas, Auzins, Schechter and Sela [1967].

The most extensive work with radiolabelled antigens has been that of Nossal, Ada *et al.*, employing Salmonella adelaide flagella, or the purified flagellin in polymerized or unpolymerized form. These are very potent immunogens, 0.01 μg or less being sufficient to elicit a detectable primary response in rats [Nossal, Ada and Austin, 1964a]. After injection into the footpad of normal rats the great majority passes through the draining nodes, but about 0.1% is retained there. It is localized in medullary macrophages and on dendritic reticular cells in germinal centres and in primary follicles. The amount in the medullary macrophages decreases quite rapidly, though—as judged by radioactivity—a small amount persists for several weeks; that on the reticular cells of the germinal centres persists for many weeks with only a gradual diminution in radioactivity. Electron microscopic autoradiographic studies have shown that in the medullary macrophages most of these antigens are in phagocytic vacuoles or lysosomes, whereas in the case of the germinal centre reticular cells the antigens are apparently on the surface rather than within the cells [Nossal, Abbot and Mitchell, 1968; Nossal, Abbot, Mitchell and Lummus, 1968]. When flagella or flagellin are injected into primed rats the localization in medullary macrophages is somewhat increased and on germinal centres greatly so. A representative, though not exhaustive, summary of studies with various antigens in various species is given in table I. This includes both normal, primed and tolerant animals and animals passively immunized with homologous or heterologous antiserum against the antigen under study. The main points which emerge are as follows:

1. Uptake by medullary macrophages occurs to a variable extent with all antigens, even in tolerant animals, and tends to be somewhat greater when the recipients have been immunized actively or passively against the antigens.

2. a) Uptake onto reticular cells in the germinal centres occurs extensively with all antigens in primed or immunized animals. In normal animals flagella or flagellin localize in germinal centres, but some other antigens do not do so to any detectable extent—until the recipient animals have themselves begun to make antibodies against the injected antigen. In truly tolerant animals localization on germinal centres does not occur at all.

b) When rats are subjected to chronic thoracic duct drainage or are germ free, localization of flagella in germinal centres is diminished or absent. This is almost certainly attributable to the absence of natural opsonins or cross reacting antibodies in rats so treated.

Table I. Localization of antigen

Antigen	Species	Immunological status	Medullary macrophages	Germinal centre	Reference
Flagella	Rat	Normal[1]	++	++	Nossal, Ada and Austin [1964b]
Homologous IgG	Rat	Normal	+	+	Ada, Nossal and Austin [1964]
Horse ferritin	Rat	Normal	+	±	Ada, Nossal and Austin [1964]
BSA	Rat	Normal	+	±	Ada, Nossal and Austin [1964]
Heated HSA	Rat	Normal	+++	—	Lang and Ada [1967b]
HSA } Haemocyanin }	Rabbit	Normal	+	—	Humphrey and Frank [1967]
TGAL	Mouse	Normal	++	±	McDevitt, Askonas, Humphrey, Schechterl and Sela [1966]
D-TGA } L-TGA }	Mouse	Normal	+++	—	Janeway and Humphrey [1968]
Heterologous IgG	Mouse	Normal	+	+	B.M. Balfour [unpublished]
All antigens	All species	Primed	++	+++	e.g. Nossal, Ada, Austin and Pye [1965]
All antigens	All species	Passively immunized	++	+++	e.g. Lang and Ada [1967a]
Flagella	Rat	Thoracic duct drainage	++	±	Williams [1966]
Flagella	Rat	Germ free	++	—	Miller, Johnsen and Ada [1968]
HSA } Haemocyanin }	Rabbit	Tolerant	+	—	Humphrey and Frank [1967]
D-TGA	Mouse	Tolerant	+++	—	Janeway and Humphrey [1968]
Heterologous IgG	Mouse	Tolerant	+	+	B.M. Balfour [unpublished]

[1] i.e. before antibody production had occurred

c) Heterologous (and homologous) immunoglobulins localize in germinal centres, even in animals tolerant of the heterologous immunoglobulin.

The Significance of Antigen in Germinal Centres

When taken in conjunction with the demonstration that the distribution of antigen and of antibody on the germinal centre reticular cells coincides completely [Balfour and Humphrey, 1966] it is evident that localization of antigen in germinal centres depends upon its being trapped by pre-existing specific or cross reacting antibody on the surface of the reticular cells. Such cells appear to take up immunoglobulin reversibly from the surrounding fluid; both IgG and IgM are present on them as judged by immunofluorescent staining, but whether there is a selective uptake of a special cytophilic fraction is uncertain. It seems probable that once antigen has also combined, attachment of the resultant complex with immunoglobulin to the reticular cells becomes largely irreversible.

Although excellent immunogens such as flagella show primary localization in germinal centres of unprimed animals, other reasonably good immunogens such as haemocyanin do not. Such localization cannot therefore be a *necessary* condition for a *primary* response. An experiment performed by my colleagues Drs. B. A. Askonas and I. Auzins demonstrated that such localization is also not a *sufficient* condition. They primed mice with a hapten-protein conjugate NIP-BGG [Brownstone, Mitchison and Pitt-Rivers, 1966] adsorbed on alum, and measured the binding power of the serum for the hapten using NIP-ovalbumin. After three weeks, when anti-NIP elicited by the primary stimulus was still present in the blood, the mice were given a further injection via the footpad, one half receiving 1 μg soluble ^{125}I labelled NIP-BGG and the other half 1 μg soluble labelled NIP-HSA. Both antigens became rapidly and extensively localized in germinal centres, by virtue of the anti-NIP present. However, eight days later the mice injected with NIP-HSA showed no rise in anti-NIP antibodies, whereas those injected with NIP-BGG showed a large secondary response to the NIP hapten. This is, of course, an example of the well recognized "carrier" effect—but it demonstrates that for a response to occur cells primed to respond to the specific antigen must be present and that antigen localized in germinal centres has no special capacity to evoke them.

Even though antigen trapping in germinal centres is not necessary for the initiation of a primary immune response, this striking phenomenon is unlikely to be without biological importance. The sequence of events in the chicken spleen after a primary injection of soluble antigens could provide a hint of what this might be. In the chick large numbers of antibody-producing cells are found in the medulla of the spleen as early as the second day after administration of human albumin or diphtheria toxoid, and they persist there for a further 6 days or so. Meanwhile, after the first antibody has appeared, reticular macrophages with trapped antigen on their surface migrate into the white pulp, and appear to act as a focus for germinal centre formation; in some of these centres, *after* antibody producing cells have largely disappeared from the medulla, clusters of antibody producing cells eventually appear intimately associated with the antigen-retaining reticular cells [WHITE, FRENCH and STARK, 1966]. This sequence suggests that antigen trapped in germinal centres may be particularly well situated to stimulate cells already primed elsewhere to go on to produce antibody. Direct evidence is lacking however that primed cells do enter germinal centres of lymph nodes, or that they are stimulated there to proliferate and differentiate into the antibody containing cells which are readily detected in the medulla. A current experiment to test the suggestion, by transfusing ³H-labelled lymphocytes from mice primed with human albumin or lysozyme into isogeneic tolerant mice, whose axillary lymph nodes contained one or the other antigen complexed with antibody in their germinal centres, has not so far shown any evidence of selective attraction of the primed cells to the node containing the appropriate antigen nor of their stimulation there to form antibody [BALFOUR, PARROTT and HUMPHREY, unpublished].

NOSSAL [1967], despite the objections which he recognizes, does not exclude a role in the induction of primary antibody responses for the antigen trapped on reticular cells of primary follicles and of germinal centres. However, he proposes that a more important role for such antigen may be in the induction of immunological memory, and suggests that the cells which proliferate in the germinal centres give rise to primed or "memory", rather than to antibody-producing cells. A quite different, but not necessarily contradictory hypothesis is that antigen trapped in germinal centres causes specific immunological paralysis of unprimed but competent lymphocytes which first come into contact with antigen at these sites. This possibility has been suggested by ADA and PARISH [1968] to explain the remarkable observation that administration to adult rats of so few as 10^8 molecules of a partially degraded preparation of flagellin results in a very considerable degree of specific tolerance. Since an adult rat contains some 4×10^9 lymphocytes, any or all of which must presumably have an opportunity to come into contact with the antigen for tolerance to occur, and since most of the antigen is known rapidly to be degraded, there is a clear implication that some molecules of antigen must contact many lymphocytes. Degraded flagellin localizes, as does the parent molecule, strongly in germinal centres in normal rats. Conceivably it could, in the course of time, there contact all the available lymphocytes so as to make unprimed but competent cells tolerant. Unfortunately, as mentioned earlier, too little is known about what happens to cells in germinal centres to allow any clear decision whether either of these hypotheses about the function of antigen there is correct.

The Significance of Antigen Uptake by Macrophages

If the immunological role of antigen on the reticular cells in the germinal centres is still a mystery, can we be more definite about that of antigen taken up by macrophages elsewhere in the lymphoid tissues? Because all antigens are taken up more or less rapidly by these cells it is difficult *in vivo* to disentangle effects due to antigen which is free from that which is associated with macrophages. The difficulty can be overcome by deliberately introducing antigen already taken up by macrophages and comparing its effects with those of a similar quantity of antigen introduced by the same route in the free form (even though much of this is also destined to be taken up by macrophages).

For technical reasons the cells used to study macrophage associated antigen are commonly obtained from the peritoneal cavity, whereas the cells in which the antigen is mainly found in lymphoid tissues of unprimed animals are the macrophages lining the medullary and marginal sinuses. Peritoneal macrophages are morphologically similar to those in the tissues, and they can be shown in mice to migrate to the medullary areas of spleen and lymph nodes after passive transfer [ROSER, 1965; RUSSELL and ROSER, 1966]; furthermore the time courses of uptake, degradation and retention of some antigens by normal lymph nodes and by peritoneal macrophages have been shown to be broadly similar [ASKONAS, AUZINS and UNANUE, 1968]. It is probably reasonable to infer that the observed effects of antigen associated with peritoneal macrophages will reflect those of antigen in lymphoid tissue medullary macrophages in a qualitative manner, while bearing in mind when such effects involve close interaction between lymphocytes and macrophages, those *in situ* in the lymphoid tissues may be more effective than those in the peritoneal cavity, the liver or elsewhere.

"Superantigens"

It has been known for many years that macrophages of the liver, bone marrow and lymphoid tissue not only ingest both inert and living particulate and macromolecular materials but also break most of these down rather rapidly. Nevertheless, small amounts of the ingested foreign materials may be retained for weeks or months, and can be recovered in a form which retains both antigenic and immunogenic properties [HAUROWITZ, 1960; CAMPBELL and GARVEY, 1963] and, as extracted, appears to be associated with RNA [CAMPBELL and GARVEY, 1963]. Interest in the possible immunological significance of RNA-associated antigen from macrophages was much stimulated by FISHMAN and ADLER's [1963] observation that RNA extracts from macrophages which had ingested T_2 bacteriophage for a brief period, when added to normal lymph node cells induced these to make specific phage neutralizing antibody—whereas contact between lymph node cells and T_2 phage alone was ineffective.

It has now been confirmed in several laboratories that during the first hours after macrophages have been exposed to a variety of different antigens, phenol extracted RNA prepared from the cells contains small amounts of antigen, and that these are considerably more immunogenic than the corresponding amount of native antigen [e.g. ASKONAS and RHODES, 1965]. However, there is no indication that the complexes present involve antigen and any special RNA newly synthesized as a result of contact with it; nor that any specific informational RNA is formed, apart from a report by ADLER, FISHMAN and DRAY [1966] that following immunization with macrophage RNA extracts the early IgM antibody first had the allotype of the macrophage donor whereas later IgG antibody had the allotype of the host. At the risk of later being proved quite wrong, I am prepared to guess that this last observation, fascinating though it be, is irrelevant to the question of how antigen normally interacts with immunocompetent cells so as to stimulate a specific response. Furthermore, although antigen-RNA complexes extracted from macrophages have markedly increased immunogenicity, this observation need imply no more than does the fact, for example, that the RNA virus "turnip yellow mosaic" is a much better immunogen than is the protein component by itself [Markham, 1959]. It cannot be decided at present whether the antigen-RNA complexes result from the extraction procedure used or whether they can play a part in the immune response. The problem has been discussed more fully by Askonas *et al.* [1968]. However, the biological interaction between antigen, macrophages and lymphocytes certainly seems to be important for the initiation of at least some immune responses. Some recent work by my colleagues Dr. Unanue and Dr. Askonas may throw light on some of the factors involved, and I shall discuss these briefly.

A Persistent Immunogenic Fraction of Antigen in Macrophages

Their studies were done in CBA mice using as antigens haemocyanin from the spider crab Maia squinado (MSH), or haemocyanin from keyhole limpets (KLH). MSH at pH 7.5 consists mainly of a 26S component. In the native state it is not a very potent immunogen and a single i.p. injection of 1 μg gives no detectable or only a minimal primary antibody response, although it primes the mice to give a good secondary response to reinjection of 1 μg of MSH three weeks later. The size of the secondary response to a 1 μg challenge dose is proportional to the amount of MSH used for priming, and it could therefore be used to compare the immunogenicity of known amounts of ^{131}I-labelled MSH administered in various forms as a priming dose. KLH in the native form is a very large molecule (S value about 93) and is a good immunogen, so that 1–5 μg i.p. gives a reliable primary 19S antibody response, as well as priming for a secondary response. KLH dissociates at mildly alkaline pH values to a smaller form whose general immunogenic properties resemble those of MSH.

The macrophages used were obtained from the peritoneal cavity three days after injection of peptone, when 80–90% of the cell population consisted of typical macrophages and—in contrast to normal peritoneal cells—immunologically competent lymphocytes were largely absent. Labelled antigen was added to the macrophages for 1 h either *in vivo* or *in vitro;* the cells were then washed and the amount of antigen taken up was assessed in terms of protein-bound radioactivity. In some experiments the antigen-containing macrophages were further incubated *in vitro* so as to observe how the antigen was degraded (by analysis of the cell contents after various time periods) and the effect of this upon its immunogenicity. Graded amounts of antigen in known numbers of macrophages, or free antigen, were administered to syngeneic recipient mice. The recipients were either normal or irradiated with 600r (nonlethal) or 660–700r (near lethal) whole body radiation one or two days before transfer. Recipients irradiated at the higher level were given in addition 5×10^6 normal lymph node cells, either simultaneously with the antigen or at various time intervals later. In all cases the mice were challenged with 1 μg soluble haemocyanin at three weeks, and the antibody response was measured eight days later. These experiments are reported in full elsewhere [UNANUE and ASKONAS, 1967; 1968 (a); 1968 (b); UNANUE, ASKONAS and ALLISON, 1968] and I shall summarize here only the main findings relevant to my theme.

First let me consider those relating to the smaller haemocyanin antigen, MSH. After uptake by macrophages into phagolysosomes about 90% is rapidly degraded to small fragments and the associated radioactivity is lost from the cells. However, the remaining 10% escapes degradation for at least several days, and possibly much longer. About half this is membrane bound, and electron microscopy combined with autoradiography suggests that much of this "stable" antigen in macrophages is held at or near the cell membrane—i.e. at a site which would be advantageous for interaction with the surface of immunologically competent lymphocytes. MSH associated with macrophages was much more immunogenic than native MSH, the difference being the more marked the smaller the quantities compared. The smallest amounts of macrophage-associated MSH which would prime mice were about 0.002 μg; at this level they primed for a 19S antibody response only, whereas larger amounts primed for both 7S and 19S antibody responses. The interesting finding emerged that the immunogenicity of macrophage-associated MSH was correlated not with the total amount of MSH originally taken up but with the fraction which persisted undegraded. When macrophage-associated

MSH was transferred to heavily irradiated mice the recipients were not primed unless normal lymph node cells were also transferred either simultaneously or later. However, lymph node cells and corresponding amounts of free MSH transferred to irradiated recipients did not result in priming. This demonstrates that the transferred macrophage population must somehow interact with lymphocytes, and that it neither made antibody itself nor contained a significant number of immunologically competent cells capable of being primed. Antigen in living syngeneic macrophages was more effective than in dead or foreign macrophages, but pre-irradiation of the donors with 750r did not affect the capacity of their macrophages to take up MSH or diminish its subsequent immunogenicity. When macrophage-associated MSH was administered to mice which had already been primed by injection of 1 μg soluble antigen three weeks previously, it elicited a secondary response more comparable in size to that elicited by an equivalent quantity of free MSH.

Now let me consider the findings relating to the larger haemocyanin antigen, KLH. As already mentioned, native KLH is a potent immunogen, and it elicits a substantial primary antibody response in mice which, as in rats and rabbits has an unusually large 19S component [Dixon, Jacot-Guillarmod and McConahey, 1966]. After uptake by macrophages, however, this antigen was much *less* immunogenic than the corresponding amount of the native form; in fact macrophage-associated KLH resembled macrophage-associated MSH so far as its immunogenicity was concerned. Furthermore, macrophage-associated KLH behaved immunogenically as though it were the dissociated form of KLH, giving rise on subsequent challenge to antibodies of which a considerable proportion were specific for determinants concealed in the native (associated) form of KLH and revealed only in the dissociated form. The two sets of findings can be reconciled if it is assumed that native KLH, which is a very large and immunogenic molecule, can stimulate immunologically competent cells to make a primary 19S antibody response by interacting directly with these cells, independently of any pathway involving presentation via macrophages. Dr. Unanue has in fact found that antibody is produced when KLH is incubated with lymphocytes without macrophages, in diffusion chambers in the peritoneal cavity of irradiated mice, even though the titres have not been very impressive [Unanue, 1968]. In addition to the postulated direct interaction with lymphocytes, KLH is taken up by macrophages, where part is retained in a macromolecular form which is perhaps too small to interact effectively with lymphocytes except when presented via macrophages, but nevertheless is efficient at priming for a secondary response.

The Significance of Macrophage-Retained Antigen for Priming

It has been proposed that direct interaction of antigen with immunologically competent lymphocytes, without stimulation of cell division and differentiation, leads to immunological tolerance [DRESSER and MITCHISON, 1968]. In the case of certain large and highly immunogenic antigen, such as KLH [UNANUE and ASKONAS, 1967] and sheep erythrocytes [PERKINS and MAKINODAN, 1965] direct interaction may also lead to primary antibody formation. The special effectiveness of the retained macrophage-associated antigens which I have been discussing appears to be mainly in priming—i.e. increasing the number of memory cells able to respond to subsequent contact with the antigen. This phenomenon is not peculiar to haemocyanins, but has been demonstrated to apply to other antigens, such as BSA, which are only weakly immunogenic when administered in soluble form [MITCHISON, 1967], and it seems likely to be of general significance, though its importance may vary from antigen to antigen. The mechanism is still quite obscure. It might depend upon the retention of antigen at a surface in or on the macrophages peculiarly well suited for direct interaction with competent lymphocytes, and upon the opportunity provided by repeated contact over a prolonged period of time for continued recruitment and subsequent stimulation of unprimed cells. Such a function resembles that postulated by NOSSAL for the antigen retained on reticular cells in germinal centres of lymphoid tissues. Although there is no proof that the macrophages with which I have been concerned in this last section are to be found in the medullary areas, the probabilities seem to me to be more in that direction.

Despite the strongly suggestive evidence outlined above that antigens associated with macrophages possess increased immunogenicity, retention in macrophages is certainly not a sufficient condition for immunogenicity. Some antigens which are insusceptible, or almost so, to digestion by macrophages are rapidly and completely taken up by these cells and retained within them for periods of several months. Such antigens are pneumococcal polysaccharides [FELTON, PRESCOTT, KAUFFMAN and OTTINGER, 1955] or synthetic polypeptides composed of D-amino acids [JANEWAY and SELA, 1967; JANEWAY and HUMPHREY, 1968]. Although these antigens administered in small quantities are potent immunogens in mice, they are also powerful inducers of immunological paralysis. It appears that the antigens retained in macrophages are continuously liberated into the circulation [JANEWAY and HUMPHREY, 1968; J.G. HOWARD, personal communication] and thereby induce and maintain a "low zone" paralysis [MITCHISON, 1964], despite the fact that the great majority is retained in macrophages in what should be, on the basis of our discussion, a highly immunogenic form capable of overriding "low zone" paralysis. Furthermore although even potent immunogens with no marked tendency to produce paralysis, such as flagellin, are retained (in small amounts) in lymph nodes for long periods, the retained antigen loses its immunogenicity after some days [NOSSAL, AUSTIN and ADA, 1965] even though it remains capable of reacting with antibody. Such a loss could partly be attributable to gradual masking by antibody, but in the case of the D-amino acid polypeptides no circulating antibody was detectable, even by the sensitive criterion of localization of the antigen in germinal centres. These considerations, and others relating to the temporary effect of some adjuvants such as vitamin A [DRESSER, 1968], suggest that the efficiency of immunogens associated with macrophages may depend not only upon the presentation of retained antigen to lymphocytes in a specially effective way but also upon some local, temporary and probably nonspecific consequence of the activation of macrophages accompanying the ingestion of antigen, which alters the reactivity of neighbouring lymphocytes, making them more responsive to immunogenic stimulation. Some evidence for a non-specific adjuvant effect of activated macrophages has been obtained by UNANUE, ASKONAS and ALLISON [1968].

This again emphasizes the probable importance of the local environment in which antigen and lymphocytes meet for determining the outcome of their interaction. The more I have studied the complicated architecture of lymphoid tissues the more I have been impressed by the variety of environments provided and the uneven distribution of antigen within them, and the likelihood that the behaviour of individual cells will be determined by these factors.

References

ADA, G.L.; NOSSAL, G.J.V. and AUSTIN, C.M.: Antigens in immunity V. The ability of cells in lymphoid follicles to recognize foreignness. Aust. J. exp. Biol. med. Sci. *42:* 331–346 (1964).

ADA, G.L. and PARISH, C.R.: Antigen localization in immunity and tolerance a role for antigen in lymphoid follicles. Proc. Nat. Acad. Sci. (submitted).

ADLER, F.L.; FISHMAN, M. and DRAY, S.: Antibody formation initiated *in vitro*. III. Antibody formation and allotype specificity directed by ribonucleic acid from peritoneal exudate cells. J. Immunol. *97:* 554–558 (1966).

ASKONAS, B.A.; AUZINS, I. and UNANUE, E.: Role of macrophages in the immune response. Bull. Soc. chim. Biol. *50:* No. 5–6, 1113 (1968).

ASKONAS, B.A. and RHODES, J.M.: Immunogenicity of antigen containing ribonucleic acid preparations from macrophages. Nature (Lond.) *205:* 470–474 (1965).

BALFOUR, B.M. and HUMPHREY, J.H.: Localization of labeled antigen in germinal centres and its relationship to the immune response. In: Germinal centres in immune responses, pp. 80–85 (Springer-Verlag, Berlin 1966).

BOYDEN, S.V.: Natural antibodies and the immune response. (Eds.) F.J. DIXON and J.H. HUMPHREY Adv. Immunology *5:* 1–28 (Academic Press, New York 1966).

BROWNSTONE, A.; MITCHISON, N.A. and PITT-RIVERS, R.: Chemical and serological studies with a synthetic immunological determinant 4-hydroxy-3-iodo-5-nitro-phenylacetic acid (NIP) and related compounds. Immunology *10:* 465–479 (1966).

CAMPBELL, D.H. and GARVEY, J.S.: Nature of retained antigen and its role in the immune response. (Eds.) F.J. DIXON and J.H. HUMPHREY Adv. Immunology *3:* 261–313 (Academic Press, New York 1963).

CRUMPTON, M.J.: An antigenic site on sperm whale myoglobin. Nature (Lond.) *215:* 17–20 (1967).

DIXON, F.J.; JACOT-GUILLARMOD, H. and McCONAHEY, P.: The antibody responses of rabbits and rats to hemocyanin. J. Immunol. *97:* 350–355 (1966).

DRESSER, D.W.: Adjuvanticity of vitamin A. Nature (Lond.) *217:* 527–529 (1968).

DRESSER, D.W. and MITCHISON, N.A.: The mechanism of immunological paralysis. In: Adv. Immunology (Eds.) F.J. DIXON and H.J. KUNKEL. Vol. 8, pp. 129–181 (1968).

FELTON, L.D.; PRESCOTT, B.; KAUFFMAN, G. and OTTINGER, B.: Pneumococcal antigenic polysaccharide substances from animal tissues. J. Immunol. *74:* 205–213 (1955).

FISHMAN, M. and ADLER, F.L.: Antibody formation initiated *in vitro*. II. Antibody synthesis in x-irradiated recipients of diffusion chambers containing nucleic acid derived from macrophages incubated with antigen. J. exp. Med. *117:* 595–602 (1963).

GILL, T.J. III.; PAPERMASTER, D.S. and MOWBRAY, J.M.: Synthetic polypeptide metabolism. I. The metabolic fate of enantiomorphic polymers. J. Immunol. *95:* 794–803 (1965).

HAUROWITZ, F.: Immunochemistry. Ann. Rev. Biochemistry *29:* 609–634 (1960).

HENNEY, C.S.; STANWORTH, D.R. and GELL, P.G.H.: Demonstration of the expose of new antigenic determinants following antigen-antibody combination. Nature (Lond.) *205:* 1079–1081 (1965).

HUMPHREY, J.H.; ASKONAS, B.A.; AUZINS, I.; SCHECHTER, I. and SELA, M.: The localization of antigen in lymph nodes and its relation to specific antibody-producing cells. II. Comparison of iodine-125 and tritium labels. Immunology *13:* 71–86 (1967).

HUMPHREY, J.H. and FRANK, M.M.: The localization of non-microbial antigens in the draining lymph nodes of tolerant, normal and primed rabbits. Immunology *13:* 87–100 (1967).

JANEWAY, C.A. Jr. and HUMPHREY, J.H.: Synthetic antigens composed exclusively of L- or D- amino acids. II. Effect of optical configuration on the metabolism and fate of synthetic polypeptide antigens in mice. Immunology *14:* 225–234 (1968).

Janeway, C.A. Jr. and Sela, M.: Synthetic antigens composed exclusively of L- or D-amino acids. I. Effect of optical configuration on the immunogenicity of synthetic polypeptides in mice. Immunology *13:* 29–38 (1967).

Kluthe, R.; Hageman, V. and Kleine, N.: The turnover of a_2 macroglobulins in the nephrotic syndrome. Vox. Sang. *12:* 308–311 (1967).

Lang, P.G. and Ada, G. L.: Antigen in tissues IV. The effect of antibody on the retention and localization of antigen in rat lymph nodes. Immunology *13:* 523–534 (1967a).

Lang, P.G. and Ada, G.L.: The localization of heat denatured serum albumin in rat lymph nodes. Aust. J. exp. Biol. med. Sci. *45:* 445–448 (1967b).

Leduc, E.H.; Avrameas, S. and Bouteille, M.: Ultrastructural localization of antibody in differentiating plasma cells. J. exp. Med. *127:* 109–118 (1968).

Markham, R.: The biochemistry of plant viruses. In: The viruses. (Eds.) F.M. Burnet and W.R. Stanley *2:* 102 (Academic Press, New York 1959).

McDevitt, H.; Askonas, B.A.; Humphrey, J.H.; Schechter, I. and Sela, M.: The localization of antigen in relation to specific antibody-producing cells. I. Use of a synthetic polypeptide [(T, G)-A-L] labelled with Iodine-125. Immunology *11:* 337–351 (1966).

Miller, J.J.; Johnsen, D.O. and Ada, G.L.: Differences in localization of Salmonella flagella in lymph node follicles of germ-free and conventional rats. Nature (Lond.) *217:* 1059–1061 (1968).

Mitchell, J. and Nossal, G.J.V.: Mechanism of induction of immunological tolerance. I. Localization of tolerance-inducing antigen. Aust. J. exp. Biol. med. Sci. *44:* 211–224 (1966).

Mitchison, N.A.: Induction of immunological paralysis in two zones of dosage. Proc. roy. Soc. (Lond.) Ser. B *161:* 275–292 (1964).

Mitchison, N.A.: Immunological paralysis as a dosage phenomenon. In: Regulation of the antibody response (Ed.) B. Cinader (C.C. Thomas, Springfield, Ill., Chapter II, pp. 54–67, 1967).

Nossal, G.J.V.: Inductive steps in antibody formation and tolerance. In: Nobel Symp. 3. Gamma globulins. Structure and control of biosynthesis (Ed.) J. Killander (Almqvist and Wiksell, Stockholm 1967).

Nossal, G.J.V.; Abbot, A. and Mitchell, J.: Antigens in immunity XIV. Electron microscopic radioautographic studies of antigen capture in the lymph node medulla. J. exp. Med. *127:* 263–276 (1968).

Nossal, G.J.V.; Abbot, A.; Mitchell, J. and Lummus, Z.: Antigens in immunity XV. Ultrastructural features of antigen capture in primary and secondary lymphoid follicles. J. exp. Med. *127:* 277–290 (1968).

Nossal, G.J.V.; Ada, G.L. and Austin, C.M.: Antigens in immunity, II. Immunogenic properties of flagella, polymerized flagellin and flagellin in the primary response. Aust. J. exp. Biol. med. Sci. *42:* 283–294 (1964a).

Nossal, G.J.V.; Ada, G.L. and Austin, C.M.: Antigens in immunity IV. Cellular localization of [125]I- and ^{131}I-labelled flagella in lymph nodes. Aust. J. exp. Biol. med. Sci. *42:* 311–330 (1964b).

Nossal, G.J.V.; Ada, G.L.; Austin, C.M. and Pye, J.: Antigens in immunity VIII. Localization of ^{125}I-labelled antigens in the secondary response. Immunology *9:* 349–357 (1965).

Nossal, G.J.V.; Austin, C.M. and Ada, G.L.: Antigens in immunity II. Analysis of immunological memory. Immunology *9:* 333–348 (1965).

Perkins, E.H. and Makinodan, T.: The suppressive role of mouse peritoneal phagocytes in agglutinin response. J. Immunol. *94:* 765–777 (1965).

Rajewsky, K.; Rottländer, E.; Peltre, G. and Müller, B.: The immune response to a hybrid protein molecule. Specificity of secondary stimulation and of tolerance induction. J. exp. Med. *126:* 581–606 (1967).

ROSER, B.: The distribution of intravenously injected peritoneal macrophages in the mouse. Aust. J. exp. Biol. med. Sci. *43:* 553–562 (1965).

RUSSELL, P. and ROSER, B.: The distribution and behaviour of intravenously injected pulmonary alveolar macrophages in the mouse. Aust. J. exp. Biol. med. Sci. *44:* 629–636 (1966).

SELIGMANN, M. et MIHAESCO, C.: L'importance de la conformation moléculaire dans la structure antigénique. Rev. franc. Et. clin. biol. *12:* 851–854 (1967).

UNANUE, E.R.: Properties and some uses of anti-macrophage antibodies. Nature (Lond.) *218:* 36–38 (1968).

UNANUE, E.R. and ASKONAS, B.A.: Two functions of macrophages and their role in the immune response. J. Reticuloendothelial Soc. *4:* 440 (1967).

UNANUE, E.R. and ASKONAS, B.A.: Persistence of immunogenicity of antigen after uptake by macrophages. J. exp. Med. *127:* 915–926 (1968a).

UNANUE, E.R. and ASKONAS, B.A.: The immune response of mice to antigen in macrophages. Immunology *15:* 287–296 (1968b).

UNANUE, E.R.; ASKONAS, B.A. and ALLISON, A.C.: In preparation (1968).

WELLENSIEK, H.J. and COONS, A.H.: Studies on antibody production IX. The cellular localization of antigen molecules (ferritin) in the secondary response. J. exp. Med. *119:* 685–695 (1964).

WHITE, R.G.; FRENCH, V.I. and STARK, J.M.: Germinal center formation and antigen localization in Malpighian bodies of the chicken spleen. In Germinal centers in immune responses. pp. 131–142 (Ed.) COTTIER, H. (Springer, Berlin 1966).

WILLIAMS, G.M.: Antigen localization in lymphopaenic states I. Localization pattern following chronic thoracic duct drainage. Immunology *11:* 467–474 (1966).

Author's address: Dr. J.H. HUMPHREY, National Institute for Medical Research, Mill Hill, *London, N.W. 7* (England).

Antibiotica et Chemotherapia, vol. 15, pp. 24–39 (Karger, Basel/New York 1969)

Recognition Mechanisms in the Chicken Spleen

R. G. WHITE

Department of Bacteriology and Immunology, University of Glasgow, Glasgow

In a previous study [WHITE, 1963] of the fate of a protein antigen which was injected intravenously into chickens and subsequently traced by means of the fluorescent antibody method applied to sections of spleen, I was impressed by the fact that by this relatively insensitive method antigen could be detected in association with cells which were then termed *dendritic macrophages* and remained in association with them for up to 21 days within the germinal centres of the red pulp. These cells are functionally and cytologically distinct from the reticular, sinus lining and free amoeboid macrophages of the red pulp of the spleen. They are cells which become loaded with antigen and migrate by a well-defined path through the white pulp to end within the lymphocytopoietic or germinal centres (fig. 1). This communication will outline these cellular events as they happen in response to some typical protein antigens and then draw a comparison with the cellular fate of some non-antigenic particles.

A justification for using such particles as possible models for a soluble protein antigen such as human serum albumin (HSA) is that previous work undertaken with Dr. VALENTINE FRENCH and Dr. MARSHALL STARK had indicated that the entity which localizes to the dendritic macrophages is an antigen/antibody complex. The evidence for this conclusion is briefly as follows [—experiments of FRENCH, STARK and WHITE, to be published]:

(i) Using fluorescein-labelled rabbit anti-HSA on frozen (cryostat) sections of chicken spleen, no localization can be seen after an intravenous injection of 1–10 mg of HSA during the first 25–30 h.

(ii) The start and increase of antigen localization to dendritic macrophages coincides with the first appearance and rise of antigen/

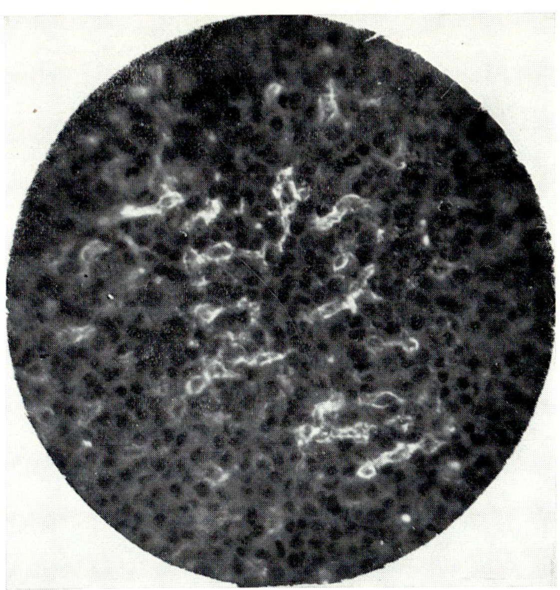

Fig. 1. Fluorescence micrograph. Scattered antigen-loaded dendritic macrophages within a germinal centre of the white pulp of the chicken spleen at 6 days after a single intravenous injection of 10 mg of human serum albumin (HSA). Single layer technique with fluorescein-labelled rabbit anti-human serum albumin. × 350.

antibody complexes in the serum. Figure 2 shows the curve of elimination of an intravenous dose of ^{125}I-HSA from the circulation of the bird, and the subsequent rise in antibody determined by the Farr technique. The curve of ^{125}I-counts which are precipitable with 40% saturated ammonium sulphate represents available antigen/antibody complexes in the blood. No complexes are detectable in the first 30 h; the rise occurs from the third to the fifth day, which coincides well with the period of antigen localization to dendritic macrophages.

(iii) At the time of the first localization (approximately 30 h) already antibody-containing plasma-cell precursors, as revealed by the "sandwich" modification of the fluorescent antibody technique for detection of antibody to HSA [Coons, Leduc and Connolly, 1955] are present in the red pulp of the spleen. These presumably provide the source for the serum anti-HSA. Antigen localization has not been seen before such antibody-containing cells occurred.

(iv) Antigen localization determined by the fluorescent antibody method (and autoradiography, see below) does not occur in chickens which are rendered specifically tolerant to HSA. Tolerance was

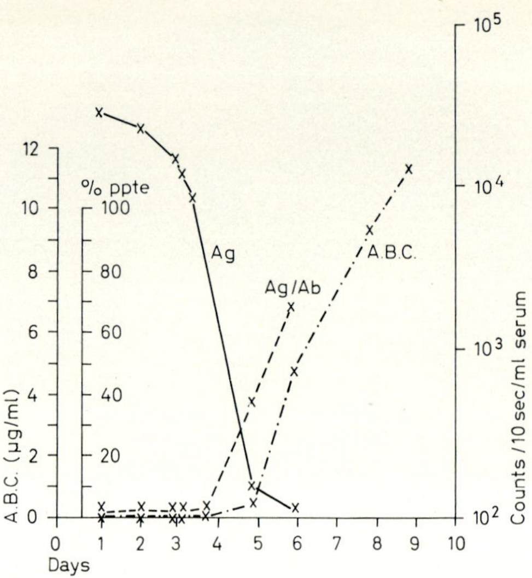

Fig. 2. Kinetics of removal of HSA from the blood of a chicken, of the subsequent rise of anti-HSA and of the presence of complexes of HSA/anti-HSA. ^{125}I-HSA levels are expressed as iodine counts per 10 sec per ml serum. Anti-HSA is expressed as antigen-combining capacity (ABC) as estimated by a Farr test. AG/AB complexes are estimated as the percentage of the antigen counts which are precipitable from serum by 40 % saturated ammonium sulphate solution. [Data from French, White and Stark, to be published.]

achieved by injecting HSA on the day after hatching and maintained by regular dosage of antigen for six weeks. Birds which were tested at 4 weeks and found tolerant, i.e. responding to a test intravenous dose of ^{125}I-labelled-HSA by a straight-line elimination on a semi-log plot, were unable to localize to dendritic macrophages a test dose of 10 mg HSA.

(v) By treating spleen sections with fluorescein-labelled anti-chicken γ-globulin, a similar pattern of fluorescence results to that of localised antigen in the germinal centre (fig. 3).

The details of the time course of localization of antigen-antibody complexes to cells in the white pulp of the spleen are as follows. The first localization as seen by the use of fluorescent antibody to HSA occurs at about 30 h to cells which are scattered along and around certain arterioles of the white pulp. There is no localization at this early time to the germinal centres. This early phase of localization has more recently been studied by the preparation of auto-radiographs of spleen sections after injecting a small dose (40 μg)

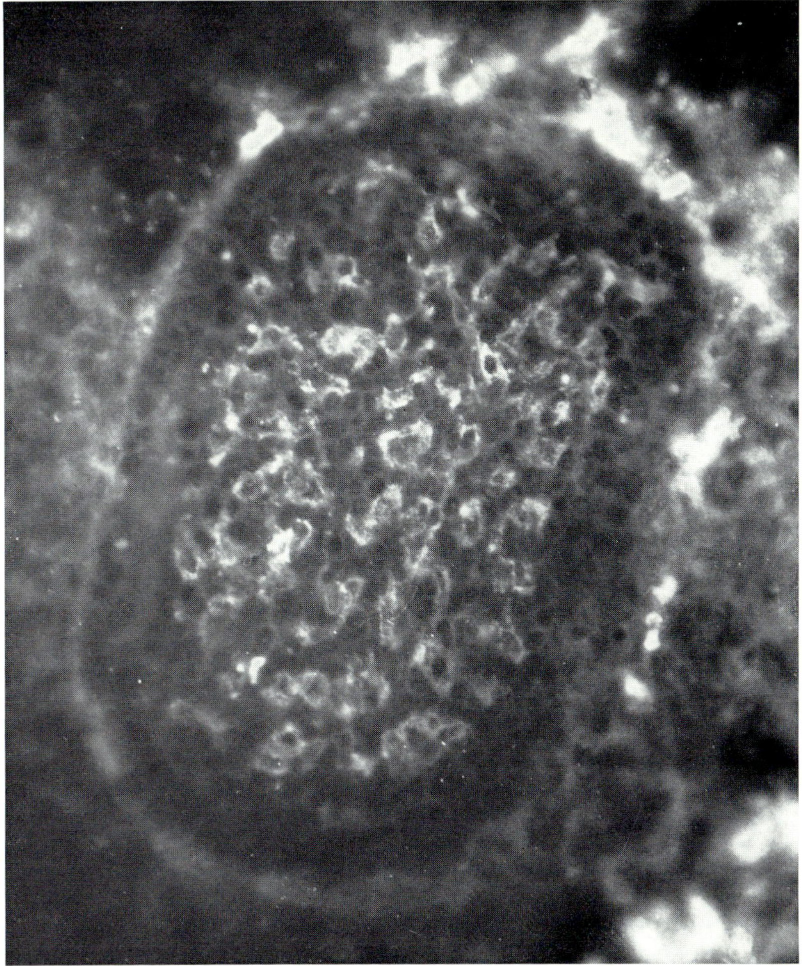

Fig. 3. Fluorescence micrograph. Frozen section of germinal centre of chicken spleen treated with fluorescein-labelled anti-chicken γ-globulin. The pattern of chicken γ-globulin on dendritic macrophages closely resembles the pattern of antigen-loaded cells shown in figure 1. $\times$ 700.

of HSA heavily-labelled with [125]I. The initial localization takes place to cells which are at the margin of the white pulp closely surrounding the Schweigger-Seidel sheaths of the penicillary arterioles before the latter enter the red pulp (fig. 4). Similar foci of antigen localization occur back along the penicillary arterioles as far as the bifurcation of the central artery of the white pulp (fig. 5).

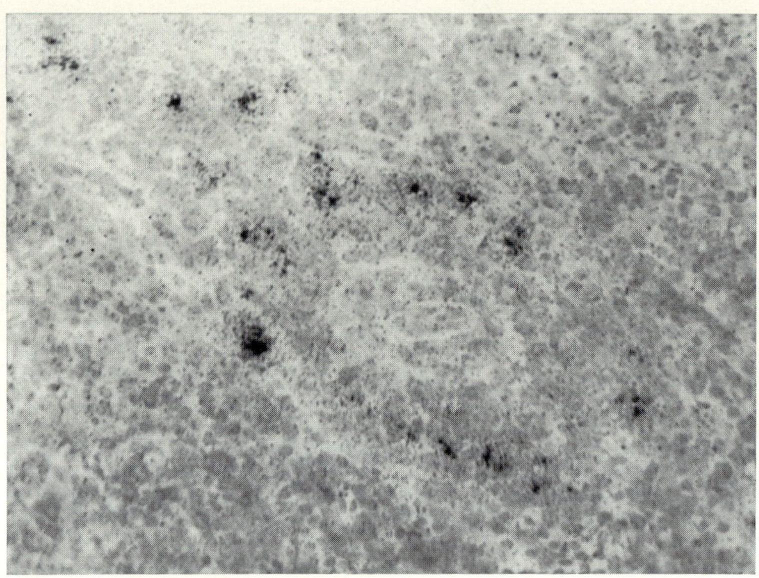

Fig. 4. Autoradiograph. Schweigger-Seidel sheath of chicken spleen after a single intra-venous injection of 40 μg of ^{125}I-HSA 3 days previously. There is a ring of increased grain density due to ^{125}I-HSA around the periphery of the sheath, and foci of higher density denoting localization of antigen to macrophages at the periphery of the sheath (which is shown dotted). [Preparation of Dr. MARSHALL STARK.]

Later auto-radiographs—from 3 days after injection show the presence of antigen-bearing cells within the germinal centres. At 3 days (fig. 6) these are seen as small, vaguely circular aggregates of cells including about 15–20 antigen-bearing cells. At this stage there is no sharp demarcation between the cells of the germinal centre and surrounding white pulp lymphoid cells. The process of inclusion of antigen-bearing cells into germinal centres proceeds progressively between the third and the sixth days. Sections taken at the sixth day (fig. 7) show that all antigen-bearing cells are within well formed germinal centres which now have a distinct general pyroninophilia of their included cells, some of which demonstrate mitotic figures. The circular outline of the centre is now well demarcated from the surrounding white pulp.

These appearances suggest that antigen-bearing cells first make their appearance at the periphery of the Schweigger-Seidel sheaths of the penicillary arterioles and subsequently migrate back along the penicillary arterioles to enter a germinal centre situated in the angle

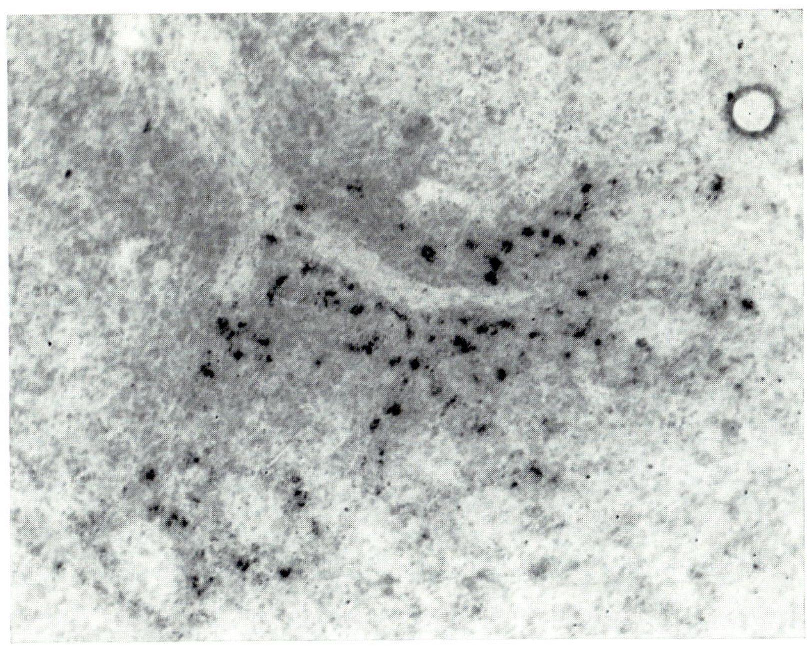

Fig. 5. Autoradiograph. Chicken spleen 88 h after intravenous injection of 40 μg of
125I-HSA. *Note* leash of vessels spreading downwards from the central arteriole of white
pulp (top left corner). The two branches of the latter are penicillary arterioles which
pass to the periphery of the white pulp in the direction of several Schweigger-Seidel
sheaths, which are shown as pale ovals with peripheral black foci of grains denoting
125I-HSA localized to macrophages. Similar grain foci extend along the penicillary vessels
to the point of bifurcation of the central arteriole of the white pulp. [Preparation of
Dr. MARSHALL STARK.]

of bifurcation of two penicillary arterioles at their site of origin
from the central artery of the white pulp.

The auto-radiographic data also suggest that the HSA antigen,
presumably in the form of antigen-antibody complexes, enters the
spleen at the periphery of the Schweigger-Seidel sheaths. Thus, at
the third day a ring of increased grain density appears at the periphery
of the sheath. Superimposed on this are foci of more intense radioactivity, suggesting that the ring of segregated antigen/antibody complexes is localized to, or picked up by, the carrier macrophages at
this site (fig. 4).

The auto-radiographic appearances from day 3 to day 6 indicate
that in the later part of their journey the antigen-bearing macrophages
become associated with surrounding lymphocytes to form mixed

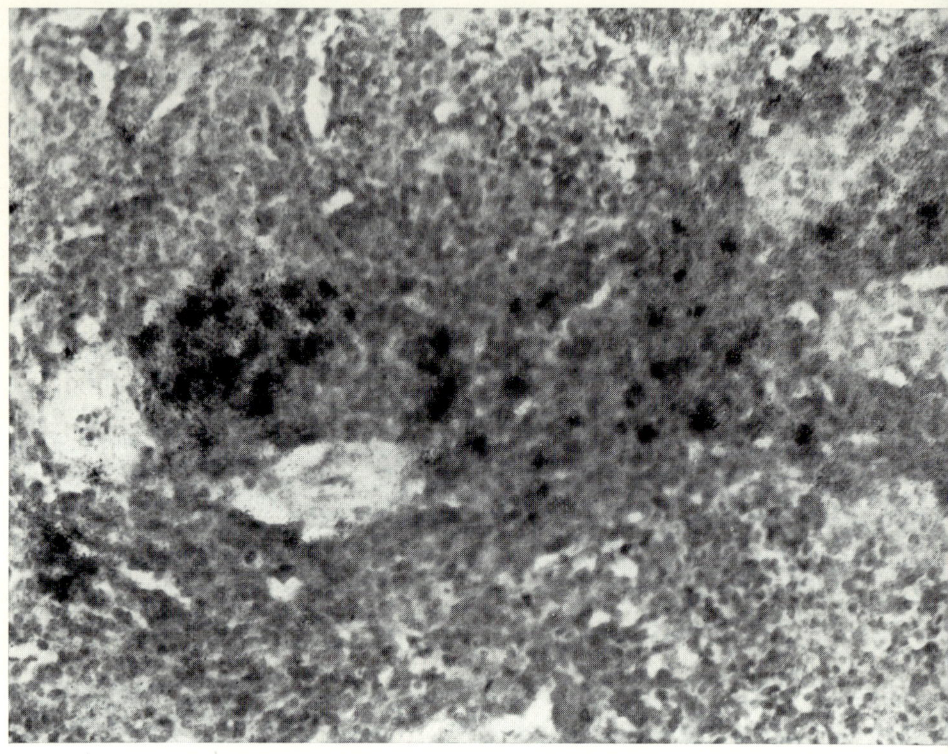

Fig. 6. Autoradiograph. Chicken spleen at 3 ½ days after an intravenous injection of 40 μg of ^{125}I-HSA. At left, in angle between two diverging penicillary arterioles is an early germinal centre. At right are three Schweigger-Seidel sheaths seen as pale ovals. Grain foci due to ^{125}I-HSA localized to macrophages are distributed along the penicillary arterioles between the germinal centre (left) and the sheaths (right). [Preparation of Dr. MARSHALL STARK.]

clumps of dendritic cells and dendritic macrophages. Such early centres appear to grow by the arrival of more antigen-bearing cells, and lymphocytes until, at the sixth day, the supply of antigen-bearing macrophages stops. This early formation of the germinal centre might represent a simple agglutinative reaction between antigen-bearing dendritic cells and small lymphocytes with a complimentary recognition molecule to antigen at their cell surface. The demonstration by SELL and GELL [1965] that anti-allotype antisera can induce transformation of rabbit peripheral blood lymphocytes to dividing pyroninophilic large "blast" forms indicates that the necessary immunoglobulin may be present at the lymphocyte surface. It could be

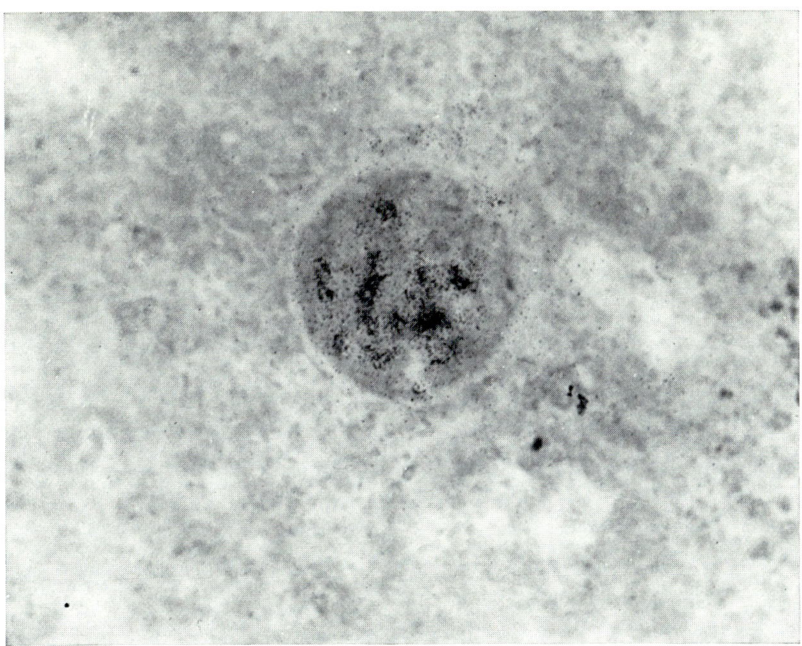

Fig. 7. Autoradiograph. Chicken spleen 6 days after a single intravenous injection of 40 µg of ^{125}I-HSA. Grain foci denoting localized antigen on dendritic macrophages are present in foci within the area of the germinal centre. *Note* complete absence of antigen in white pulp outside this centre. [Preparation of Dr. Marshall Stark.]

argued that the dendritic cells bearing antigen/antibody complexes over their long branching cytoplasmic processes would provide an efficient net for filtering off selected immunoglobulin-bearing small lymphocytes as the latter circulated through the splenic white pulp.

In the germinal centre reaction, antigen reacting with homologous antibody at the surface of the small lymphocytes would be the stimulus for the pyroninophilic transformation and subsequent mitosis which is seen in the developing germinal centre. The centre would not therefore represent a *clone,* but would be the product of the division of the original small number, say 20–40 lymphocytes which were netted by the dendritic cells.

It was considered that the process of inclusion of HSA into germinal centres represented a recognition mechanism and would be specific for immunogenic particles. It was therefore of interest to compare the localization of non-immunogenic particles such as indian ink (carbon particle size 250 Å diameter) and saccharated iron oxide (particle size 125 Å diameter). In experiments carried out by Mr. J. S. ANDERSON and Dr. MARIA DE SOUSA, these particles after intravenous injection were found to segregate rapidly to form dense rings round the periphery of the Schweigger-Seidel sheaths (fig. 8). Birds which were killed only seconds after injection showed the iron oxide or carbon outlining the peripheral cells of the sheaths. At higher microscope magnification it seemed that the iron oxide or carbon lay around and between the peripheral sheath cells. The carbon gradually leaves the periphery of the sheaths and after a day or so there are only small specks of carbon in this area. The subsequent migration follows a path which resembles that described for the antigen/antibody complexes. One obvious difference is that large deposits of carbon are found in the red pulp in clumps of reticular macrophages. In the white pulp a migration takes place along the penicillary arterioles to the region where the germinal centres normally form,

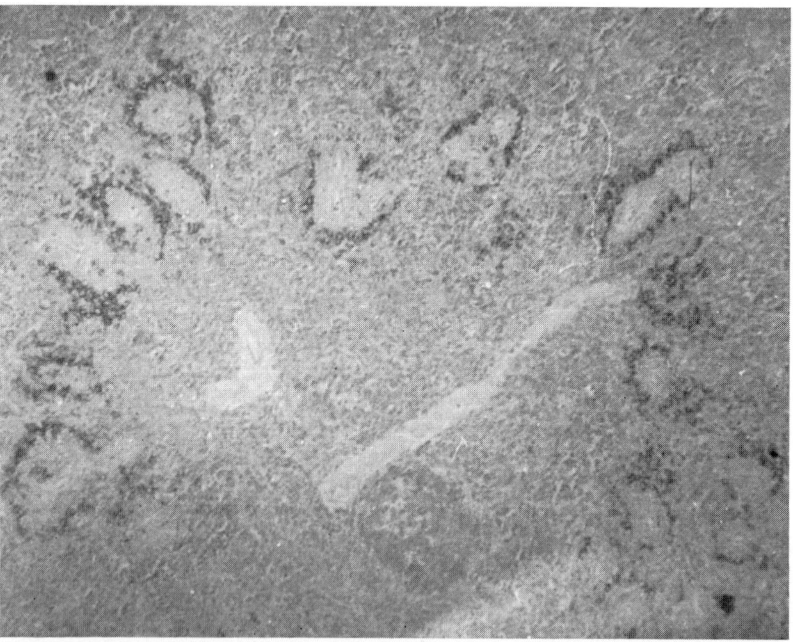

Fig. 8. Section of spleen of chicken killed 10 min after an intravenous injection of indian ink. Island of white pulp with germinal centre (below), central arteriole and penicillary vessels. In the marginal zone between red and white pulp are the Schweigger-Seidel sheaths which are outlined by indian ink which has segregated from the bloodstream to the periphery of the sheaths. × 150.

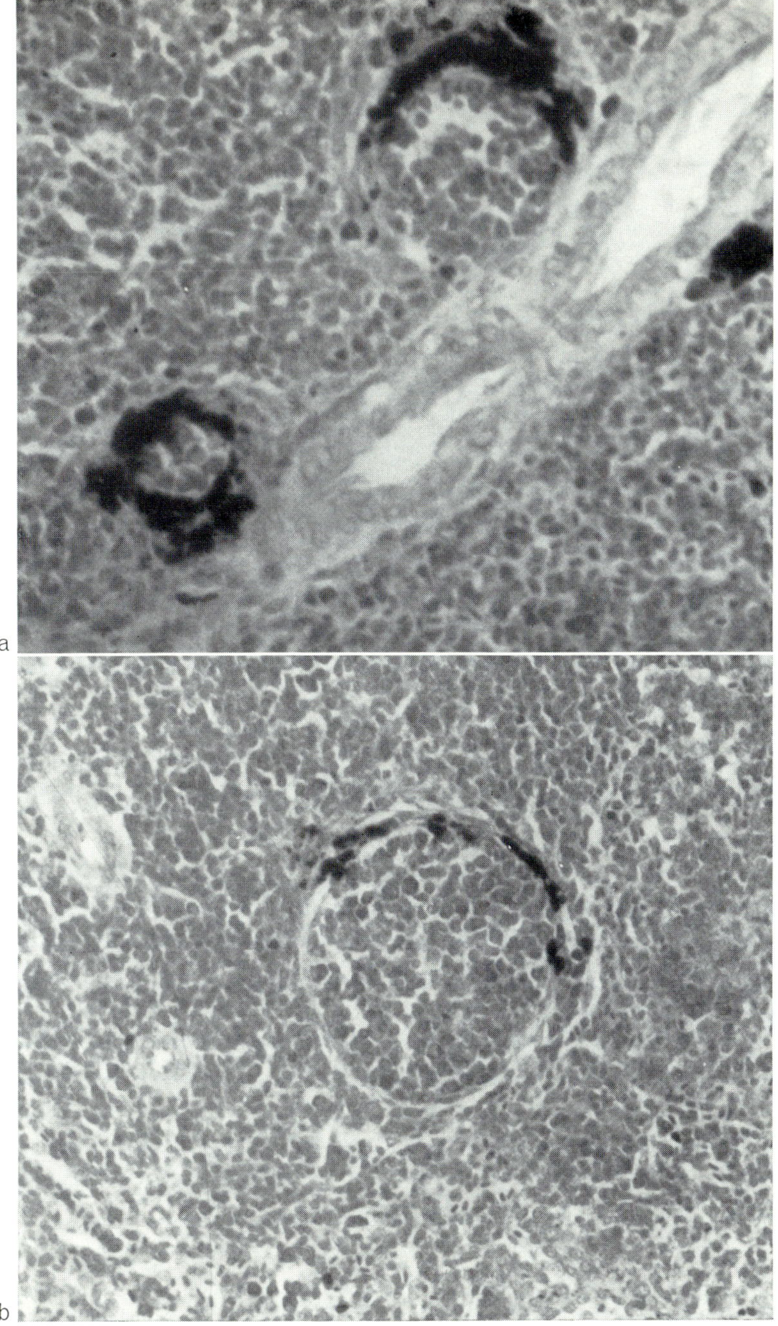

Fig. 9. (a) Section of spleen of chicken at five days after a single intravenous injection of indian ink. Carbon-laden macrophages have migrated to the vicinity of the angle between two diverging penicillary arterioles, and have accumulated at the periphery of the developing germinal centres. (b) Same section as above showing more mature germinal centre with peripheral accumulation of carbon-laden macrophages.

i.e. in the angles of bifurcation between the penicillary arterioles at their origin from the central artery of the white pulp. However, neither carbon nor saccharated iron oxide becomes incorporated into the germinal centre in a pattern which in any way resembles that of antigen on or in dendritic macrophages. Most of the carbon or iron oxide becomes left outside the circle of the germinal centre and forms a dense rim around part of the circumference (fig. 9a and 9b).

These findings support the hypothesis that the inclusion of antigen within the developing germinal centre is the manifestation of a specific recognition mechanism. The earlier process of uptake of carbon or antigen at the periphery of the Schweigger-Seidel sheaths is presumably a non-specific process, although this is a matter which requires further investigation. For the present it seems reasonable to conclude that similar cells take up carbon as take up antigen-antibody complexes.

Presumably the segregative role of the Schweigger-Seidel sheath is also a non-specific process. We have, rather hopefully for the present, accepted indian ink as a model for antigen-antibody complexes in order to study the route and cellular destination within and outside the sheaths. A few seconds after intravenous injection of indian ink, the chickens were killed and sections prepared for election microscopy after embedding in araldite, and post-staining with a 50% alcoholic solution of uranyl acetate and lead citrate. The ink can be seen to segregate as a concentrated suspension of particles in the space between adjacent cells of the outer layer of the Schweigger-Seidel sheath (fig. 10).

The structure of the sheath in cross section can be seen in figure 11. Surrounding the central lumen is a single layer of high endothelial cells. The cells of this inner layer rest at their outer borders on a loosely textured basement membrane made up of individual membrane profiles 200–250 Å thick. Club-like small cytoplasmic processes appear to protrude from these endothelial cells, outwards through small gaps in the basement membrane. External to the basement membrane is

---

Fig. 10. Electron micrograph of cross section of a Schweigger-Seidel sheath of a chicken killed a few seconds after a single intravenous injection of indian ink. At centre, the lumen contains a nucleated erythrocyte. A single layer of high endothelial cells is surrounded by a loosely-organized basement membrane. The outer layer of sheath cells is partly visible. *Note* the cytoplasmic extension of a macrophage containing carbon particles in vesicles extends inwards (from top left corner) to the outer surface of the basement membrane (arrows). × 18,000. [Preparation of Dr. J. Gordon.]

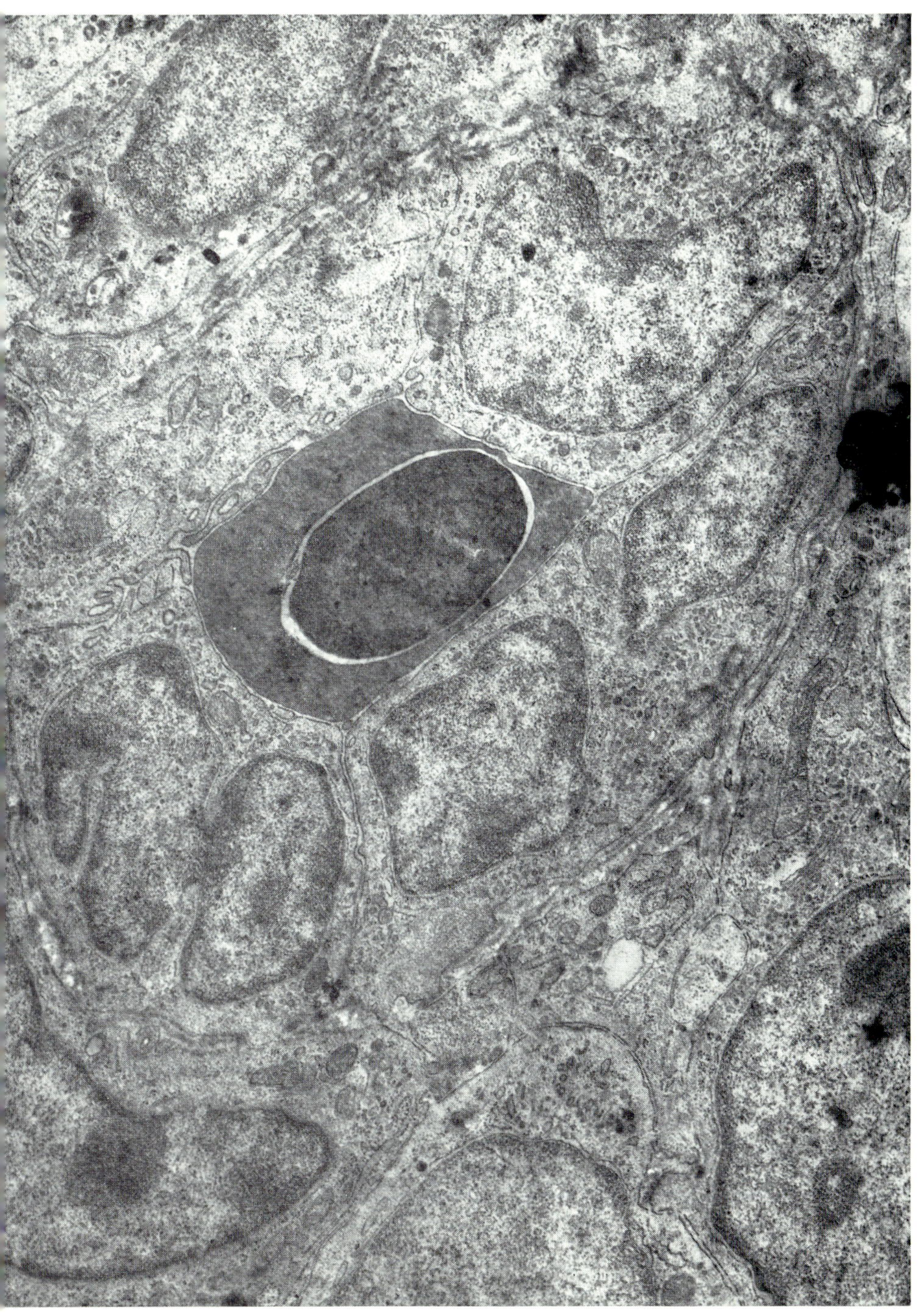

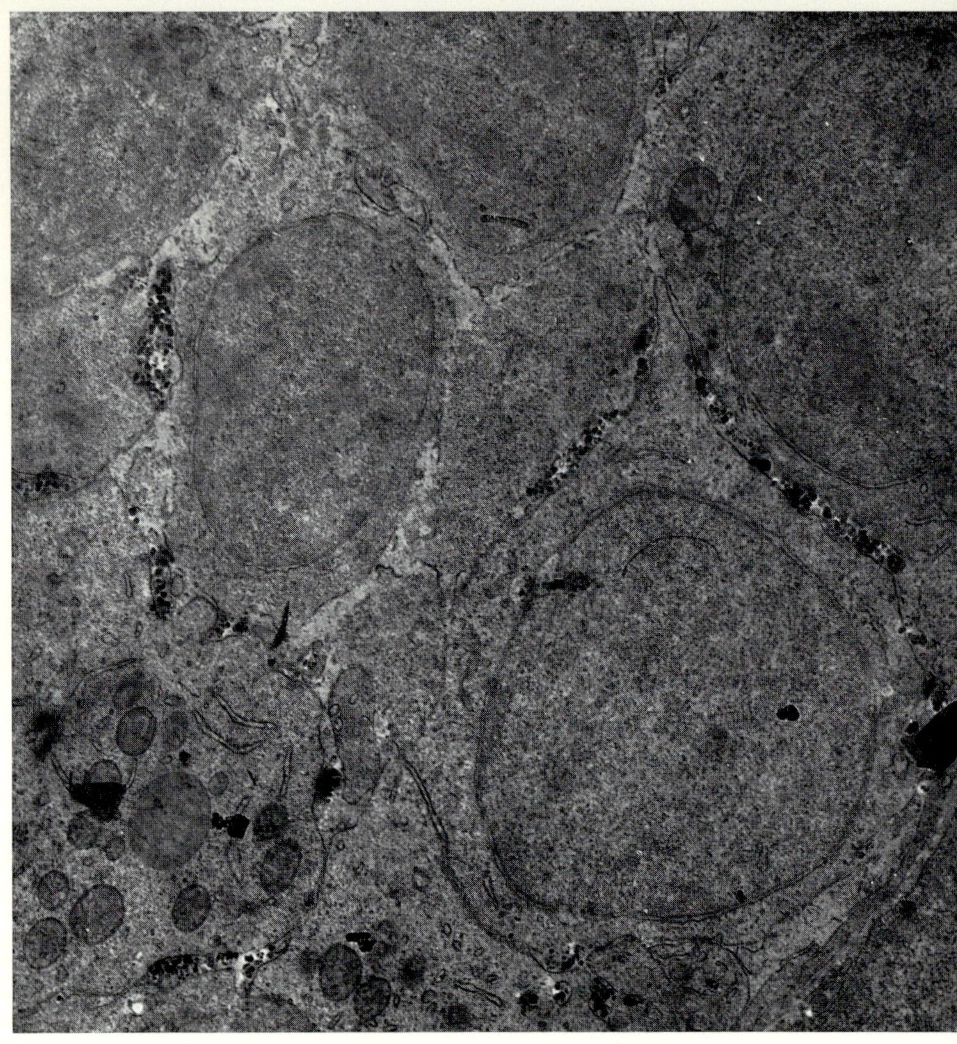

Fig. 11. Electron micrograph. Section of outer cells of a Schweigger-Seidel sheath a few seconds after an intravenous injection of indian ink. Carbon particles are closely packed in the spaces between adjacent sheath cells. Across the bottom left-hand corner is a part of the cytoplasm of a macrophage which has included carbon particles within pinocytotic tubules and vesicles. × 26,000. [Preparation of Dr. J. Gordon.]

Fig. 12. Electron micrograph. Section of sheath endothelium. At left is the lumen with parts of two chicken erythrocytes. The vertical line of endothelial cells (centre) is bounded (right) by basement membrane. *Note* highly convoluted channel between adjacent endothelial cells which extends from the lumen to the inner surface of the basement membrane. Arrows indicate carbon particles. × 26,000. [Preparation of Dr. J. Gordon.]

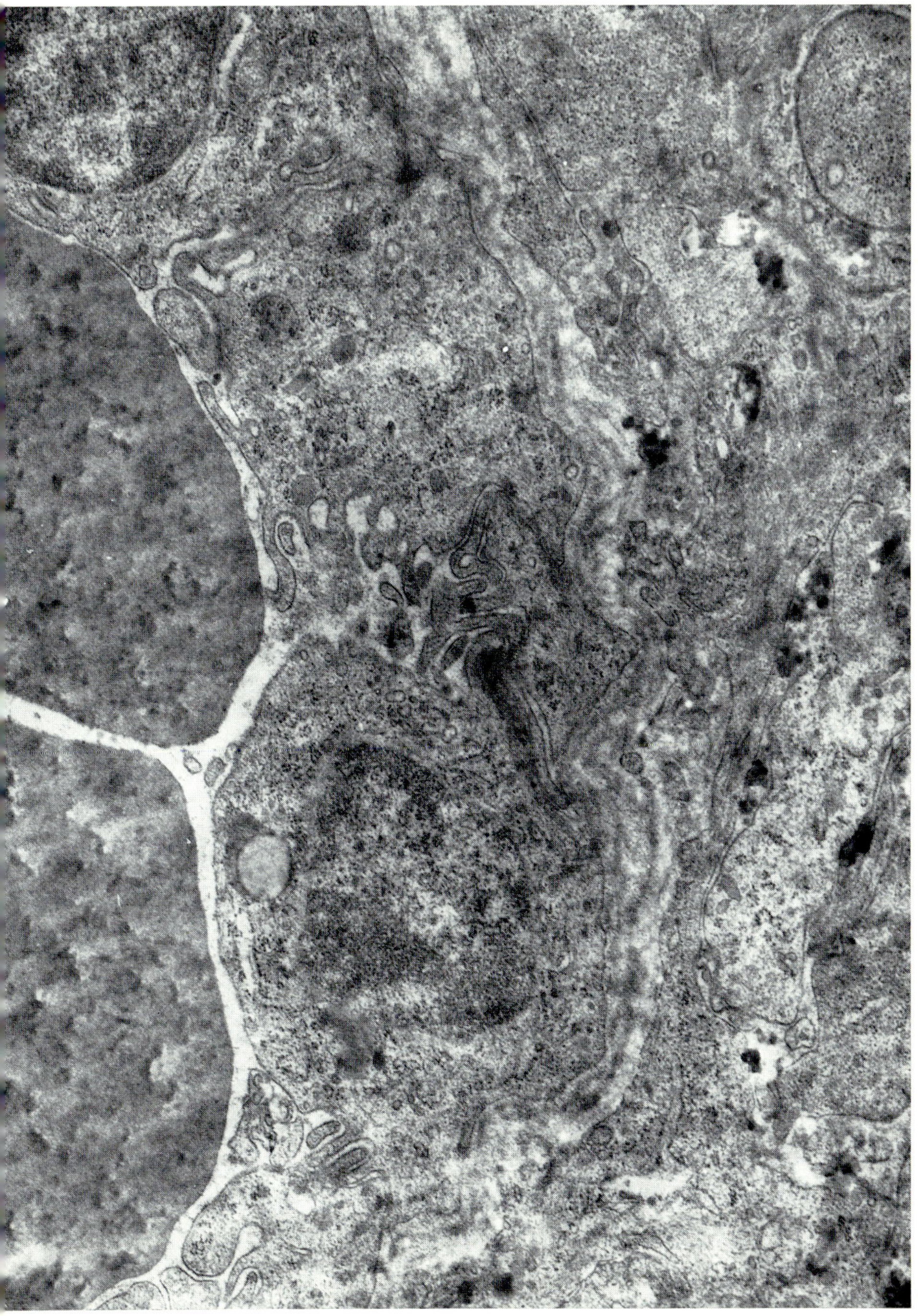

a double layer of sheath cells, and beyond this are the closely applied cell bodies and elongated pseudopodia of peripheral macrophages. As seen from figure 12 the cytoplasmic processes of the macrophages penetrate between the cells of the outer layer of sheath cells to reach the basement membrane. Carbon particles can be seen to segregate to the outer side of the basement membrane and extend as a closely packed suspension in the spaces between the outer sheath cells, from which position the carbon is taken up, within a few seconds, into the surface pinocytotic vesicles of the macrophages.

No carbon particles have been observed in or between the cells of the inner layer (or endothelium), and at present it remains uncertain how the particles are able to penetrate to the spaces between the cells of the outer layer of the sheath. Electron micrographs reveal a space between adjacent endothelial cells which runs a remarkably convoluted course towards the basement membrane (fig. 12). Several observers have in the past recorded the existence of lateral channels passing outwards through the wall of the sheath [quoted by Solnitzky, 1937].

On the basis of these models for the segregation of particulate matter from the blood of the chicken, the following summary of the sequence of events which follows the injection of a protein antigen into the bloodstream has been constructed. In the presence of newly synthesized antibody, antigen/antibody complexes are formed, which rapidly segregate through the Schweigger-Seidel sheaths. The complexes are then taken up by the peripheral macrophages of the sheath, which migrate with their load of antigen/antibody complex along the side of the penicillary arterioles. In the course of this migration they encounter small lymphocytes which are in process of circulation through the splenic white pulp. At the beginning of the fourth day after antigen injection sufficient numbers of selected lymphocytes have been netted and co-agglutinated with the antigen-bearing dendritic macrophages to form the recognizable anlage of the germinal centre. The process of agglutinative growth of the centre by addition of further macrophages and lymphocytes proceeds up to the sixth day. At this time all the antigen-bearing dendritic macrophages have been included within germinal centres.

On the above hypothesis for the formation of the germinal centre practically all of the included small lymphocytes would be expected to carry a surface specificity which is complementary to the antigen localized to the surface of the dendritic macrophages. Some support for this hypothesis is provided by the finding that at a later time

(14–35 days), some of the germinal centres in the spleen can be shown to include cells almost all of which contain antibody to the injected antigen [White, 1963].

References

Coons, A.H.; Leduc, E.H. and Connolly, J.M.: Studies on antibody production 1. A method for the histochemical demonstration of specific antibody and its application to a study of the hyperimmune rabbit. J. exp. Med. *102:* 49 (1955).

Schweigger-Seidel, F.: Untersuchungen über die Milz. Virchow Archiv *23:* 526 (1862).

Schweigger-Seidel, F.: Untersuchungen über die Milz. Virchow Archiv *27:* 460 (1863).

Sell, S. and Gell, P.G.H.: Studies on rabbit lymphocytes *in vitro*. I. Stimulation of blast transformation with an anti-allotype serum. J. exp. Med. *122:* 423 (1965).

Solnitzky, O.: The Schweigger-Seidel sheath (ellipsoid) of the spleen. Anat. Rec. *69:* 55 (1937).

White, R.G.: Functional recognition of immunologically competent cells by means of the fluorescent antibody technique. In: The immunologically competent cell, p. 6 (eds. G.E.W. Wolstenholme and J. Knight) (Churchill, London 1963).

Author's address: Prof. R.G. White, Dept. of Bacteriology and Immunology, University of Glasgow, *Glasgow* (Scotland).

Antibiotica et Chemotherapia, vol. 15, pp. 40–55 (Karger, Basel/New York 1969)

The Origin of Antibody Forming Cells from Lymphocytes

Susan T. Ellis, J. L. Gowans and J. C. Howard

Cellular Immunology Research Unit, Sir William Dunn School of Pathology,
Oxford University, Oxford

Introduction

At the cellular level the simplest view of the induction of antibody formation is that the cell which initiates the response (the antigen sensitive cell) is also the cell from which the antibody forming cells are derived. An alternative view, recently suggested by Mitchell and Miller [1968], is that these two cell lines are distinct and that the antigen sensitive cell, having reacted with antigen, collaborates in some undefined way with the precursor of the antibody forming cell which is derived originally from the bone marrow. The aim of the present study was to identify antigen sensitive cells and precursor cells in a primary and a secondary antibody response in the rat.

The analysis is based on two simple observations. First, lymphocytes from the thoracic duct of normal (non-immune) rats will restore primary immune responsiveness to sheep erythrocytes in recipients whose immunological activity has been destroyed by a heavy dose of radiation. Second, lymphocytes from rats immunized some weeks previously with a single dose of alum precipitated tetanus toxoid will confer secondary immune responsiveness on heavily irradiated recipients; that is, the recipients respond in a secondary manner when challenged for the first time with antigen. In each of these experiments we have sought the answers to four questions. (a) Is it the small lymphocyte or the large lymphocyte in lymph which restores or transfers immunological responsiveness? (b) Is the restorative cell type also the cell which initiates the response; is it an antigen sensitive cell? (c) Is the restorative cell also the precursor of the cells which eventually synthesize specific antibody in the host? (d) Are (b) and (c) one and the same cell?

Small Lymphocytes

In connection with the first of the questions listed above it is necessary to define what is meant in these experiments by small and large
lymphocytes. The cells in thoracic duct lymph from the rat are almost
exclusively lymphocytes. Erythrocytes may contaminate the lymph
during the immediate postoperative period, presumably because lymph
drains from the site of operation into the thoracic duct, but they soon
disappear. Eosinophils may be present in small numbers (<0.1 %),
particularly following prolonged drainage of lymph. The remainder
of the cells are non-phagocytic, non-chemotactic, motile cells which in
the presence of serum do not adhere to glass or plastic surfaces and
which, despite their variation in size, all show the same characteristic
mode of locomotion when observed in the living state [Lewis, 1931,
1933; Gowans, 1957]. When examined in smears 90% or more of
these lymphocytes have cell diameters of <8 μ and when freshly isolated from lymph they never incorporate tritiated thymidine into their
DNA *in vitro*. These two criteria define "small" lymphocytes in the
context of the present experiments.

The remainder of the lymphocytes are larger, show a great variation in size and can be readily labelled with tritiated thymidine. No
complete picture can yet be drawn of the origin, fate and function of
these "large" lymphocytes in the rat but there is no doubt that some
of them give rise to plasma cells and others to small lymphocytes
[Gowans and Knight, 1964]. There are no macrophages in rat thoracic duct lymph, nor have macrophage precursors yet been detected
in it [Volkman and Gowans, 1965 a and b].

In recent years it has become apparent that small lymphocytes, as
defined by conventional microscopy, make up a heterogeneous collection of cells. This idea is based on studies in the rat which point
to the coexistence in thoracic duct lymph [Caffrey, Rieke and
Everett, 1962] and in blood [Robinson, Brecher, Lourie and
Haley, 1965] of two types of small lymphocytes with either short
or long life-spans; on the existence in bone marrow of small lymphocytes which are apparently formed in the marrow [Osmond and
Everett, 1964] but which lack the dramatic immunological properties of small lymphocytes from lymph and blood; and on the demonstration that under certain experimental conditions in the mouse,
small lymphocytes can develop into macrophages [Boak, Christie,
Ford and Howard, 1968]. Thoracic duct lymph from the mouse does

not apparently contain the precursors of erythrocytes or granulocytes [GESNER and GOWANS, 1962]. Heterogeneity of small lymphocytes must be sharply distinguished from pluripotentiality for which there is no decisive evidence.

Small lymphocytes, in the context of the present experiments with rat thoracic duct cells, will accordingly comprise a mixture of long and short lived cells but on present evidence no other sub-divisions can yet be defined. The long lived small lymphocytes are members of the recirculating pool and according to EVERETT, CAFFREY and RIEKE [1964] they make up about 90 % of the cells in rat thoracic duct lymph.

Methods

In order to determine whether the immunological performance of cells from thoracic duct lymph could be attributed to its content of small lymphocytes two kinds of inocula were prepared: (1) Washed cells from freshly collected lymph which contained up to 10 % of the large, dividing lymphocytes, the remainder being small lymphocytes. (2) Suspensions of thoracic duct cells which had been incubated *in vitro* at 37° for 24 h before their injection into the recipients. The large lymphocytes die more rapidly than small lymphocytes during incubation *in vitro* and the technique yields populations of small lymphocytes in which the proportion of large cells is reduced up to about 100-fold [GOWANS, 1962; GOWANS and UHR, 1966]. Comparisons of the activities of fresh and incubated thoracic duct cells provided the grounds for deciding whether the restoration or transfer of immunological responsiveness could be attributed to the small lymphocytes alone. It has not yet been determined whether the relative proportions of short and long lived small lymphocytes is changed following incubation for 24 h *in vitro*.

Most of the experiments have employed highly inbred strains of rat: AO (albino), HO (hooded) and DA (agouti) strains together with (AO × HO) and (HO × DA) F_1 hybrids. Rats from a non-inbred albino colony were used in one experiment.

The general plan of the experiments was as follows. (1) Fresh or incubated lymphocytes from the thoracic duct of normal (non-immune) rats, together with 1 ml of 1 % sheep erythrocytes, were injected intravenously into recipients which had received varying doses of γ-radiation from a Co^{60} source 24 h previously. The titres of serum haemolysin and the number of plaque forming cells (PFC) in the spleens were determined at various intervals after cell-transfer. (2) Inocula of fresh or incubated lymphocytes were prepared from the thoracic duct of rats immunized two to three months previously with a single intraperitoneal injection of 20 Lf of alum precipitated tetanus toxoid. The lymphocytes, together with 20 Lf of fluid tetanus toxoid, were injected intravenously into syngeneic recipients given varying doses of γ-radiation 24 h previously. Antibody was assayed by passive haemagglutination and antibody-containing cells were identified in smears of spleen cells by immunofluorescence. The techniques employed in these experiments are described in detail elsewhere [ELLIS, GOWANS and HOWARD, 1967].

Mouse-anti-rat and rat-anti-mouse sera were prepared by injecting members of one species with pooled spleen, thymus and lymph node (cervical and mesenteric) cells from donors of the other species. Three intraperitoneal injections, each of $50-75 \times 10^6$ cells, were given at intervals of two weeks and the animals were bled for the preparation of sera two weeks after the last injection.

Rat isoantisera were prepared by injecting members of one strain of rat with lymphoid cells from another strain. A number of different regimes of immunization were employed and sera giving the highest cytotoxic titres by trypan blue staining were selected for use in determining the origin of antibody forming cells in chimeric spleens. AO-anti-HO serum: AO rats were given three injections at intervals of two weeks, each of about 9×10^8 pooled cells from the thymus and lymph nodes of HO donors; half each dose was injected intraperitoneally, half subcutaneously. Sera were prepared from blood taken two weeks after the last injection. DA-anti-HO serum: a DA female, which had borne six litters by an HO male, was given three injections at intervals of one month, each of about 2×10^8 pooled cells from the spleen and lymph nodes of HO donors. Blood for the preparation of serum was taken eight days after the last injection.

Incubation of spleen cells with antisera. In order to discriminate between cells of donor and host origin suspensions of spleen cells were first incubated with an appropriate antiserum before assaying for the presence of antibody forming cells. Alliquots of about 4×10^7 washed spleen cells were incubated at 37° for one hour in volumes of 0.4 ml made up of fresh guinea pig serum (1 part), antiserum diluted one in four in foetal calf serum (2 parts) and cell suspension in 1:1 medium 199/foetal calf serum (1 part). The subsequent manoeuvres depended upon the technique for identifying antibody forming cells and are described in the text.

Primary Response to Sheep Erythrocytes

Lymphocytes from the thoracic duct of normal rats will restore to heavily irradiated rats primary responsiveness to sheep erythrocytes as assayed either by the titres of serum haemolysin or by the Jerne plaque technique. Figure 1 shows that the restored response differs from the normal response only in the time after immunization at which the peak number of PFC is achieved; in all other respects the tempo and magnitude of the responses are identical. Figure 1 also shows that purified populations of small lymphocytes (80-fold reduction in proportion of large lymphocytes) were effective as lymphocytes

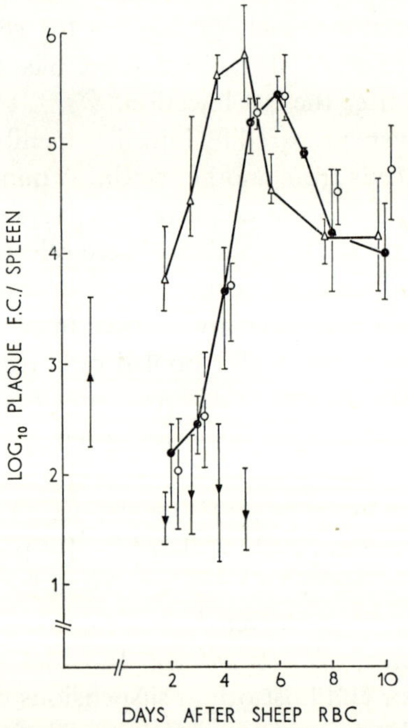

Fig. 1. Restoration of primary splenic PFC response in irradiated AO rats by 2.5×10^8 fresh (●) or incubated (○) thoracic duct lymphocytes (TDL) from normal syngeneic donors. Mean and range for 3–14 rats at each interval. △: response of normal rats to 1 ml 1 % sheep erythrocytes intravenously. ● and ○: response of rats given TDL and antigen 22 and 24 h respectively after 600 rad γ-irradiation. ▲: background PFC in normal, non-immunized AO rats; ▼: response of AO rats given antigen 24 h after 600 rad, but not TDL [from Ellis, Gowans and Howard, 1968].

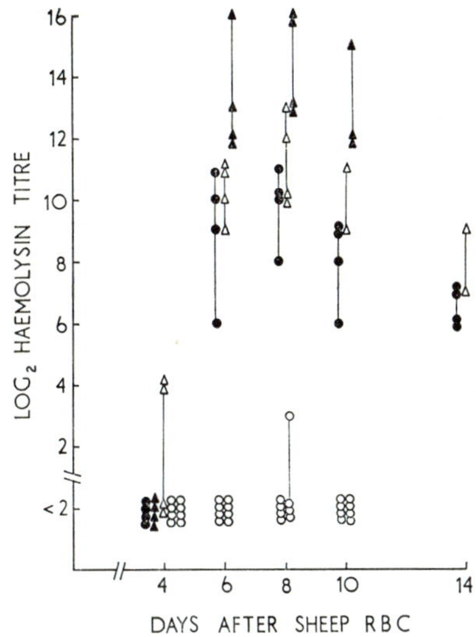

Fig. 2. Restoration of haemolysin response in irradiated rats by either thymocytes (Thy) or 2.4×10^8 fresh thoracic duct lymphocytes (TDL) given intravenously with 1 ml 1 % sheep erythrocytes 24 h after γ-irradiation. ●: 4 rats given TDL after 600 rad; △: 4 rats given TDL after 850 rad; ▲: 4 rats given TDL after 1000 rad; ○: 8 rats given Thy after 850 rad: 4 given 2.5×10^8 cells, 4 given 10^9 cells. ○ and ▲: syngeneic transfers; other cell transfers between non-inbred albino rats. Deaths occurred after 8 days.

from fresh lymph in restoring the response. Restoration with lymphocytes could be achieved equally well in rats given a lethal dose of 1000 rad of γ-irradiation but large doses of syngeneic thymocytes left the irradiated recipients completely unresponsive (fig. 2).

These results made it very likely that the injected small lymphocytes had given rise to the antibody forming cells because it is hard to see how host cells, after receiving 1000 rad, could differentiate, divide and synthesize normal amounts of antibody. This conclusion was tested by restoring irradiated DA rats with (HO × DA) F_1 lymphocytes and determining the survival of PFC after incubating spleen cells from the recipients with an isoantiserum directed against the unshared tissue antigens of the donor. Table I shows that, in terms of PFC numbers per spleen, F_1 hybrid lymphocytes restored a satisfactory immune response in parental strain rats given 1000 rad 24 h previously. Incubation of the spleen cells with an anti-donor serum (DA-anti-HO) resulted in a reduction of 82–99 % in the number of PFC in comparison with the number surviving in control suspensions incubated in normal DA serum. The results suggest that PFC were more readily eliminated by antiserum early in the response; this phenomenon is not

Table I. Origin of PFC in lethally irradiated parental strain rats restored with lymphocytes from F_1 hybrid donors

Recipient	PFC assay on recipient spleens		% PFC reduction after incubation with antidonor serum[2]
	Days after cells and antigen	Initial PFC/spleen	
1	3.75	2540	97.3
2	3.75	2200	98.2
3	4	[1]	99.3
4	4	[1]	98.5
5	5	140,000	84.0
6	5.5	277,500	82.0
7	6	825,000	86.0
8	6	465,000	85.0

Assay of PFC in spleens of DA rats given 1000 rad γ-irradiation and then, 24 h later, 1 ml 1 % sheep erythrocytes together with 2.5×10^8 lymphocytes from the thoracic duct of normal (HO $\times$ DA) F_1 donors. PFC assayed before and after incubation for 1 h at 37° with either normal DA serum or DA-anti-HO serum.

[1] no estimates made.

$$^2 \; \% \text{ reduction} = \left(1 - \frac{\text{PFC after incubation in antiserum}}{\text{PFC after incubation in normal serum}}\right) \times 100$$

related to the chimeric status of the animals since it was also observed when spleen cells from normal immunized rats were treated with a specific isoantiserum. An unresolved difficulty which complicates the technique is the variable survival of PFC in control cultures containing normal serum: reductions of up to 40 % in the number of PFC sometimes occurred. A similar but less serious loss has been described by MITCHELL and MILLER [1968] in their experiments on PFC in mice.

The results of this preliminary study provide strong evidence that the PFC were exclusively donor in origin, that is, derived from the inoculum of small lymphocytes. Admittedly, the design of the experiment was not ideal since it requires, in addition, the formal demonstration that a specifically anti-host serum does not reduce the PFC number. However, the dramatic effect of the DA-anti-HO serum cannot be explained by an effect on host (DA) cells.

Secondary Response to Tetanus Toxoid

Small lymphocytes from rats immunized some months previously with a single injection of bacteriophage ϕX 174 will confer secondary responsiveness to this antigen on heavily irradiated syngeneic recipients [Gowans and Uhr, 1966]. The recipients yielded a brisk antibody response if, and only if, they were challenged with antigen. The small lymphocytes were not secreting antibody at the time of transfer but they apparently carried the property of immunological memory.

A similar transfer of secondary responsiveness can be achieved with lymphocytes from rats immunized with tetanus toxoid. Figure 3 shows that thoracic duct cells from primarily immunized donors will confer on irradiated rats the ability to mount secondary responses which rival in magnitude those shown by normal immune animals; and that purified suspensions of small lymphocytes are as efficient as cells from freshly collected lymph in transferring responsiveness. Control experiments with irradiated recipients showed that the transfer of immune cells yielded no response unless antigen was also injected and that cells from normal (non-immune) donors conferred no reactivity to the challenging dose of antigen (fig. 3). Thus, irradiated rats acquired secondary responsiveness only after receiving cells from im-

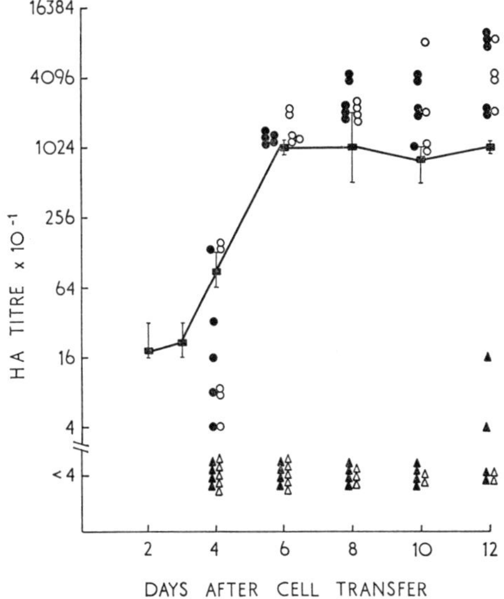

Fig. 3. Transfer of secondary responsiveness to irradiated rats by syngeneic thoracic duct lymphocytes (TDL) from donors given single dose of alum precipitated tetanus toxoid (APTT) 3 months before. Recipients given 2×10^8 fresh (●) or incubated (○) TDL and 20 Lf fluid tetanus toxoid (FTT) intravenously 24 h after 850 rad γ-irradiation. For comparison, secondary response to 20 Lf FTT in 4 normal rats given APTT six months before (■: range and mean). ▲: 4 irradiated rats (850 rad) given 2×10^8 fresh TDL from immunized donors but no antigen. △: 4 irradiated rats (850 rad) given $2.5-3 \times 10^8$ fresh TDL from non-immunized donors together with 20 Lf FTT.

mune donors and they only formed antibody after cell transfer if they were challenged with antigen.

Stimulation of lymphocytes with antigen in vitro. In the previous experiments the recipients were challenged with antigen *in vivo* at the time of cell transfer and it is possible that macrophages in the irradiated host contributed in some way to the initiation of the response. To examine this possibility lymphocytes from immune donors were challenged with antigen *in vitro*, thoroughly washed and then injected into the irradiated recipients. The production of antibody in the recipients, in the absence of antigenic challenge *in vivo,* would support the idea that macrophages are not essential for the inductive stages of this response.

Cells from the thoracic duct of immunized donors were washed once and resuspended at a concentration of about 50×10^6/ml in medium 199 to which had been added 20% v/v phosphate buffered saline, pH 7.3 (Dulbecco "A") and 1% normal inactivated rat serum. Fluid tetanus toxoid without preservative was added to the cell suspension to give a final concentration of 0.02 Lf/ml. The cells were incubated in corked flasks at 37° with constant shaking for periods ranging from 30 min to 24 h. After incubation, the cells were washed five times before resuspension into a convenient volume for intravenous injection into the irradiated rats. Attempts were made to detect the presence of residual antigen in lymphocytes incubated for 12 h in this way. No antigen could be detected by applying a specific fluorescent antibody to smears of these cells nor by disintegrating an aliquot of the cells ultrasonically, injecting them into a normal immune rat and assaying for the appearance of a secondary response.

A comparison of figures 3 and 4 shows that equally good responses could be obtained in heavily irradiated recipients with immune lymphocytes which had been challenged *in vitro*. In the first experiments of this kind the lymphocytes were incubated *in vitro* for 24 h with antigen in order to combine stimulation with antigen with the destruction of the large lymphocytes in the suspension. The responses transferred by such suspensions differed in no way from those which could be achieved by incubating lymphocytes for only 30 min at 37°.

Origin of the antibody forming cells. Two experiments have shown conclusively that the transferred lymphocytes develop into antibody forming cells.

In the first experiment lymphocytes from immune donors were incubated with antigen *in vitro* for 24 h, washed five times and injected

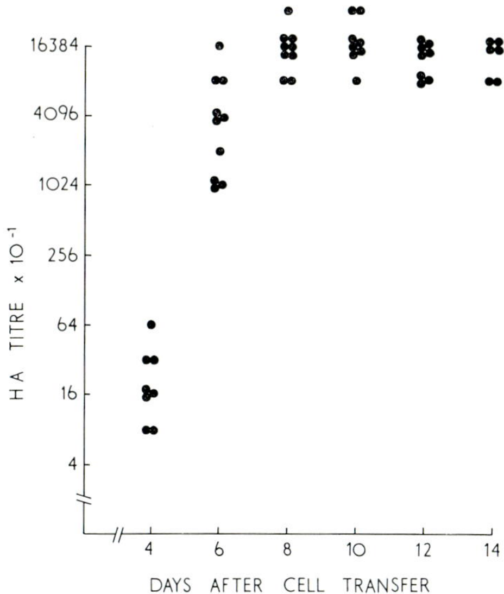

Fig. 4. Stimulation of lymphocytes with antigen *in vitro*. Thoracic duct lymphocytes (TDL) incubated *in vitro* for 30 min–24 h with 0.02 Lf/ml fluid tetanus toxoid, then washed and given intravenously to syngeneic rats 24 h after 850 rad γ-irradiation. No *in vivo* challenge with antigen. ●: 10 rats given 1.7–2.7×10^8 stimulated TDL. Deaths occurred after 6 days.

intravenously in doses of 1–2×10^8 cells into lethally irradiated CBA mice (1000 rad 250 KVP X-rays 24 h previously). Smears of spleen cells were prepared from those mice which survived for five days after cell transfer. The smears were fixed in cold ethanol and treated in turn with fluid tetanus toxoid and a fluorescein-conjugated horse anti-tetanus toxoid serum in order to identify the antibody-containing cells [ELLIS, GOWANS and HOWARD, 1967]. Large numbers of fluorescent cells were present in these preparations and the problem was to determine whether they were "rat" or "mouse" in origin. This was achieved by carrying out the above procedure on suspensions of spleen cells which had first been incubated *in vitro* with either mouse-anti-rat or rat-anti-mouse sera. The application of trypan blue to cell suspensions which had been incubated with mouse-anti-rat serum showed that the mouse spleens were composed almost exclusively of rat cells (table II). Fluorescent cells of normal morphology were present after incubating the spleen cell suspensions in either normal mouse serum, normal rat serum or in rat-anti-mouse serum. In contrast, incubation in mouse-anti-rat serum severely damaged the fluo-

Table II. Origin of antibody-containing cells in lethally irradiated mice given rat lymphocytes

		% all cells surviving[1]		% intact fluorescent cells[2]
		Pool 1	Pool 2	Pool 1
Serum in incubation mixture	Mouse-v-rat	1.4	3.8	3.6
	Normal mouse	100	91	93
	Rat-v-mouse	88	86	95
	Normal rat	95	86	97
No. spleens in pool		4	4	4

Overall survival of cells and proportion of morphologically intact fluorescent cells in spleen suspensions after incubation for one hour at 37° with various sera. Spleens taken from lethally irradiated mice injected 5 days previously with small lymphocytes from rats immunized with tetanus toxoid. Lymphocytes challenged with antigen *in vitro* (see text).

[1] by exclusion of trypan blue.

[2] antibody-containing cells identified by immunofluorescence. 250 fluorescent cells examined.

rescent cells so that none of them was morphologically normal: many were fragmented and those which were intact were swollen, showed an irregular and indistinct cell margin, and a stippled rather than a uniform cytoplasmic fluorescence (figs. 5 and 6). These experiments left little doubt that all the fluorescent cells in the spleens of the irradiated mice were rat in origin.

In the second experiment an attempt was made to determine the origin of the fluorescent cells in the spleen when both the lymphocyte-donor and the recipient were rats. For this purpose thoracic duct cells from (HO $\times$ AO) F_1 immunized donors were injected together with antigen into AO strain recipients which had received 1000 rad of γ-irradiation 24 h previously. Secondary responses of normal magnitude developed in these rats as judged by titres of serum antibody. Five days after cell-transfer the spleens of some recipients were removed, teased into a single cell suspension and aliquots incubated with normal serum or an isoantiserum. After incubation, the spleen cells were centrifuged, smeared, and treated with antigen and conjugate in order to identify antibody-containing cells.

Fluorescent cells of normal morphology were observed after incubation with normal rat serum but after incubation with an AO-anti-

Table III. Origin of antibody-containing cells in lethally irradiated parental strain rats given lymphocytes from immunized F_1 hybrid donors

		% all cells surviving[1]		% intact fluorescent cells[2]	
		Recipient		Recipient	
		1	2	1	2
Serum in incubation mixture	AO-anti-HO	27	15	0	0.5
	Normal AO	91	94	99	92

Overall survival of cells and proportion of morphologically intact fluorescent cells in spleen suspensions after incubation in normal and anti-donor serum for one hour at 37°. Spleens taken from AO rats given 1000 rads of γ-irradiation and then, 24 h later, 20 Lf fluid tetanus toxoid together with 2×10^8 lymphocytes from the thoracic duct of (HO $\times$ AO) F_1 donors immunized with alum precipitated tetanus toxoid 3 months previously.

[1] by exclusion of trypan blue.

[2] antibody containing cells identified by immunofluorescence. 500 fluorescent cells counted in each spleen. See Figs. 5 and 6.

HO serum virtually all the fluorescent cells were severely damaged and showed the same range of morphological changes which were described in the analysis of the rat/mouse chimeras (table III; figs. 5 and 6). These experiments provide strong evidence that the antibody-forming cells in the parental strain recipients arose from the inoculum of F_1 hybrid lymphocytes.

Discussion

Primary response to sheep erythrocytes. Thoracic duct cells from normal rats are extremely efficient at restoring primary responsiveness to sheep erythrocytes in rats given even lethal doses of irradiation. Thus, an inoculum of 2.5×10^8 cells, which probably amounts, at the most, to 20% of the number of lymphocytes lost from the recipient as a result of radiation, restores a response which rivals in magnitude and tempo that of a normal animal, as judged either by the titres of serum haemolysin or by the number of plaque-forming cells in the spleen. On the other hand, syngeneic thymus cells in very large numbers failed to restore any measure of responsiveness. This contrasts sharply with the results in neonatally thymectomized mice in which thymocytes and thoracic duct cells were equally effective in restoring antibody formation to sheep erythrocytes [MITCHELL and MILLER, 1968].

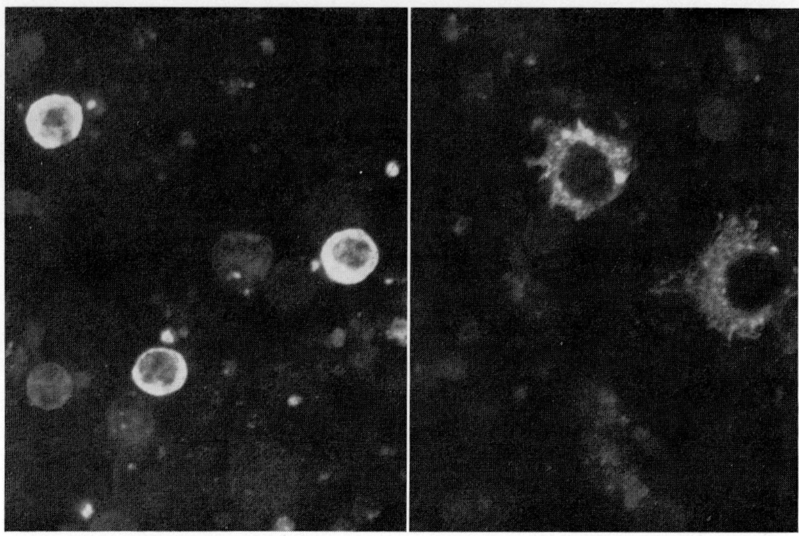

Figs. 5 and 6. Donor origin of fluorescent cells in spleen of irradiated parental strain rat given F$_1$ hybrid thoracic duct lymphocytes (TDL). AO rats given 1000 rad γ-irradiation and then, 24 h later, injected intravenously with 20 Lf fluid tetanus toxoid together with 1.8×10^8 TDL from an (AO × HO) F$_1$ donor immunized three months before with alum precipitated tetanus toxoid. AO recipient killed after six days and spleen cells incubated for one hour in either normal AO serum (fig. 5) or AO-anti-HO serum (fig. 6). Antibody identified in spleen cell smears by immunofluorescence. Fluorescent cells in figure 5 are intact; those in figure 6 are swollen, show indistinct and irregular cell margins, and the cytoplasmic fluorescence is speckled rather than uniform (see text). Both figures × 700.

These studies on the restoration of the response to sheep erythrocytes have led to the following conclusions. (a) We are confident that the restorative cell type in thoracic duct lymph is a small lymphocyte as defined by its size and by its initial lack of DNA synthesis. The magnitude and tempo of the restored response are not perturbed by varying up to about 80-fold the proportion of large, dividing lymphocytes in a standard inoculum of small lymphocytes. In addition, the main seat of the restored response is the spleen but we know that less than 1 % of an inoculum of large lymphocytes localizes in the spleen [McGREGOR, McCULLAGH and GOWANS, 1967]. (b) We think that small lymphocytes are antigen sensitive cells in this response. The strongest reason for this conclusion is the failure of lymphocytes from immunologically tolerant donors to restore the response [McGREGOR, McCULLAGH and GOWANS, 1967]. (c) The analysis with isoantisera of spleens from parental strain rats restored with F$_1$

hybrid lymphocytes has shown that the antibody forming cells are of donor origin, that is, derived from the injected small lymphocytes. Indeed, the lack of a host contribution in recipients receiving 1000 rad is not surprising. The magnitude of the restored response in lethally irradiated rats raises the further point that if induction by antigen involves the activity of host macrophages, then this activity in the rat must be highly radioresistant. There are suggestions from studies *in vitro* that macrophages may be essential for initiating the immune response to sheep erythrocytes [FORD, GOWANS and McCULLAGH, 1966; MOSIER, 1967] but nothing is known about requirements *in vivo*.

Secondary responsiveness to tetanus toxoid. Thoracic duct cells from rats primarily immunized with tetanus toxoid enabled irradiated rats to respond in a secondary manner to their first injection of antigen. The responses were at least equal in magnitude to those given by normal immune animals. As in the experiments with bacteriophage $\emptyset$ X 174 [GOWANS and UHR, 1966] the small lymphocytes were not secreting detectable quantities of antibody at the time of transfer and they only mediated a response when the recipients were challenged with antigen.

The conclusions emerging from this study are as follows: (a) The performance of incubated thoracic duct cells points to a small lymphocyte as the cell type transferring responsiveness; it carries the immunological memory. (b) Lymphocytes from immune donors, after a brief incubation with antigen *in vitro,* mediated substantial secondary responses in irradiated recipients without any antigenic challenge *in vivo*. The efficiency of stimulation with antigen *in vitro* is evidence that small lymphocytes are antigen-sensitive cells in this system and suggests that a preliminary processing of antigen by macrophages is not essential for the response. Possibly, the ease with which secondary responses can be carried to completion *in vitro* [DUTTON, 1967], in contrast to primary responses, is related to the relative importance of macrophages in the two responses. (c) An analysis of recipient spleens with antisera directed against donor tissue showed that the cells making antibody to tetanus toxoid were derived from the injected lymphocytes. Experiments of two kinds were performed. In one, antibody-forming cells of rat origin were identified in the spleens of lethally irradiated mice; in the other, which employed a rat to rat transfer of lymphocytes, antibody-forming cells from F_1 hybrid donors were identified in the spleens of lethally irradiated parental strain recipients.

In the primary and the secondary immune response examined in the present study it has been concluded that thoracic duct lymph from the rat contains small lymphocytes which can interact with antigen to initiate the response and also small lymphocytes whose progeny synthesize the specific antibody. The final problem is whether these two functions are performed by one and the same small lymphocyte. This would be the simplest view but unfortunately we have no evidence which bears upon it. The alternative view, following Mitchell and Miller [1968], would be that thoracic duct lymph contains two kinds of small lymphocytes: antigen sensitive cells of thymus origin and precursor cells of marrow origin, and that these collaborate to put the response into effect. The long and short lived small lymphocytes respectively are obvious candidates for these two cell lines but there is no information about their respective roles in antibody formation.

The idea that two cell lines collaborate in antibody formation does not, in itself, rule out the most plausible hypothesis: that antigen-sensitive cells generate antibody forming cells. One cell line (thymus-derived) might be concerned with the cell-mediated immunities and the other (marrow-derived) with the production of circulating antibody, and each might be independently stimulated by antigen. The dividing thymus-derived cells [Davies, Leuchars, Wallis, Marchant and Elliott, 1967] might exert their effect on the other cell line by providing a stimulus for cell division or by increasing the inductive influence of antigen by concentrating it at cell surfaces [Mitchison, 1968]. Speculations of this kind seem inherently more plausible than a transfer from cell to cell of the information for specific protein synthesis, but the available evidence leaves matters completely open.

Summary

Small lymphocytes from the thoracic duct of non-immunized and immunized donors respectively conferred primary responsiveness to sheep erythrocytes and secondary responsiveness to tetanus toxoid on rats given heavy doses of γ-irradiation.

Small lymphocytes carrying immunological memory to tetanus toxoid could be stimulated with antigen *in vitro*. Macrophages were not essential for the induction of the secondary response.

The use of antisera directed against the tissue antigens of the donor showed that the cells making antibody to sheep erythrocytes and to tetanus toxoid were the descendants of the injected lymphocytes. In these two immune responses in the rat the antigen-sensitive cells and the precursors of the antibody-forming cells are morphologically both small lymphocytes. The possibility that these two activities are performed by one and the same small lymphocyte is discussed.

References

Boak, J.L.; Christie, G.H.; Ford, W.L. and Howard, J.G.: Pathways in the development of liver macrophages: alternative precursors contained in populations of lymphocytes and bone-marrow cells. Proc. roy. Soc. B. *169:* 307 (1968).

Caffrey, R.W.; Rieke, W.O. and Everett, N.B.: Radioautographic studies of small lymphocytes in the thoracic duct of the rat. Acta haemat. *28:* 145 (1962).

Davies, A.J.S.; Leuchars, E.; Wallis, V.; Marchant, R. and Elliott, E.V.: The failure of thymus-derived cells to produce antibody. Transplantation *5:* 222 (1967).

Dutton, R.W.: *In vitro* studies of immunological responses of lymphoid cells. Adv. Immunol. *6:* 253 (1967).

Ellis, S.T.; Gowans, J.L. and Howard, J.C.: Cellular events during the formation of antibody. Cold Spr. Harb. Symp. quant. Biol. *32:* 395 (1967).

Everett, N.B.; Caffrey, R.W. and Rieke, W.O.: Recirculation of lymphocytes. Ann. N.Y. Acad. Sci. *113:* 887 (1964).

Ford, W.L.; Gowans, J.L. and McCullagh, P.J.: The origin and function of lymphocytes. In: The Thymus; Experimental and clinical studies. Ciba Foundation Symposium, p. 58 (Churchill/London 1966).

Gesner, B.M. and Gowans, J.L.: The fate of lethally irradiated mice given isologous and heterologous thoracic duct lymphocytes. Brit. J. exp. Path. *43:* 431 (1962).

Gowans, J.L.: The effect of the continuous re-infusion of lymph and lymphocytes on the output of lymphocytes from the thoracic duct of unanaesthetized rats. Brit. J. exp. Path. *38:* 67 (1957).

Gowans, J.L.: The fate of parental strain small lymphocytes in F_1 hybrid rats. Ann. N.Y. Acad. Sci. *99:* 432 (1962).

Gowans, J.L. and Knight, E.J.: The route of re-circulation of lymphocytes in the rat. Proc. roy. Soc. B. *159:* 257 (1964).

Gowans, J.L. and Uhr, J.W.: The carriage of immunological memory by small lymphocytes in the rat. J. exp. Med. *124:* 1017 (1966).

Lewis, W.H.: Locomotion of lymphocytes. Bull. Johns Hopk. Hosp. *40:* 29 (1931).

Lewis, W.H.: Locomotion of rat lymphocytes in tissue cultures. Bull. Johns Hopk. Hosp. *53:* 147 (1933).

McGregor, D.D.; McCullagh, P.J. and Gowans, J.L.: The role of lymphocytes in antibody formation. 1. Restoration of the haemolysin response in X-irradiated rats with lymphocytes from normal and immunologically tolerant donors. Proc. roy. Soc. B. *168:* 229 (1967).

Mitchell, G.F. and Miller, J.F.A.P.: Immunological activity of thymus and thoracic duct lymphocytes. Proc. nat. Acad. Sci., Wash. *59:* 296 (1968).

Mitchison, N.A.: Personal communication (1968).

Mosier, D.E.: A requirement for two cell types for antibody formation *in vitro*. Science *158:* 1573 (1967).

Osmond, D.G. and Everett, N.B.: Radioautographic studies of bone marrow lymphocytes *in vivo* and in diffusion chamber cultures. Blood *23:* 1 (1964).

Robinson, S.H.; Brecher, G.; Lourie, I.S. and Haley, J.E.: Leukocyte labeling in rats during and after continuous infusion of tritiated thymidine: implications for lymphocyte longevity and DNA reutilization. Blood *26:* 281 (1965).

Volkman, A. and Gowans, J.L.: The production of macrophages in the rat. Brit. J. exp. Path. *46:* 50 (1965a).

Volkman, A. and Gowans, J.L.: The origin of macrophages from bone marrow in the rat. Brit. J. exp. Path. *46:* 62 (1965b).

Authors' address: Dr. Susan T. Ellis, Prof. J.L. Gowans and Dr. J.C. Howard, Cellular Immunology Research Unit, Sir William Dunn School of Pathology, Oxford University, *Oxford* (England).

Antibiotica et Chemotherapia, vol. 15, pp. 56–63 (Karger, Basel/New York 1969)

Macrophages, Lymphocytes and Antibody Formation

M. FELDMAN

Department of Cell Biology
The Weizmann Institute of Science, Rehovoth, Israel

The studies reviewed in the present paper were designed to test whether the processing of antigen by macrophages is an essential step in the induction of antibody production. They were initiated following our observations on the kinetics of the induction of tolerance to human serum albumin (HSA) in x-irradiated rabbits [17–20]. Rabbits exposed to 550 r total body x-irradiation, then injected during the recovery period with otherwise immunogenic doses of HSA, acquired specific immunological tolerance to HSA. The animals remained susceptible to tolerance induction four weeks following exposure to x-rays [16, 20]. Furthermore, it seemed that smaller amounts of antigen are required for the induction of tolerance when antigen treatment is begun four weeks after irradiation, than when the same treatment is initiated after 24 h [20]. The histogenetic regeneration of the antibody-forming organs is practically complete at four weeks after x-irradiation, and the circulating lymphocytes, which decreased sharply after x-irradiation, regained normal levels within three weeks following exposure [16, 20]. In fact, they rose above the mean normal in the second month post-irradiation. It was therefore inferred that the lymphoid system *per se* may recover in advance of the recovery of immunocompetence. Accordingly, the regeneration of immune competence following exposure to total body irradiation depends not exclusively on the regeneration of lymphocytes, but most probably also on the post-radiation recovery of another cell type, which is thus essential for the induction of antibody production. The obvious candidate was the macrophage.

Experiments were therefore carried out in our Laboratory, aimed at testing whether x-rays can suppress immunological reactivity by inactivating the immunogenic function of macrophages. These were made in mice, using *Shigella paradys.* as the antigenic material [5, 6, 9–11]. The first series of experiments tested whether macrophages from normal mice, after interacting *in vitro* with Shigella antigen, will evoke antibody production in mice exposed to sublethal doses of total body x-irradiation. Peritoneal exudate cells of normal C57BL mice were incubated *in vitro* with Shigella antigen, then inoculated into mice exposed two days previously to 550 r total body irradiation. The inoculation of such antigen-treated macrophages elicited the formation of antibody in irradiated animals, which could not respond to the injection of the antigen alone [9–11].

The peritoneal cell populations used in the previous experiments consisted of 80% macrophages, yet they also contained about 10% lymphocytes. To test whether the macrophages *per se* were the cells which, following interaction with the antigen, triggered the production of antibody, further experiments were carried out in which pure populations of macrophages were obtained by culturing peritoneal cells *in vitro*. These macrophages were exposed to Shigella in culture, then injected into x-irradiated mice. The results showed that lymphocyte-free macrophage populations, obtained following *in vitro* culturing of peritoneal cells, induced the production of antibody in the x-rayed recipients [6, 11].

Experiments were then carried out to define the cells which produce antibody following the inoculation of antigen-treated macrophages into x-rayed animals. To test whether the recipient lymphocytes are the cells which respond to the macrophage "signal"—different groups of mice were subjected to different doses of total body x-irradiation which were expected to cause different levels of lymphoid depletion. Each of these groups was then inoculated with antigen-treated macrophages. The results showed that there was an inverse relationship between the levels of total body irradiation and the levels of antibody produced following injection of the "primed" macrophages. It was therefore inferred that normal macrophages, following interaction with Shigella antigen, can "instruct" cells of the sublethally irradiated mice to produce antibodies [6, 11].

Macrophages were found to be capable of inducing antibody production across genetic barriers. Macrophages from C57BL mice (H-2b), which had interacted *in vitro* with Shigella antigen, elicited antibody production in x-irradiated BALB/C animals (H-2d), and vice versa [6]. It appears that their capacity to signal antibody production depends upon their function as living cells within the recipient animals. This was deduced from experiments in which normal C57BL or BALB/C animals were immunized against the iso-antigens of the prospective macrophage donors by three weekly intraperitoneal injections of spleen cell suspension. The iso-immunized mice were then exposed to 550 r, and inoculated with "primed" macrophages of the genotype against which they were immunized. The results showed that primed macrophages can elicit antibody production in x-irradiated mice across H-2 barriers; their immunogenic effect is, however, completely inhibited if the recipients were previously sensitized against the prospective donors [6].

To further substantiate the participation of two cell types in the production of antibodies to Shigella, and the lymphoid nature of the cells responding to the macrophage "signal", reconstruction experiments were attempted. Mice were exposed to a lethal dose of total body x-irradiation (850 r). One group was inoculated with antigen-treated macrophages, a second with antigen-treated lymphocytes of either thoracic duct or lymph node origin, and a third group with a mixed cell population composed of antigen-treated macrophages and nontreated lymphocytes. Only animals of the third group produced a significant titer of agglutinating antibody [6]. Experiments were then performed to test directly whether x-irradiation does in fact inactivate the capacity of macrophages to process antigen. Macrophages from mice exposed to total body x-irradiation were incubated *in vitro* with antigen, then tested for their immunogenic activity in other x-irradiated recipients. The results showed that x-irradiation suppressed the capacity of the peritoneal cells to elicit agglutinin production in other sublethally irradiated mice [6, 11]. To test whether the effect of x-irradiation on the immunogenic function of macrophages is a direct one, macrophages from normal animals were exposed to x-rays *in vitro,* then incubated with Shigella antigen and tested for their immunogenic effect in mice exposed to 550 r. The result was that the *in vitro* irradiation, similar to the irradiation of the whole animal, abolished the capacity of macrophages to signal antibody production [6]. The inactivation of the processing capacity of macrophages by x-rays cannot be attributed to the suppression of the capacity of macrophages to take up antigenic material [6]. It thus appears that x-irradiation impairs the processing of antigen within the cells in an as yet unknown manner.

The cells responding to the immunogenic signal of the macrophages in the experiments reported in the present review could either be lymphocytes which had survived depletion caused by total body x-irradiation, or lymphocytes which had regenerated following exposure to x-rays. To differentiate between these two possibilities experiments were carried out, in collaboration with A. GLOBERSON, using the organ culture system for the induction of a primary antibody response *in vitro,* developed by GLOBERSON and AUERBACH [12]. Preliminary experiments were made to test whether organ cultures of spleen explants from normal donors will produce antibodies to Shigella. These have indicated that cultures of spleen explants when challenged *in vitro* with Shigella antigen produced agglutinating antibodies which could be demonstrated both in the culture medium and on the millipore filter supporting the spleen explant [to be published]. When, however, cultures of spleen explants from x-irradiated donors were similarly treated with Shigella, no antibodies were formed. Neither could antibodies to Shigella be produced when spleen explants of x-rayed donors were treated with Shigella in the presence of macrophages. On the other hand, when thymus explants were added to culture containing irradiated spleens, macrophages and Shigella, agglutinating antibodies were produced. These preliminary results may suggest that the spleen cells of x-rayed donors responding *in vitro* to the immunogenic signal of macrophages are cells which have achieved immunocompetence following irradiation due to an inductive effect of the thymus.

According to this concept, then, a bicellular mechanism is operating in the induction of a primary immune response to Shigella, based on the interaction, first of macrophage and antigen (processing stage), then of macrophage and lymphoid cell. This is obviously in accord with previous demonstrations of the immunogenic role of macrophages [1, 2, 7, 13]. The impairment, by x-irradiation, of the capacity to produce antibodies may thus depend not only on the depletion of the lymphoid cells per se, but also on the impairment of the immunogenic function of macrophages.

In a subsequent series of studies [H. GERSHON and M. FELDMAN, to be published], we tested whether the immune response to sheep red blood cells (SRBC) in sublethally irradiated mice can also be reconstituted with "primed" macrophages. The first series of experiments with SRBC aimed at testing whether peritoneal macrophages from normal mice, that had interacted *in vitro* with SRBC, will elicit antibody to this antigen in sublethally irradiated mice. Recipient mice were exposed to 500 r total body irradiation. Forty-eight hours later macrophages from normal mice were incubated *in vitro* with intact SRBC. After incubation, the macrophage-RBC mixture was gently centrifuged once, the RBC were then selectively lysed by dispersing the pellet in a small volume of Hanks' solution to which an equal volume of cold distilled water was added with rapid shaking. Immediate reconstitution to isotonicity was achieved by adding two volumes of 1 ½ times concentrated Hanks' solution. The macrophages remained intact, as attested by cytological smears made before and after the treatment. The "ghosts" of the lysed SRBC were then washed from the macrophages by repeated gentle centrifugations. The washed macrophages were injected intraperitoneally into the irradiated recipients. No detectable anti-RBC response was obtained. Having found that the minimum dose of irradiation which eradicated all but the slightest suggestion of a response to RBC fell between 400 and 450 r (whereas to obliterate the anti-Shigella response x-ray doses of 550 r or more had to be used), the previous experiment was repeated with recipient mice exposed to 400–450 r. Negative results were obtained.

It could be assumed that the hypotonic treatment of the macrophage-SRBC suspension is physiologically damaging to the macrophages even though no morphological changes were detected. Therefore, to eliminate the potentially detrimental step of hemolysis for the removal of the SRBC antigen, an immunogenically equivalent dose of RBC "ghosts" in isotonic solution was substituted for whole SRBC in the incubation mixture. "Ghosts", substituted in our protocol using 400 r irradiation, did not ameliorate our results.

Throughout these experiments, cytological smears of the macrophage suspensions were examined for phagocytosis of RBC. Depending upon the experiment, 0–5 % of the macrophages incubated with RBC in Hanks' solution exhibited phagocytosis. We therefore thought that the application of specific antibodies to SRBC to the *in vitro* incubation medium might improve phagocytosis [6] and concomitantly, perhaps, the processing of antigen for the immune response. On the basis of the enhancement of phagocytosis, 20 % C57BL normal serum and 1 % 5-day and 11-day[1] antisera were chosen as media for

---

[1] Mouse anti-SRBC serum obtained five days after a single i. p. injection of 10^9 SRBC ($1/\log_2$ agglutinin titer $= 10$); mouse anti-SRBC serum obtained 11 days after a single i. p. injection of 10^9 SRBC [$1/\log_2$ agglutinin titer $= 16$].

the incubation of macrophages with "ghosts". After incubation, the macrophages were washed thoroughly and injected into mice exposed to 400 r 48 h previously. None of the irradiated groups was capable of an immune response to SRBC under these experimental conditions.

Were the macrophage indeed the intermediary cell in the immune response to erythrocytes which was damaged by the sublethal irradiation, one should have been able to reconstitute the immune response of such irradiated mice by a simultaneous injection of macrophages plus antigen. Such a procedure might ensure a completely physiological incubation of the macrophages with antigen in the peritoneal fluid of the recipient mouse. The experiment performed demonstrated the ability of such a simultaneous injection to reconstitute the response to Shigella but not to SRBC.

It is a well-established fact that bacterial endotoxins function as adjuvants of the immune response [3] and afford some level of protection against irradiation [22]. In an attempt to solve the enigma of the different behavior of the anti-Shigella and anti-RBC responses, experiments were made to determine whether the endotoxin in the Shigella preparation might function nonspecifically to enhance the immune response in sublethally irradiated mice. Mice irradiated with 550 r were inoculated with well-washed samples of macrophages which had been incubated with "ghosts" plus Shigella. Anti-Shigella agglutinins were observed in the sera of mice which had been injected with macrophages preincubated with Shigella plus "ghosts", whereas no response to SRBC was detectable.

The experiments reported here indicated significant differences between anti-Shigella and anti-SRBC responses in sublethally irradiated mice. Yet, these need not indicate that the macrophage-lymphocyte interaction, which was demonstrated to be an essential step for the anti-Shigella response, is not so for the anti-SRBC reaction. The bicellular interaction in the response to RBC antigens has been demonstrated both *in vivo* [8] and *in vitro* [15]. Our *in vitro* experiments with Shigella have suggested that normal macrophages triggered the production of anti-Shigella antibodies by lymphocytes which, following irradiation, had regenerated and achieved immune competence due to the inductive effect of the thymus. The regeneration of immune competence towards different antigens may take place at different time intervals following irradiation. Indeed, a stepwise development of immune competence has been described by Silverstein *et al.* [21] in the normal ontogeny of adaptive immunity in the fetal lamb. The post-irradiation time interval required for the regeneration of the capacity of lymphocytes to respond to RBC may be longer than that for Shigella.

Whether the macrophage-lymphocyte interaction is an *essential* stage in the induction of a primary production of antibodies to *every* antigen is still an open question. Some observations indicate that a bicellular mechanism of macrophage-lymphocyte interaction is required to trigger a primary immune response to protein antigens as well. Thus, lymphocytes from adult donors did not confer immune reactivity to protein antigen on newborn rabbits [4], yet peritoneal macrophages when injected into newborn animals rendered otherwise immunologically incompetent rabbits immunologically reactive [14]. These experiments suggest that in normal ontogeny the immunological maturation of lymphocytes precedes that of macrophages, similar to the stagewise process of postradiation recovery of immunological reactivity, as demonstrated in our experiments.

References

ADLER, F. L.; FISHMAN, M. and DRAY, S.: Antibody formation initiated *in vitro*. III. Antibody formation and allotypic specificity directed by ribonucleic acid from peritoneal exudate cells. J. Immunol. *97:* 554–558 (1966).

ASKONAS, B. A. and RHODES, J. M.: Immunogenicity of antigen-containing ribonucleic acid of antigen-containing ribonucleic acid preparations from macrophages. Nature (Lond.) *205:* 470–474 (1965).

BRAUN, W. and NAKANO, M.: Influence of oligodeoxyribonucleotides on early events in antibody formation. Proc. Soc. exp. biol. Med. *119:* 701–717 (1965).

DIXON, F. J. and WEIGLE, W. O.: The nature of the immunologic inadequacy of neonatal rabbits as revealed by cell transfer studies. J. exp. Med. *105:* 75–83 (1957).

FELDMAN, M. and GALLILY, R.: The function of macrophages in the induction of antibody production in x-irradiated animals (Eds.) SMITH, R. T.; GOOD, R. A. and MIESCHER, P. A. In: Ontogeny of immunity, pp. 39–46 (Univ. of Florida Press, Gainesville 1967).

FELDMAN, M. and GALLILY, R.: Cell interactions in the induction of antibody formation. Cold Spr. Harb. Symp. quant. Biol. *32:* 415–421 (1968).

FISHMAN, M.: Antibody formation *in vitro*. J. exp. Med. *114:* 837–856 (1961).

FORD, W. L.; GOWANS, J. L. and McCULLAGH, P. J.: The origin and function of lymphocytes. In: Ciba Foundation Symp.: The thymus: experimental and clinical studies. Melbourne 1965, pp. 58–78 (Churchill, London 1966).

GALLILY, R. and FELDMAN, M.: The induction of antibody production in x-irradiated animals by macrophages that interacted with antigen. Israel J. med. Sci. *2:* 358–361 (1966).

GALLILY, R. and FELDMAN, M.: The cellular components in the induction of antibody by x-irradiated animals. Proc. Symp. on germinal centers in immune responses, Bern, 1966, pp. 333–336 (Springer, Berlin 1967).

Gallily, R. and Feldman, M.: The role of macrophages in the induction of antibody in x-irradiated animals. Immunology (Lond.) *12:* 197–206 (1967).

Globerson, A. and Auerbach, R.: Primary antibody response in organ cultures. J. exp. Med. *124:* 1001–1016 (1966).

Gottlieb, A.A.; Glisin, V.R. and Doty, P.: Studies on macrophage RNA involved in antibody production. Proc. nat. Acad. Sci., Wash. *57:* 1849–1856 (1967).

Martin, W.J.: The cellular basis of immunological tolerance in newborn animals. Austr. J. exp. Biol. med. Sci. *44:* 605–608 (1966).

Mosier, D.E.: A requirement for two cell types of antibody formation *in vitro*. Science, *158:* 1573–1575 (1967).

Nachtigal, D.: Lymphoid regeneration following x-ray treatment and the susceptibility to the induction of immunological tolerance. Proc. Symp. on germinal centers in immune responses, Bern 1966, pp. 329–332 (Springer, Berlin 1967).

Nachtigal, D. and Feldman, M.: Immunological unresponsiveness to protein antigens in rabbits exposed to x-irradiation or 6-mercaptopurine treatment. Immunology (Lond.) *6:* 356–369 (1963).

Nachtigal, D. and Feldman, M.: The immune response to azo-protein conjugates in rabbits unresponsive to the protein carriers. Immunology (Lond.) *7:* 616–625 (1964).

Nachtigal, D.; Eschel-Zussman, R. and Feldman, M.: Restoration of the specific immunological reactivity of tolerant rabbits by conjugated antigens. Immunology (Lond.) *9:* 543–551 (1965).

Nachtigal, D.; Greenberg, E. and Feldman, M.: The kinetics of immune tolerance to human serum albumin induced in sublethally x-irradiated rabbits. Immunology (Lond.) (in press).

Silverstein, A.M.; Uhr, J.W. and Kraner, K.L.: Fetal response to antigenic stimulus. II. Antibody production by the fetal lamb. J. exp. Med. *117:* 799–812 (1963).

Smith, W.W.; Alderman, I.M. and Gillespie, R.E.: Increased survival in irradiated animals treated with bacterial endotoxins. Amer. J. Physiol. *191:* 124–130 (1957).

Author's address: Prof. M. Feldman, Department of Cell Biology, The Weizmann Institute of Science, *Rehovoth* (Israel).

Antibiotica et Chemotherapia, vol. 15, pp. 64–81 (Karger, Basel/New York 1969)

Some Molecular Aspects of Antibody Formation

Brigitte A. Askonas and A. R. Williamson

National Institute for Medical Research, London

Introduction

This discussion is limited to cells and their precursors which are involved in the formation and secretion of immunoglobulins; it does not cover cells responsible for cell mediated immune reactions since much less is known at a molecular level about the latter.

Immunoglobulins (Ig) are multichain proteins, each molecule consisting of light and heavy chains, linked by disulphide bonds. The heterogeneous spectrum of Ig molecules found in the serum of an individual is derived from a heterogeneous plasma cell population throughout lymphoid tissues; each clone of differentiated cells appears to be limited to the formation of a single variant of light and a single variant of heavy chain, with each chain carrying a single allelic determinant.

Present views on the origin of molecular variability of Ig molecules within an individual and the question of limitation in expression of Ig genes during development of the lymphoid cells will be briefly discussed. It is known that antigenic stimulation leads to cell proliferation and differentiation of antigen sensitive cells; it is not clear as yet whether the antigen exerts any choice in gene expression or whether genotype and phenotype are fixed before a cell becomes "antigen sensitive"; whether the stimulation with antigen is direct or via macrophages is being discussed by other speakers.

At the level of the Ig forming cells the control of formation of light and heavy chains and steps in their assembly into Ig molecules will be discussed. In normal tissue there is overall a balanced synthesis of heavy and light chains whereas in neoplastic plasma cells defects in structural and regulatory genes often occur.

Genes and their Expression in Antibody Formation

The tremendous variability in amino acid sequence of immuno-globulin molecules, which an individual can make, has been a challenging problem for the geneticist. The large genome which would be required to code for all possible variants of heavy and light chains in an individual has brought the view into favour that at least a large part of the variability arises by somatic processes such as recombination (scrambling) and point mutation during the life of the animal.

A number of theories have been proposed based on somatic recombination between two similar but not identical genes coding for the variable region of each type of chain [Smithies, 1967] or between a small set of such duplicated genes [Edelman and Gally, 1967]. Recent data on the amino acid sequence of the variable region of light chain is not compatible with the minimal gene theory of Smithies, involving recombination between two genes coding for the variable section of the molecule [Milstein, 1967]. Therefore additional genetic events such as somatic mutation or additional genes coding for variable regions have to be involved.

Some type of somatic genetic event would imply that the stem cells, or primitive cells on division "scramble" their genes ending up with daughter cells possessing structural genes coding for a variety of different amino acid sequences in the variable parts of the Ig molecule. Presumably a large number of such divisions must be possible to account for the diversity of the Ig molecules and the cell population forming them.

At the other end of cell development, it is known that the differentiated plasma cells which are actively forming and secreting immunoglobulin molecules and antibody, have a potentiality limited to a single class of Ig molecules carrying a single allelic specificity on light chains and a single one on heavy chains. Evidence for this comes from fluorescent staining of Ig producing cells in lymphoid tissue of immunized animals using antisera specific for a given class or subclass of Ig, or a given allelic determinant [Cebra, Colberg and Dray, 1966; Pernis, Chiappino, Kelus and Gell, 1965]. Single cell studies in animals immunized with two non cross reacting antigens have shown furthermore that the majority of single cells form a single antibody specificity and occasional cells producing two different antibodies tend to be attributed to methodology [see discussion Lennox and Cohn, 1967 or Cohn, 1967]. At the molecular level, it is not yet possible to study the physicochemical properties of the Ig product of a single antibody forming cell. However neoplastic plasma cells in myelomatosis in mouse and human have provided us with cells derived from single cell clones which form molecular species of Ig representative of the spectrum of Ig molecules found in the serum of normal and immunized animals. Analyses of the products of myeloma cells have confirmed that a differentiated plasma cell forms a single variant of heavy chain and a single variant of light chain [see Mårtensson, 1966]. Allelic exclusion of autosomal genes has not so far been found in other mammalian cells. The mouse plasmacytomas have also established that Ig formed by each plasma cell tumour line remains constant over many transplant generations covering many years [Potter and Fahey, 1960; Askonas, 1961]. Thus, once a cell is differentiated to an Ig forming and secreting cell, the Ig phenotype and genotype are fixed, although cell proliferation takes place rapidly. This must be true also at the level of the antigen sensitive cell which is stimulated by exposure to antigen to proliferate for a limited number of cell divisions into further cells forming antibody with the same specificity. This is in contrast to the stem cells described earlier where gene "scrambling" and point mutations during cell division could be responsible for creating variability of Ig molecules.

This raises a number of questions: at what stage in cell development does the genome become fixed? Every cell possesses genes for the different Ig classes (α, μ, γ) and subclasses of heavy chains, and $\varkappa$ and λ type light chains and their subclasses; one must ask therefore at what stage in cell development does selection of one type of light chain and one type of heavy chain take place?—and in addition when is the choice of allele made? Two alternatives come to mind.

Freshly divided stem cells can in the right environment (e.g. lymphoid tissue) under influence of other factors, such as thymus, "mature" so as to limit the expression of their Ig genes to a single class or subclass or a single allele per chain, and to start forming small amounts of this species of Ig or antibody which would serve as cellular "receptor" for recognition and interaction with antigen. Following interaction with the antigen, the cells divide and differentiate always forming the same "receptor type" antibody molecules. This would be the simplest model, in which interaction with antigen would have no role other than stimulation of cell division and differentiation. The alternative is that the early cells can still express several Ig genes (several classes of heavy chain, types of light chain, both alleles) and form a few molecules of each Ig for which they still have a synthetic potentiality; antigen then would have the role, on inter-action with its specific receptor, to ensure that more of the specific antibody alone is formed, with the exclusion of the other Ig molecules. Whereas the first model mentioned above is simpler, further studies are required to establish this point. Purely on a quantitative basis, some findings are difficult to explain unless antigen sensitive cells possess more than a single potentiality. Considering the large number of antibodies with different specificities which an animal can make, an amazingly high proportion of cells (1 per 1000 peritoneal cells) have been found to be able to make 19S antibody to sheep red blood cells *in vitro* on exposure to sheep red blood cells in the presence of mitotic inhibitors [BUSSARD, 1967]. Observations of similar nature but involving cell mediated immune responses have been made by others [see discussion by COHN, 1967].

It can be concluded that fixation of genotype and phenotype, limitation in gene expression and allelic exclusion must occur during development of the cells, but further elucidation of the stages at which these events occur, whether before or after the cells have become antigen sensitive, is required. Whatever the chronology, however, the end result is that the differentiated plasma cell appears to have limited its potentiality to forming a single variant of heavy and light chains even on cell division. A simplified outline of the questions discussed above is presented in figure 1.

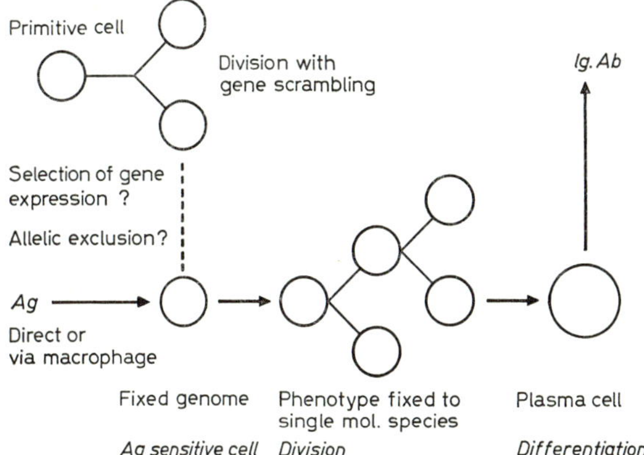

Fig. 1. Cellular and genetic events leading to antibody formation. Simplified schematic presentation.

Cellular Events Leading to Antibody Secretion

Other speakers are discussing antigenic stimulation including the mode of presentation of antigen possibly via the macrophage, and the experimentally elusive interaction between antigen and the potential antibody forming cells. Once the cells are triggered off by exposure to antigen, they respond by cell proliferation and differentiation and these stages of the response lend themselves to experimental study. It has been established that although some antibody can be formed and secreted during the first 24–48 h after exposure to antigen without cell division [Sterzl, Vesely, Jilek and Mandel, 1965; Bussard and Lurie, 1967] a full antibody response relies on cell proliferation which has a lag period of 24 h; Dutton and Mishell [1967], using their elegant *in vitro* system in which spleen cells exposed to sheep red blood cells, proliferate into large numbers of antibody forming cells which can then be assayed by their ability to form plaques, have been able to show that ^{3}H-thymidine at very high specific activities (15 c/mM) kills cells actively forming DNA. During the first 24 h after exposure to sheep red blood cells such a "hot pulse" (blocked after 24 h with cold thymidine) had no effect on the final number of plaque forming cells—whereas the same "hot pulse" administered 24 or 48 h later reduced the number of plaque forming cells to less than 3% of the stimulated control. The potential antibody forming cells were completely blocked since later addition of sheep red blood cells did not lead to increases in plaque forming cells. By this technique, the fact was also established that in this system, the cell population able to respond to sheep red blood cells was different from that able to respond to a non-cross reacting antigen, burro red blood cells. Thus the population responsive to sheep red blood cells could be knocked out with a "hot pulse" in the presence of sheep red blood cells. Subsequent addition of burro red blood cells in the absence of a "hot pulse" resulted in the usual number of cells able to form antibody to burro red blood cells. A similar result had been obtained by O'Brien and Coons [1963] studying the secondary response *in vitro* in lymph nodes from doubly immunized animals. DNA inhibitors such as bromodeoxyuridine, added with antigen A, blocked response to antigen A only. Removal of the inhibitor and subsequent addition of antigen B led to the usual antibody response. This requirement of a full antibody response for cell division and DNA synthesis within 48 h after antigenic stimulation may be the most likely step at which metabolic inhibitors of DNA synthesis will be specifically effective in blocking cells with this particular antibody potential, but not all antigen sensitive cells.

Less is known about the following stage, the actual differentiation of antigen-sensitive cells which involves cytoplasmic organization of the endoplasmic reticulum for secretion of the protein and active RNA and ribosome synthesis. Inhibitors of phospholipid or RNA synthesis would be expected to block at this stage. It does appear that some differentiation can occur without recent cell division [i.e. STERZL et al., 1965; BUSSARD, 1967] but during the normal course of an antibody response, most of the antibody forming cells will be derived from recently divided cells as mentioned above.

Control of Heavy and Light Chain Synthesis

Formation of Subunits Each as Single Polypeptide Units

Experimental findings so far indicate that the light and heavy chains are formed separately on polyribosomes of different size, each chain being formed as a single unit. Final proof is not available but this view is based on (a) studies of polyribosomes of Ig forming cells; (b) examination of relative labelling of peptides along the light and heavy chain following pulse labelling and (c) pattern of inheritance of genetic groupings located on different parts of the heavy chain.

a) *Polyribosomes.* By the use of an IgG forming murine plasmacytoma (5563 tumour line) as a model system and antisera specific for light and heavy chain, it was possible to characterize nascent heavy and light chains on different sized polyribosomes each of sufficient size to carry messenger RNA with the expected size to code for complete light and heavy chains [WILLIAMSON and ASKONAS, 1967]. Recently the size of polyribosomes in the relevant sucrose gradient fractions was examined by Dr. DE PETRIS by electron microscopy. The heavy polyribosomes of which 30–40% were precipitable with antisera to heavy chain contained up to 16–18 ribosomes. Polyribosomes of the expected sizes for complete light and heavy chain on RNA molecules have been found in lymph nodes of immunized rabbits [BECKER and RICH, 1966] and in another plasmacytoma (MPC 11) forming light and heavy chains [SHAPIRO, SCHARFF, MAIZEL and UHR, 1966a] whereas the very large polyribosomes were found to be missing in a plasma cell tumour line forming only light chains [SHAPIRO *et al.*, 1966a].

b) *Pulse labelling patterns of peptides.* The rate of synthesis of different portions of the heavy chain from the N- to the C-terminus was examined following pulse labelling of Ig forming cells for different time periods.

Peptides isolated from the heavy chain of rabbit antibody after degradation with cyanogen bromide followed a gradient of specific radioactivity from the N-terminal to the C-terminal end compatible with a single initiation point in the synthesis of heavy chain—with the exception of one black sheep peptide, which may not have been pure [FLEISCHMAN, 1967]. Further data has been obtained for tryptic peptides of light chain and for the Fd (N-terminal part) and Fc fragment (C-terminal half) of heavy chain of a mouse G_{2a}-myeloma protein [LENNOX, KNOPF, MUNRO and PARKHOUSE, 1967]. Difficulties in purification of peptides and chain fragments are considerable in all these studies; contamination of Fd by light chain is the most likely explanation for the finding that the Fd/Fc radioactivity ratios at the shortest time pulses (30 and 60 sec) are too high for agreement with a single growing point per chain. Overall the data is consistent with a single initiation point for each chain but final proof awaits solution of the technical problems.

c) *Linkage of genetic groupings.* Thus at the translational level, separate messenger RNA molecules appear to code for the entire heavy or light chains. On the basis of normally accepted relationships this implies that one structural gene determines the entire light, and one the entire heavy chain. In the human, inheritance of genetic factors located on different parts of the γ_1 heavy chain (e.g. Gm (a) on Fd and Gm (z) on Fc fragments) as a single gene complex in a given population have made it extremely likely that only one gene is required to code for each class of heavy chains [LITWIN and KUNKEL, 1967], although exact localization of the groupings in the chain are still missing. However, the paradoxical observation that three classes of rabbit immunoglobulin (IgG, IgA and IgM) carry identical allotypic markers on the Fab fragments, i.e. Fd part of the rabbit heavy chain [see reviews, OUDIN, 1966; KELUS and GELL, 1967] is responsible for the suggestion that the variable and constant regions of the heavy chain are under control of different cistrons, and that fusion of genes might precede transcription of the gene [see review LENNOX and COHN, 1967]. This would add further complexity to the problem of the Ig gene control. However, the observations on rabbit allotypes are based entirely on serological work using anti-allotypic sera which may have unknown complexity, and too little is known about the actual structure of heavy chains and allotypic determinants to reach any conclusions. It is even possible that the allotypic determinant represents a carbohydrate or other grouping which is attached to the α, μ and γ heavy chains following synthesis of the peptide chain [PERNIS *et al.*, 1968]. Not all of the IgM molecules appear to carry the allotypic determinants present on IgG, and heavy chains of IgM do have allotypic markers specific for the μ chains which may occur on different IgM molecules [KELUS and GELL, 1967]. If the allotypic determinant turns out to represent a constant amino acid sequence on the different heavy chains, mutational events leading to the different allotypic determinants must have preceded duplication and evolution of the different classes of heavy chain, and the preservation of the region carrying the allotypic determinant must be favoured by being important for light-heavy chain interaction as other regions of the Ig chains appear to be preserved in evolution, even between mouse and man.

Intermediates in Assembly

Pool of free light chains. A number of steps in the assembly of the completed heavy and light polypeptide chains into IgG can now be defined (fig. 2). Our previous findings [ASKONAS and WILLIAMSON, 1966; 1967a] have shown that completed light chains are autonomously released from polyribosomes into an intracellular pool of free light chains. This pool is small relative to the intracellular pool of IgG (molar ratio approximately 1:4). Free light chains in the pool turn over rapidly as intermediates in IgG assembly thus maintaining the pool at a constant size. Evidence for the intermediate role of free light chains comes from the time course of labelling (30 sec to 10 min) of free light chains and of light chains in assembled IgG, as well as from "pulse chase" experiments; in the latter experiment lymph node cells are incubated for brief periods (5–10 min) with radioactive amino acids, and then during subsequent incubation with non-radioactive amino acids the radioactivity in the free light chain pool is "chased" i.e. decreases with concomitant increase in radioactivity of IgG. The labelling of light chain relative to IgG at various

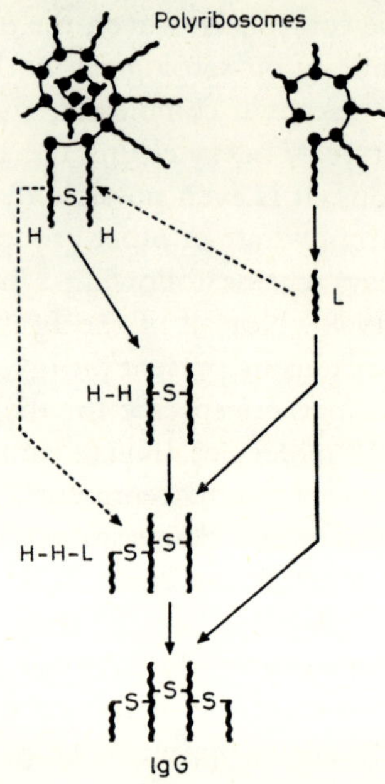

Fig. 2. Polyribosomal synthesis of light and heavy chains and assembly of IgG; schematic summary: L, light chains of IgG; H, heavy chains of IgG. Light and heavy chains are formed on separate polyribosomes, clusters containing 5–7 ribosomes forming light chains, and other containing 16–18 ribosomes are responsible for heavy chain synthesis. Light chains are rapidly released from polyribosomes. There are two alternative modes of assembly; (1) one represented by the broken arrows - - - - - → indicates possible inter-action of chains at the polyribosomal level, but there is no direct evidence for this release mechanism of heavy chains, (2) the presence of heavy chain dimers in the cell suggests early formation of the interheavy chain disulphide bond, release of the heavy chain dimer from polyribosomes and final assembly of the molecule with light chains.

times of incubation of lymph node pieces in the presence of radio-active amino acids and after a "chase" experiment are illustrated in figure 3. The existence of this small light chain pool does not conflict with the evidence for balanced synthesis of heavy and light chains discussed below. Indeed the pool of free light chains may play a role in maintaining balanced synthesis by interacting with heavy chains while still on polyribosomes, and aiding their release, but no direct evidence is available to prove this.

Disulphide bond formation. In discussing the assembly of IgG we must distinguish between the order of non-covalent interaction be-tween the four chains and the order in which the interchain disulphide bonds are then formed. In view of the pool of light chains, association

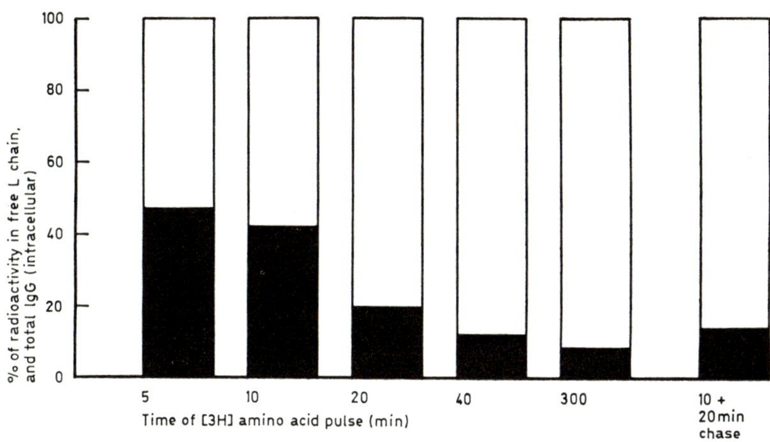

Fig. 3. Relative labelling of light chains and immunoglobulin-G within the cells after various time periods of pulse labelling. Pieces (1 mm³) of lymph node were incubated from 5–40 min with 10 μc ³H-labelled valine and leucine, and the intracellular proteins were extracted. Radioactivity of IgG and light chains within the cells was determined by sucrose gradient centrifugation followed by precipitation of IgG and light chains with antibodies specific for (a) IgG or (b) light chains [ASKONAS and WILLIAMSON, 1966]. The radioactivity in IgG plus light chains at any given time point represents 100 % radioactivity. ■ Percentage of radioactivity in light chains, ⊓ percentage of radioactivity in IgG. In the last column, lymph node pieces were incubated for 10 min with ³H-amino acids and then radioactivity in light chains was "chased" into IgG by continuing incubation for 20 min with non-radioactive amino acids.

between heavy and light chains might be expected to occur at or near the heavy chain synthesizing polyribosomes; if disulphide bond formation accompanied the interaction then half molecules (L-H) should be intermediates in assembly. Experiments designed to look for covalently linked intermediates, in which purified IgG determinants from pulse labelled cells were analysed by polyacrylamide gel electrophoresis under conditions which dissociate non-covalently linked subunits, did not reveal the presence of half molecules. Two other covalently linked intermediates of IgG were however found to be labelled; these were heavy chain dimer (H-H) and heavy chain dimer with a single light chain (L-H-H) attached to it. The relative labelling of these components with time suggests that they are intermediates in IgG assembly [ASKONAS and WILLIAMSON, 1967b and in preparation].

These data are summarized in figure 2. Two alternatives are indicated on the Figure since they cannot at present be distinguished.

Dimerization of heavy chains may occur at the polyribosome level with subsequent stepwise addition of light chains; alternatively heavy chain dimerization may take place after completion and release of heavy chain into the cisternae of the endoplasmic reticulum, with subsequent interaction with light chain, and formation of the inter light-heavy chain disulphide bond.

Normal Balance of Light and Heavy Chain Production

Overall balanced synthesis of equal numbers of light and heavy chains occurs in differentiated plasma cells forming IgG in lymphoid tissue of immunized animals and in some plasmacytomas, e.g., murine plasma cell tumour 5563 [ASKONAS and WILLIAMSON, 1966; 1967b]. In studies on myeloma globulin-A synthesis by plasma cells from peripheral blood of a patient (Dur) exhibiting myelomatosis, CIOLI and BAGLIONI [1967] found balanced synthesis of light and α heavy chains.

The question of balance can be posed at two levels: (1) is intracellular synthesis of subunits blanced? and (2) what are the secretory products of the cell? Do they represent only the final multichain protein, or are subunits or "intermediates" also secreted? The second question can usually be studied (a) by examination of immunoglobulin in the serum and urine and (b) by analysis of radioactive immunoglobulin determinants secreted by the cells during incubation of appropriate tissue *in vitro* in the presence of radioactive amino acids. For plasma cell tumour 5563, which we have studied extensively, and lymphoid tissue from immunized mice at the peak of the secondary response, i.e. five to six days after a booster injection, the results clearly indicate a balance of secretory products [ASKONAS and WILLIAMSON, 1966; 1967b]. Labelled proteins, secreted by these cells during *in vitro* incubation with radioactive amino acids for not longer than 3 h to ascertain preservation of the cells, were fractionated on sucrose gradients and characterized immunologically with specific antisera. The only specific secretory product was 7S IgG with no detectable excess of any Ig subunits [ASKONAS and WILLIAMSON, 1967b].

In all of these experiments, highly stimulated lymph nodes were chosen, with IgG representing 50% of the total protein synthesized. We have more recently examined light and heavy chain synthesis in lymphoid cells from mice primed two months previously with haemocyanin (HCY) during the course of a secondary response. The progression of IgG production before (0 days) and after a booster injection of 10 μg HCY in saline (2, 4.5 days) is shown by the relative incorporation of radioactive amino acids into intracellular and secreted IgG during a 3 h incubation of similar amounts of lymph node tissue *in vitro* (table I). Analyses of the labelled secretory products present in the incubation fluid by polyacrylamide gel electrophoresis followed by immune precipitation show no significant excess of light chains. Figure 4 shows the radioactivity of secreted IgG and no more than a trace amount of radioactivity in the light chain region of the polyacrylamide gel column. The trace amounts of radioactivity limit possible excess light chain production to less than 3–4% of the total radioactivity incorporated into IgG. For the purpose of this analysis polyacrylamide gel electrophoresis was carried out in phosphate buffer pH 7.2 containing 0.1% SDS and 0.5 M urea. The columns of gel (5% acrylamide) were sliced and the gel dispersed by a mechanical cutter [MAIZEL, 1966]. The radioactive protein was eluted with saline overnight, and radioactive Ig determinants were precipitated with antiserum specific for IgG and its light chains. The method will be fully described elsewhere [ASKONAS and WILLIAMSON, in preparation]. In parallel examination of the intracellular IgG determinants (not illustrated) a balance of light and heavy chain synthesis similar to that

Table I. IgG Formation by lymph nodes at various time intervals following antigenic booster

Group	Days after Ag boost	Radioactivity (CPM) Intracellular IgG (Ab/Ag ppt)		Intracellular IgG % of total protein formed	Radioactivity (CPM) Extracellular IgG	
			Corr^n. for isotope conc[+]			Corr^n. for isotope conc[+]
1	0	11,500	3,630	9	9,000	3,000
2	2	15,000	7,500	9.7	15,200	7,100
3	4.5	29,500	29,500	31	16,800	16,800[1]

C57/B1 mice were primed in the footpad with 10 μg haemocyanin (HCY) in Freund's adjuvant eight weeks previously.

Boost: 10 μg soluble HCY. Twenty pieces of lymph node (flank) from each group of animals were incubated with different amounts of ^{3}H-L-valine and ^{3}H-L-leucine for 3 h at 37° as follows: group 1, 30 μc; group 2, 20 μc and group 3, 10 μc of each amino acid.
[+] The correction for the same isotope concentration at each time point is approximate.

[1] Some material lost on concentration of fluid.

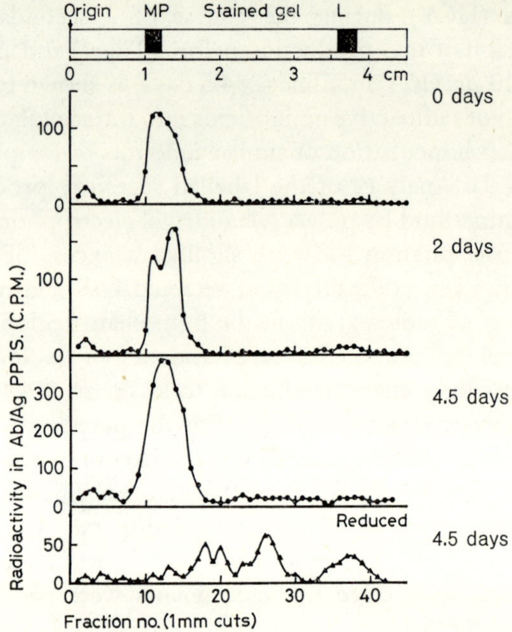

Fig. 4. Analysis of immunoglobulins secreted by lymph node cells at various stages during a secondary response. Lymph nodes from mice primed in the footpad with 10 μg HCY in Freund's adjuvant 2 months previously were tested: 0 days (no further treatment), and 2 or 4.5 days following a booster injection of 10 μg soluble HCY (as indicated in the figure). Pieces of lymph nodes were incubated for 3 h at 37° with ³H-valine and leucine (see table I): the extracellular fluids were collected and radioactivity of IgG and possible light chains analyzed by electrophoresis on columns of 5 % acrylamide gels followed by immunological identification of radioactive IgG determinants (see text). Top of the figure gives position on acrylamide gel of IgG (G$_{2a}$-myeloma protein 5563) and light chain (L). The last analysis was carried out following reduction of labelled IgG with 0.1 M mercaptoethanol to indicate the position of light and heavy chains on the acrylamide gel.

previously described for hyperimmune mice [ASKONAS and WILLIAMSON, 1967b] was found at each stage of the secondary response studied. Recent examination of lymph nodes from normal mice excludes any gross overproduction and secretion of light chains by unstimulated lymphoid cells.

There are however two reports which suggest that normal balance is not universal. SHAPIRO, SCHARFF, MAIZEL and UHR [1966b] and SKVORTSOV and GURVICH [1968] have both observed that rabbit lymphoid tissue synthesizes and secretes a great excess of free light chains. The latter workers noted however that antigenic stimulation only increases the production of whole Ig molecules, whereas incorporation of radioactive amino acids into light chains remains constant during immunization.

Defects in Regulatory or Structural Genes in Neoplastic Cells

Although certain neoplastic plasma cells (see above) exhibit a balanced synthesis of light and heavy chains, imbalanced production of subunits is frequently observed in plasma cell tumours in both mouse and human. Excess light chains are often produced, leading to secretion of light chains from the cells into the circulation and excretion of light chains in the urine (Bence Jones proteinuria). Such cases have been studied in the mouse, showing linear incorporation of radioactive amino acids into both light chains and myeloma protein intracellularly and secreted into the medium [ASKONAS and FAHEY, 1961]. CIOLI and BAGLIONI [1967] described rapidly labelled light chain dimers in pulse labelled bone marrow cells from a patient (Col) with Bence Jones proteinuria. The light chain dimers (L-L) most likely represent overproduction of light chains, which can dimerize, rather than intermediates in assembly of IgG since L-L needs to be reduced before the chains can effectively assemble with heavy chains into Ig molecules. The above authors also showed that light chains can be synthesized in excess over heavy chains by neoplastic cells from patients who do not show any detectable Bence Jones protein in the urine. Clearly isotope incorporation is a more sensitive method of detecting excess light chain synthesis than the estimation of Bence Jones protein in the urine.

In many cases of myelomatosis, there is complete suppression of the expression of the structural gene for heavy chain—with the appearance of only light chains in the serum and urine. Excellent demonstrations of the suppression of heavy chain genes are provided by the isolation of tumours forming only light chains as sublines from several tumours which originally formed both heavy and light chains [POTTER and KUFF, 1964]. Polyribosomes of one such subline (47B) have been studied by us and were found to lack the large polyribosomes with heavy chain determinants present in the original 47A line.

Formation and secretion of completed excess heavy chains, or only heavy chains (with suppression of the expression of light chain genes) have not been described. This may be due to the properties of heavy chains, which are very unstable molecules and tend to aggregate and become insoluble at neutral pH. Non-secretory plasma cells and tumours thereof have been described in the literature, and may well contain insoluble heavy chains. Such tumours are now being studied by Dr. Allison and Dr. McIntyre. A Burkitt's lymphoma which forms and secretes only μ chains has been described [Finegold, Fahey and Granger, 1967]. In addition to these defects in regulation of gene expression or translation, there are many examples of faults in assembly of incompleted chains, which most likely are caused by defective structural genes, or possibly by a block in assembly due to faulty attachment of carbohydrate to the polypeptide chains or some such step.

Potter and Kuff [1964] described a plasmacytoma in mice (47A) which forms and secretes half molecules (one light chain linked to one heavy chain by disulphide bonds). This suggests that the region around the inter-heavy chain disulphide bond is defective, unless the bond formation is blocked. The latter is apt to be responsible for the observed presence within the cell and the secretion of Ig molecules, half molecules and light chains by mouse plasma cell tumour MPC-11 [Scharff, 1967]. The kinetics of labelling of intracellular half molecules are not consistent with a precursor-product relationship and one might expect their excess secretion from the cell was due to a block in disulphide bond formation. "Heavy chain disease" appears to be caused by a faulty structural gene for heavy chains; the product excreted by one such patient has been analyzed and the subunit consisted of the Fc portion of the heavy chain (the C-terminal half) and appeared to have the same N-terminal amino acids as found in human γ heavy chains (PCA-VAL-GLN) [Prahl, 1967]. This may represent a rare deletion of a large part of the Fd region of the heavy chain, resulting in a soluble product which can be secreted.

Disorders in haemoglobin synthesis provide us with an analogous situation. Normally, there is synchronized production of α and β chains of haemoglobin. In disorders, such as α and β thalassaemia, there is excess production of β or α chain respectively [see for example Fessas, 1966].

One can thus conclude that, under normal conditions, there is a synchrony in the formation of the different subunits of a given protein, with the final protein as the only product. This is the case even when the genes for the two types of chains (light and heavy) are on either different chromosomes, or at least far apart on the same chromosome; by analysis of genetic groupings on light and heavy chains it has been shown that the genes for the two types of chains are inherited separately [see review Mårtensson, 1966]. However, under abnormal conditions such as the rapid, unlimited cell division in plasmacytomas asynchrony in the transcription of structural genes develops frequently.

Summary

Recent studies have led to the following general picture of IgG biosynthesis in cells actively forming and secreting immunoglobulin.

a) The differentiated cells appear to have a limited potentiality and to express genes for a single variant of light and a single variant of heavy chain. The question as to how the variability of Ig normally formed by different cells of an individual arises and at what stage in cell development the genome becomes fixed and limitation of gene expression occurs have been briefly discussed.

b) Experimental evidence indicates that light and heavy chains are formed on separate polyribosomes each as a single polypeptide chain.

c) Light chains are rapidly released from their site of synthesis into a small intracellular pool which turns over rapidly, is limited in size by incorporation of light chains into IgG and is maintained within the cells.

d) Disulphide bonding between the heavy chains precedes the linking of light and heavy chains.

e) Overall, in lymphoid tissue from hyper-immunized animals, there is synchrony in the production of equal numbers of light and heavy chains, so that the final immunoglobulin molecules are the only secretory product of the cell and no significant secretion of excess light chains can be detected. This holds true also for lymphoid tissue from normal animals, and at all stages during the secondary response. However, in neoplastic plasma cells in the mouse and human defects in structural genes, as well as in regulatory genes, occur frequently, with resulting difficulties in assembly of the molecule and imbalance in chain production.

Despite the unique nature of immunoglobulins, no novel mechanism of protein synthesis has been uncovered—so that immunosuppression at the level of protein synthesis by cells already forming antibody can hardly be expected to specifically affect only Ig forming cells. However, antigen sensitive cells, which on exposure to antigen are stimulated to proliferate with a 24 h lag period and then to differentiate, may be very sensitive target cells to agents blocking DNA synthesis if these are administered at the time of or within 48 h after exposure to antigen. These agents would be expected to block only the cell population activated to divide by exposure to antigen, and not all of the cells sensitive to other antigens. Since strong antigens like sheep red blood cells induce some antibody without cell division, this would not block antibody formation entirely. Killing of antigen sensitive cells as an effective means of depressing the immune response will be discussed fully by other speakers.

References

Askonas, B.A.: A study on globulin formation by plasma-cell neoplasma (5563) transplantable in mice. Biochem. J. *79:* 33–43 (1961).

Askonas, B.A. and Fahey, J.L.: Formation of Bence-Jones protein and myeloma protein *in vitro* by the plasma-cell tumour MPC-2. Biochem. J. *80:* 261–268 (1961).

Askonas, B.A. and Williamson, A.R.: Biosynthesis of immunoglobulins. Free light chain as an intermediate in the assembly of γG-molecules. Nature (Lond.) *211:* 369–372 (1966).

Askonas, B.A. and Williamson, A.R.: Biosynthesis and assembly of immunoglobulin G. Cold Spring Harbor. Symp. quant. Biol. *32:* 223–231 (1967a).

Askonas, B.A. and Williamson, A.R.: Balanced heavy and light chain synthesis in immune tissue and disulphide bond formation in IgG assembly. In: Gamma globulins. Nobel Symp. 3., pp. 369–383 (Almqvist and Wiksell, Stockholm 1967b).

Becker, M.J. and Rich, A.: Polyribosomes of tissues producing antibodies. Nature (Lond.) *212:* 142–146 (1966).

Bussard, A.E.: Primary antibody response induced *in vitro* by cells from normal animals. Cold Spring Harbor. Symp. quant. Biol. *32:* 465–475 (1967).

Bussard, A.E. and Lurie, M.: Primary antibody response *in vitro* in peritoneal cells. J. exp. Med. *125:* 873–891 (1967).

Cebra, J.J.; Colberg, J.E. and Dray, S.: Rabbit lymphoid cells differentiated with respect to α-, γ- and μ-heavy polypeptide chains and to allotypic markers AA1 and AA2. J. exp. Med. *123:* 547–557 (1966).

Cioli, D. and Baglioni, C.: Studies on the synthesis of the peptide chains of human immunoglobulins. In: Gamma globulins. Nobel Symp. 3., pp. 401–420 (Almqvist and Wiksell, Stockholm 1967).

Cohn, M.: Antibody synthesis; the take home lesson. In: Gamma globulins. Nobel Symp. 3., pp. 615–640 (Almqvist and Wiksell, Stockholm 1967).

Dutton, R.W. and Mishell, R.I.: Cell populations and cell proliferation in the *in vitro* response of normal mouse spleen to heterologous erythrocytes. J. exp. Med. *126:* 443–454 (1967).

Edelman, G.M. and Gally, J.A.: Somatic recombination of duplicated genes: An hypothesis on the origin of antibody diversity. Proc. nat. Acad. Sci., Wash. *57:* 353–358 (1967).

Fessas, P.: The disturbance of haemoglobin synthesis in thalassaemia. Int. Symp. Comp. Hemoglob. Struct., Thessalonika, pp. 51–59 (1966).

Finegold, I.; Fahey, J.L. and Granger, H.: Synthesis of immunoglobulins by tumour cell lines in tissue culture. J. Immunol. *99:* 839–848 (1967).

Fleishman, J.B.: Synthesis of the γG heavy chain in rabbit lymph node cells. Biochemistry *6:* 1311–1320 (1967).

Kelus, A.S. and Gell, P.G.H.: Immunoglobulin allotypes of experimental animals. Progr. Allergy *11:* 141–184 (1967).

Lennox, E.S. and Cohn, M.: Immunoglobulins. Ann. Rev. Biochem. *36:* 365–406 (1967).

Lennox, E.S.; Knopf, P.M.; Munro, A.J. and Parkhouse, R.M.E.: A search for biosynthetic subunits of light and heavy chains of immunoglobulins. Cold Spring Harbor. Symp. quant. Biol. *32:* 66–70 (1967).

Litwin, S.D. and Kunkel, H.G.: The genetic control of γ-globulin heavy chains. Studies of the major heavy chain sub-group utilizing multiple genetic markers. J. exp. Med. *125:* 847–862 (1967).

Maizel, J.V. Jr.: Acrylamide-gel electrophorograms by mechanical fractionation: Radioactive adenovirus proteins. Science *151:* 988–990 (1966).

Mårtensson, L.: Genes and immunoglobulins. Vox Sang. *11:* 521–545 (1966).

Milstein, C.: Linked groups of residues in immunoglobulin $\varkappa$ chains. Nature (Lond.) *216:* 330–335 (1967).

O'Brien, T.F. and Coons, A.H.: The effect of 5-bromodeoxyuridine on the *in vitro* anamnestic antibody response. J. exp. Med. *117:* 1063–1074 (1963).

Oudin, J.: Genetic regulation of immunoglobulin synthesis. J. cell Physiol. *67:* 77–108 (1966).

Pernis, B.; Chiappino, G.; Kelus, A.S. and Gell, P.G.H.: Cellular localization of immunoglobulins with different allotypic specificities in rabbit lymphoid tissues. J. exp. Med. *122:* 853–875 (1965).

Pernis, B.; Torrigiani, G.; Amante, L.; Kelus, A.S. and Cebra, J.J.: Identical allotypic markers of heavy polypeptide chains present in different immunoglobulin classes. Immunology (Lond.) *14:* 445–451 (1968).

Potter, M. and Fahey, J.L.: Studies on eight transplantable plasma cell neoplasms of mice. J. nat. Cancer Inst. *24:* 1153–1163 (1960).

Potter, M. and Kuff, E.L.: Disorders in the differentiation of protein secretion in neoplastic plasma cells. J. molec. Biol. *9:* 537–544 (1964).

Prahl, J.W.: N- and C-terminal sequences of a heavy chain disease protein and its genetic implications. Nature (Lond.) *215:* 1386–1387 (1967).

Scharff, M.D.: The assembly of gamma globulin in relation to its synthesis and secretion. In: Gamma globulins. Nobel Symp., 3, pp. 385–399 (Almqvist and Wiksell, Stockholm 1967).

Shapiro, A.L.; Scharff, M.D.; Maizel, J.V. Jr. and Uhr, J.W.: Polyribosomal synthesis and assembly of the H and L chains of gamma globulin. Proc. nat. Acad. Sci. Wash. *56:* 216–221 (1966a).

Shapiro, A.L.; Scharff, M.D.; Maizel, J.V. Jr. and Uhr, J.W.: Synthesis of excess light chains of gamma globulin by rabbit lymph node cells. Nature (Lond.) *211:* 243–245 (1966b).

Skvortsov, V.T. and Gurvich, A.E.: *In vitro* synthesis of the immunoglobulin subunits. Molekulj. Biolog. *2:* 59 (1968).

Smithies, O.: Antibody variability. Science *157:* 267–273 (1967).

Sterzl, J.; Vesely, J.; Jilek, M. and Mandel, L.: The inductive phase of antibody formation studied with isolated cells. In: Molecular and cellular basis of antibody formation. Czech. Acad. Sci. Prague. pp. 463–475 (1965).

Williamson, A.R. and Askonas, B.A.: Biosynthesis of immunoglobulins: The separate classes of polyribosomes synthesizing heavy and light chains. J. molec. Biol. *23:* 201–214 (1967).

Authors' address: Dr. Brigitte A. Askonas and Dr. A.R. Williamson, National Institute for Medical Research, Mill Hill, *London, N.W. 7* (England).

Antibiotica et Chemotherapia, vol. 15, pp. 82–97 (Karger, Basel/New York 1969)

Use of Humoral or Cellbound Antibody to Achieve Depression of Immunological Reactivity

H. Wigzell

Department of Tumor Biology, Karolinska Institute, Stockholm

The induction of detectable antibody formation has as a normal prerequisite the presence of immunogen [30]. Although the action of the inducer, antigen, is largely unknown it is commonly assumed that antigen will combine with specific, antibody-receptors before potential, antibody-forming cells will be switched into immunoglobulin synthesis [13, 32]. The location of the antigen-specific receptors is unknown at the cellular level but they are tacitly considered to be present on the outer surface of the potential, antibody-forming cells. Three principal approaches to achieve immunological depression by antibody of immunocompetent cells *in vivo* or *in vitro* will be discussed in the present article, all of which are taking advantage of the above mentioned facts. A fourth possibility, that of using specific anti-lymphocytic antibody to depress the immunological capacity of lymphocytes will be adequately covered by other speakers in this symposium.

Blocking of Cellbound Receptors for
Antigen Using Anti-Immunoglobulin Antisera

If induction of immunity involves the combination between inducing immunogen and cellbound receptors having the antigenic characteristics of serum immunoglobulins blocking of that receptor with anti-immunoglobulin antibody would act in an immunosuppressive manner. That this principle is seemingly valid is indicated by the results obtained when administrating specific anti-allotype antiserum to newborn rabbits [7, 8] or mice [12] being heterozygous as to that allotype locus. Administration of antibodies directed against one of the two possible allotypes could be shown to cause a significant depression in the subsequent production of that allotype as shown in the serum [7, 8] and to reduce the number of cells producing antibodies carrying the allotype marker [3]. The inhibition could be shown to be reversible with time, the time period needed to recover being similar to that of recovery from immunological paralysis to protein antigens [27]. It is quite conceivable that both processes might revert to the normal stage by a similar process, the rate of recruitment of new, uninhibited cells into the immune system.

More direct evidence for the identity of the receptor as a protein of immunoglobulin-nature has been provided by trials to use an anti-immunoglobulin antiserum to block the induction of secondary response *in vitro* by antigen [17]. The addition of this antiserum could be shown to inhibit the induction of the secondary response in a truly competitive manner, where the blocking effect of antiserum could be overcome by using larger doses of antigen. This latter finding would exclude that the anti-immunoglobulin antiserum merely acted by exerting a cytotoxic effect on the immunological memory cells. The results are fully compatible with the concept of the immunoglobulin nature of the receptor but do not exclude that the inhibition caused by the anti-immunoglobulin antiserum was caused by steric hindrance rather than actual direct combination by the anti-immunoglobulin antibody with the receptor.

Taken together, the anti-allotype-induced suppression *in vivo* [3, 7, 8] as well as the inhibition of the induction of secondary response *in vitro* by anti-immunoglobulin antiserum [17] both argue, although in an indirect manner that the cellbound receptors for antigen are of the same or very similar immunoglobulin type as the eventual product of the cells, the serum antibody. The above described approach to cause immunosuppression by using antibody directed against antibody could conceivably lead to specific inhibition of the production of any immunoglobulin class, however, the method would not allow any specific depression of immunological reactivity against different, antigenic specificities. Major emphasis will be devoted in this lecture to two procedures allowing such a specific immunodepression.

Inhibition of Specific Antibody Synthesis by Passively Administered Antibody

It has been known for a long time that primary antibody formation can be prevented by mixing the antigen with excess antibody prior to injection [2, 28, 35]. This inhibition requires the use of specific reagents and suggest an inhibitory action of antibody by binding and blocking the antigenic specificities [19, 20, 36]. Mere blocking of the antigenic sites does not seem to be the sole explanation as only a limited number of antigenic specificities on each immunogenic unit have to be blocked by antibody in order to cause significant inhibition in several systems [6, 35]. It seems likely that this inhibition of the immune response despite only partial blocking of antigenic sites is taking place through a changed distribution pattern of the antigen-antibody complexes as compared to uncoated antigens, thus removing the antigenic sites from contact with immunologically competent cells [1]. This removal of antigen from contact with potential antibody-producing cells after *in vitro* or *in vivo* reaction with antibody will, however, be overcome with time in case of an antigen which will resist *in vivo* degradation better than the corresponding antibody partner [36]. In these cases the administration of antigen-antibody complexes will only result in the delayed appearance of an immune response [36]. Paradoxically the presence of antibody might occasionally enhance antibody production instead of causing inhibition. This is especially true for soluble protein antigens being in themselves often very weak immunogens which might be rendered more immunogenic by complexing with antibody [18]. The exact nature of this enhancing action of antibody is unknown, it has, however, been reported that administration of anti-HSA antiserum will slow down the rate of catabolism of HSA in rats in a highly significant manner [1]. Particulate antigens are mostly inhibited by antibody, however, there are reports in a mouse-anti-sheep system [11, 20] as well as in the Rh-system in man [4] that macroglobulin antibodies might enhance the antibody response.

Although antibody sometimes will enhance its own production the most frequently observed effect of passively administered antibody is inhibition. Recent findings have emphasized the importance of antibody in the regulation of the immune response *after* induction of antibody synthesis has taken place as passively administered antibody can inhibit antibody production even if not administered until several days [10, 20, 25, 36], up to a 1–2 months [40] after induction of antibody synthesis. This "feed-back" function of antibody on its own formation might take place through mere blocking of antigenic sites and/or as some authors have suggested by a direct action at the cellular or s.c. "central" level [23, 24, 36]. Especially two findings have been considered as being in support of this "central" inhibition, the first being the reports [23, 24] that incubation of normal splenic cells with anti-SRBC antiserum will render these cells incompetent to react immunologically to a subsequent treatment with SRBC. Several contradictory results to these findings [23, 24] have now been reported using the same [14, 42] or another kind of antigen [19]. McCullagh [14] using the same experimental system except that he was using thoracic duct lymphocytes instead of spleen cells found no evidence of any antibody-induced inhibition on the capacity of lymphocytes to respond to antigen. He interpreted the findings [23, 24] as being caused by cytophilic antibodies being attached to macrophages and thus being difficult to wash away. The action of the transferred cytophilic antibodies would then be by blocking and changing the distribution of the antigen in the same way as ordinary passively administered antibody. Also, in another animal species but using the same experimental system [42] the results [23, 24] could not be confirmed although there was a slight trend for inhibition after antibody contact. This inhibition could, however, be abolished by a more extended and thorough washing of the cells after antibody-contact indicating the slight effect to be due to a transfer of antibodies. Prolonged *in vivo* contact with antibodies could not be shown to induce any "central" inhibition which strongly suggests that if indeed "central" inhibition does exist at the level of potentially reactive cells this inhibition is very short-lived in the absence of antibodies [39, 42]. The finding that the inhibitory capacity of the administered antibodies reside in their Fab-fragments [33] adds further support for the view that inhibition is caused by direct combination with antigen.

A significant lag period was found to exist before any antibody-induced suppression could be demonstrated, the lag being of similar magnitude (40–70 h) in both 19S [20, 40] and early 7S [40] antibody synthesis. In conclusion, according the opinion of the author, there exist no data which will support any "central" hypothesis without being equally well explainable on the basis of antibody interacting directly with antigen. If it is accepted that antibody-induced inhibition of antibody *production* is to a major degree taking place through a blocking of antigenic determinants the impact of antibody being administered after the peak of synthesis has passed [40] could only be explained on the assumption that the majority of antibody-producing cells during the early stages of the primary immune response are short-lived in the absence of antigen. This assumption is supported by experiments using autoradiography showing that the majority of the plasma cells in the mouse [37] as well as in other rodents [5], have a life-span of the order of 48 h with a minority being capable of survival for several months [15]. The finding that the plasma cells are so short-lived even in the probable presence of antigen [5, 37] raises the possibility that presence or absence of antigen might play no role in the life-span of a plasma cell. This hypothesis might explain the resistance of 7S producing cells to antibody-induced suppression when this is tried very long time after induction of antibody synthesis [40]. At this late stage the concentration of antigen might conceivable be very low and the rate of requitement of new 7S producing cells might subsequently be minimal, in fact these "antibody resistant" antibody-producing cells might be of the type of long-lived plasma cells previously discussed [15]. Alternatively, the late 7S PFC might be cells synthesizing high avidity antibodies as systems have been described where a 1000-fold increase in avidity of the antibody being produced will take place during the 2nd and 8th week after primary immunization [9]. If one accepts the concept [32] that the antibody response is stimulated by a reaction between antigen and antibody receptors at the cell surface where the avidity of the receptor is similar to that of the antibody being produced it would follow that "high-avidity" cells might be very efficient in competing with passively administered antibodies for persisting antigenic specificities. According to this concept "high-avidity" cells would have an especially pronounced selective advantage as compare to "low-avidity" cells at very low concentrations of antigen and it has indeed been found [29] that the higher the primary dose of antigen the slower is the rise in avidity of antibody being produced. Furthermore, it has recently been found that the concentration of antigen needed to induce DNA-synthesis of preimmunized cells *in vitro* is invertly related to the affinity of antibody being produced by these cells [21]. This finding is in excellent agreement with the concept formulated above.

Both 19S and 7S antibodies have been shown capable of inhibiting the immune response in several systems [10, 19, 20, 23]. It has generally been considered that 19S antibodies are less efficient inhibitors than are 7S immunoglobulins [10, 20] although according to some calculations 19S antibodies might be comparable to "early" 7S antibodies in inhibiting capacity per molecule [23, 41]. Reports have been published showing that "late" 7S antibodies are significantly more inhibitory than "early" 7S antibody directed against the same antigen [10, 40]. This is not surprising as the possible effect of affinity should also be reflected where passively administered antibodies are used to inhibit the immune response. "High" affinity antibodies should be more efficient inhibitors than the corresponding antibodies with a lower affinity, and final proof for this postulate has recently been published [26, 38].

---

1. Specific.

2. Inhibiting capacity resides in the FAB-fragment.

3. Significant lag phase before inhibitory action of administered antibody on antibody production.

4. Acts by reducing the number of antibody forming cells, not by reducing the rate of antibody synthesis per cell.

5. Does not inhibit the "immunological memory" cell.

6. "Early" antibody synthesis more easily inhibited than "late".

7. "Late" antibodies more efficient inhibitors than "early"; positive correlation between affinity of administered antibody and capacity to inhibit antibody synthesis.

Fig. 1. Characteristics of antibody-induced inhibition of the immune response.

Figure 1 is summarizing the facts about inhibition of specific antibody synthesis by passively administered antibody. In conclusion, the results obtained have shown that administered antibody might function as an immunosuppressive agent, inhibiting formation of antibody directed against the same antigen. No evidence has been found in support of any "central" inhibitory action by the inhibiting antibody. The results are in support of the concept that administered antibody is inhibiting the antibody synthesis not by a direct action on the antibody-producing cells but rather by removing from the system the stimulus for maintenance of antibody production, the antigen(s). The curve of decay of antibody synthesis will then be dependent upon the life-span of the antibody-producing cells being induced before the administration of inhibiting antibody.

*Induction of Specific Lack of Immunological Reactivity of Cells by Passage
Through Antigen-Coated Columns*

It is speculated that immunologically competent cells do have antigen-specific receptors on their surface as discussed in the introduction [13, 32]. A direct method to test this hypothesis has been developed by the author. The test method uses antigen-coated beads making up columns through which suspensions containing immunologically reactive cells are allowed to pass. If the above concept is true one would anticipate a specific elimination or retardation of cells carrying receptors capable of binding to the bead-attached antigen(s). Several of the experiments reported have been done in collaboration with Dr. B. Andersson.

As column material was choosen beads made of glass (Type 100–5005, Minnesota Mining and Manufacturing Co., St. Paul, Minn.) or polyacrylic plastic (Degalan V 26, Degussa W., Hanau am Main, Germany). Glass beads have previously been shown to allow the passage of antibody-forming cells [22]. Both kinds of material have also been shown to display a capacity to bind antigenic molecules to their surface. Glass beads treated with boiling aqua regia for 15 min will firmly bind serum albumin in such a way that the glass beads were found suitable for using as immunoabsorbent thereafter [31]. Polyacrylic plastic particles have earlier been used for attaching protein antigens [34] and we have been able to demonstrate by the use of isotope-labelled antigens that this absorbing capacity of polyacrylic particles is not limited to protein antigens but applies to a variety of high-molecular substances.

Labelling of the beads was carried out for one hour at 45°C followed by overnight at 4°C. Antigen concentration used during labelling was 10 mg/ml fluid if not otherwise stated. After labelling at one hour for 45°C normal mouse serum was added to a final concentration of 5% for the overnight incubation. This was found to significantly increase the percentage of passing cells that would otherwise get stuck in an unspecific manner. The beads were suspended in a balanced salt solution or phosphate buffered saline during labelling, the amount of uptake of antigen being very similar in the various salt solutions tested. After the overnight incubation the beads were washed by Eagle's minimum essential medium until no antigen could be detected free in the medium. Columns were made up by filling glass columns 1.5 cm × 50 cm with the beads, a tiny piece of cotton wool was used to plug the bottom of the columns. The columns were then cooled to 4°C and were subsequently ready for use.

The first tests were designed to test whether cells producing antibody at high speed as to enable detection by haemolytic plaque assays would be selectively eliminated or retarded by passing through an antigen-coated column. A cell suspension known to contain antibody-forming cells against two or more antigenic specificities was passed through columns coated with the respective antigens and was subsequently assayed for antibody production in the agar plaque assay. Eluation of retained cells was carried out by mechanically shaking the column material in a large volume of Eagle's tissue culture medium. Table I discloses the results showing that a significant specific reduction of antibody-synthesizing cells could be obtained by passing the cells through the columns coated with the respective antigen. In some experiments complete elimination of antibody-producing cells against a given antigen was obtained by filtration through the antigen-coated column. It could also be seen from the table that retention contain a moment of unspecificity as a substantial number of relevant as well as irrelevant antibody-forming cells were found in the retained cell population. The fraction of retained antibody-forming cells of the irrelevant specificity was of a similar order of magnitude as found when using columns coated with normal mouse serum only.

Next step was to see whether cells carrying immunological memory would be retained in a similar fashion using the same separation procedures. The capacity of the cells to produce antibodies was assayed in a transfer system where the recipients had received sublethal irradiation before transfer in order to ensure space and reduce the immunological capacity of the recipient own cells. The antigens used are such that a secondary challenge of antigen administered in a soluble form will only stimulate preimmunized cells [16]. Table II shows that a specific elimination was obtained of "memory" cells by passing through the appropriate column while leaving the memory intact as regards to other antigens. In some experiments complete elimination within the sensitivity of the assay was obtained, as more than 99.7% of the specific reactivity was eliminated by passage through specific antigen-coated material. Cross-reacting antigens which cross-react at the level of serum antibodies did also cross-react at the level of column fractionation, in fact in some experiments this cross-reaction was more pronounce in separation than found at the level of serology.

Table I. The elimination of antibody-forming cells from cells passing columns coated with antigen

Exp.	Cells[1]	Column[2]	Anti-HSA cells/10^6 cells[3]	Anti-Ovalb. cells/10^6 cells	Anti-HSA cells / Anti-Ovalb. cells	
1	passed	HSA-10 mg	0 (less than 0.1)	4.1	less than	0.03
	retained	HSA-10 mg	4.2	16.0		0.26
	passed	Ovalb.-10 mg	3.3	0 (less than 0.1)	more than	33
	retained	Ovalb.-10 mg	7.0	25.3		0.28
	control	no column	5.6	30.3		0.18
2	passed	HSA-10 mg	0.9	23.6		0.04
	retained	HSA-10 mg	30.0	112.5		0.27
	passed	HSA-0.1 mg	6.3	13.1		0.48
	retained	HSA-0.1 mg	42.6	122.9		0.35
	control	no column	16.2	47.1		0.34

[1] Cells retained in column were mechanically eluted.
[2] Concentration figure of antigen during labelling of column beads (mg/ml).
[3] Assayed by indirect plaque assay detecting 7S antibody-producing cells. HSA and Ovalb. attached to SRBC by bisdiazotized benzidine.

Table II. Specific elimination of immunological memory cells by the passing through antigen-coated columns

Cells[1]	Column[2]	Anti-HSA memory[3]	Anti-Ovalb. memory[3]	Specific reduction
passed	HSA, 10 mg	more than 4.00	1.45 ± 0.18	more than 97 %
retained	HSA, 10 mg	2.07 ± 0.24	1.04 ± 0.19	—
control	no column	2.20 ± 0.33	1.20 ± 0.13	—
Cells	Column	Anti-BSA memory	Anti-Ovalb. memory	Specific reduction
passed	BSA, 10 mg	4.65 ± 0.17	2.32 ± 0.15	99.6 %
retained	BSA, 10 mg	2.47 ± 0.19	1.91 ± 0.40	—
control	no column	2.08 ± 0.17	2.18 ± 0.28	—

[1] Cells taken from animals immunized against HSA, BSA or Ovalbumin. Pools were made of anti-HSA and anti-Ovalb. cells, or of anti-BSA and anti-Ovalb. cells.

[2] mg-value denotes antigen concentration during the labelling of the columnar beads.

[3] Memory expressed as capacity to produce antibodies when transferring equal cell numbers into sublethally X-irradiated animals followed by 100 μg of antigen. Memory capacity expressed as μl of serum from recipient animals needed to bind 50 % of 1 μg of antigen, the μl being expressed in $\log_{10}$-units.

Table III. The impact of antigen concentration on the capacity of columns to eliminate immunological memory in passing cells

Concentration of antigen[1]	Anti-HSA memory[2]	Percent reduction[3]
0	1.52 ± 0.14	0%
0.1 mg HSA	1.78 ± 0.14	42%
1.0 mg HSA	2.36 ± 0.08	86%
10.0 mg HSA	4.00 ± 0.21	99%

[1] Concentration of antigen in the fluid when labelling the beads for columns.

[2] Anti-HSA memory measured as the capacity of the passing cells to produce antibodies after transfer to sublethally X-irradiated animals together with antigen. Anti-Ovalb. memory serving as control of specificity was the same in all four experimental groups. Memory expressed as in table II.

[3] Percent reduction of immunological memory as compared to cells passing a column labelled with syngeneic, normal mouse serum only.

The effectiveness of separating "memory" cells could be shown to be affected by several factors such as antigen concentration during coating of the bead material. Table III shows such experiments where the impact of antigen concentrations was investigated demonstrating a very clear and gradual decrease in effectiveness of the column separation by the reduction in antigen dose.

A theoretically more interesting observation was the preliminary results on the effect of time after immunization upon the effectivity of the separation procedure suggesting that cells taken earlier after immunization were eliminated to a less efficient degree than cells taken later. This would suggest that surface qualities, such as affinity of the receptor increasing with time after immunization, could be studied by column separations. In all the comparable groups the "younger" cells had a relatively higher frequency of memory cells passing the columns when compared to the "older" cells supporting the above mentioned concept.

Attempts have been made to fractionate unsensitized cell-populations on antigen-coated columns using antigens that would cause rapid primary responses in mice. The results obtained so far are too preliminary to be reported in detail, sufficient to say in six experiments made so far *specific* reduction has been obtained by passage through the appropriate antigen-coated columns. More work is needed to establish beyond doubt that potential antibody-forming cells from unimmunized animals can be separated under present conditions, it may be that the average binding constants between the cell bound receptor and the antigen is too low to allow as complete elimination as is the case using presensitized cells.

What is then the explanation for the elimination of antigen-sensitive cells by passing through the antigen-coated columns? At least three alternative explanations are to be considered; (i) they are eliminated because of specific receptors for antigen in such a way that they are retained in the columns; (ii) these receptors are not present only on the cells of production but also on all potential antibody-forming cells in the animal representing a class of passively absorbed, cytophilic antibodies; (iii) the cells are rendered tolerant when passing the columns. Concerning the possibility of cytophilic antibodies being produced and interfering in this system by introducing "false" specific retainment several sets of results argue against this explanation. If this was the case it might be anticipated that the cytophilic antibody would attach to a significant fraction of the cells in the lymph node or spleen cell populations of the immunized cell donor. However, when using cells taken from animals immunized with two antigens and passed through the *specific*, antigen-coated columns they show the same kind of *specific* elimination.

Considering the third alternative, immunological tolerance, several facts argue against this. It is conceivable that a low rate of antigen dissociation occurs from the antigen-coated beads and that antigen is present in the passing fluid although this could not be demonstrated by other means. Mere incubation of sensitized cells with antigenic concentrations ranging from 1 mg–0.001 microgramme per ml for varying time intervals at 4°C has not been shown to reduce the immunological capacity of the presensitized cell population when testing after washing, transfer and challenge. Moreover, preincubation of the cells with antigen followed by passing through columns coated with normal mouse serum only does not allow any reduction in the immunological memory of the passing cells arguing against the possibility that bead column will separate two cell-populations, one of which is easily inducible to a tolerant state by antigen *in vitro*. Thirdly, fractionation on antigen-coated columns in the *presence* of free antigen will block the eliminatory capacity of the column in a specific manner, allowing the memory cells to pass through. This finding, on the other hand, is in excellent agreement with the receptor hypothesis, where the cells would be retained in the antigen-coated columns due to bindings between cell-bound antibody and bead-attached antigen. The blocking by free antigen would take place through a competition with bead antigen for the cell-bound receptor.

Thus, the first explanation, for the elimination of specific memory cells by columns would be that they are retained in the columns due to the specific combination between receptors on the cell surface of the potential antibody-forming cells and antigenic specificities being present on the beads. This explanation is considered the most plausible but direct, final proof of this explanation is still lacking, the main problem is to elute the antigen-sensitive cells from the columns in a more efficient way. Mechanical elution has been tried and found capable of extracting cells trapped in the columns. When tested for immunological capacity, however, the retained cell population in an antigen-coated column show the same or less reactivity against the relevant antigen as compared to the relative efficiency of immuno-logical reaction of the cell populations towards other antigens. This is opposite to the enhanced capacity to be expected if mechanical eluation did recover all antigen-sensitive cells that had got stuck in the column according to the receptor hypothesis. It is known, how-ever, that mechanical force when getting the cells detached from the beads will kill a significant fraction of the cells as judged by supravital dyes. If the assumption is made that the stronger the attachement of the cells to the beads the more damage will have to be inflicted on the cells before mechanical detachment there would be reduction in relative terms of the recovery of specific memory cells versus the memory cells against other antigens being trapped in the column for non-immunological reasons. If the receptor of the potential anti-body-forming cell is displaying the same affinity as the serum antibody product as is suggested by the findings of several authors, the stronger binding of high avidity receptor would result in a higher frequency of damage to these cells before being detached from beads by mechani-cal elution. Specific elution by antigen has been tried but in the cell-populations obtained by this mean the relative increase in specific memory versus memory against other antigens has been very slight. The best results so far have been obtained using cross-reacting antigens and elute with the specific antigen for the cells that have got stuck in the column coated with the cross-reacting antigen. It may well be, however, that the antigens used, serum albumins with high molecular weights, are comparatively inefficient in eluting the cells and experiments are now in progress trying elution in other antigenic systems using haptens for the elution process.

Summarizing, three ways of achieving immunological depression by the use of either humoral or cellbound antibodies have been described. Of these methods passively administered antibodies against the Rh-antigens have already been shown of great value in the prevention of Rh-disease of the newborn [4] and it is conceivable that the same principle will be applied in other disorders, especially in certain diseases considered to be of auto-immune nature. The other two principles described, that of using antibodies against immunoglobulins and that of eliminating antigen-sensitive cells by passing through antigen-coated columns will seemingly both provide further important information about basic principles of the immune system. It is to be seen whether they will find any application in the clinical field.

Acknowledgements

This work was supported by grant Ca-4747, U.S. Public Health Service from the National Cancer Institute, by the Jane Coffin Childs Memorial Fund, by the Knut and Alice Wallenberg Foundation and by the Swedish Cancer Society. The technical assistance of Miss ULLA KÄLLSTRÖM is gratefully acknowledged.

Summary

Three principal ways to achieve immunological depression by using antibody have been described.

1. Antibodies against immunoglobulin(s) will under suitable circumstance inhibit the subsequent production of that (these) immunoglobulin class(es).

2. Passively administered antibody against a given antigen will inhibit the production of antibodies against the antigen in a strictly competitive manner.

3. Immunologically competent cells can be eliminated in a specific manner by passing cells through antigen-coated columns.

References

1. ADA, G. L. and LANG, P. G.: Antigen in tissues. II. State of antigen in lymph node of rats given isotopically-labelled flagellin, haemocyanin or serum albumin. Immunology (Lond.) *10:* 431–443 (1966).
2. BUXTON, J. B. and GLENNY, A. T.: The active immunization of horse against tetanus. Lancet *ii:* 1109–1111 (1921).
3. CHOU, C.-T.; CINADER, B. and DUBISKI, S.: Allotypic specificity and hemolytic capacity of antibodies produced by single cells. Int. Arch. Allergy *32:* 583–616 (1967).
4. CLARKE, C. A.: Prevention of Rh-Haemolytic Disease. Brit. med. J. *4:* 7–12 (1967).
5. COOPER, E. H.: Production of lymphocytes and plasma cells in the rat following immunization with human serum albumin. Immunology (Lond.) *4:* 219–239 (1961).
6. DIXON, F. J.; JACOT-GUILLARMOD, H. and McCONAHEY, P. J.: The effect of passively administered antibody on antibody synthesis. J. exp. Med. *125:* 1119–1136 (1967).

7. DRAY, S.: Effect of maternal isoantibodies on the quantitative expression of two allelic genes controlling gamma-globulin allotypic specificities. Nature (Lond.) *195*: 677–680 (1962).

8. DUBISKI, S. and FRADETTE, K.: The feed-back mechanism in immunoglobulin synthesis. Proc. Soc. exp. Biol. (N.Y.) *122*: 126–130 (1966).

9. EISEN, H.N. and SISKIND, G.W.: Variations in affinities of antibodies during the immune response. Biochemistry *3*: 996–1020 (1964).

10. FINKELSTEIN, M.S. and UHR, J.W.: Specific inhibition of antibody-formation by passively administered 19S and 7S antibody. Science *146*: 67–71 (1964).

11. HENRY, C. and JERNE, N.K.: The depressive effect of 7S antibody and the enhancing effect of 19S antibody in the regulation of the primary immune response. Nobel Symp. 3, pp. 421–429 (Almqvist and Wiksell, Stockholm 1967).

12. HERZENBERG, L.A.; HERZENBERG, L.A.; GOODLIN, R.C. and RIVERA, E.C.: Immunoglobulin synthesis in mice. Suppression by anti-allotype antibody. J. exp. Med. *126*: 701–713 (1967).

13. JERNE, N.K.: The natural selection theory of antibody formation. Proc. nat. Acad. Sci. (Wash.) *41*: 849–857 (1955).

14. McCULLAGH, P.: (personal communication).

15. MILLER, III, J.J.: An autoradiographic study of plasma cell and lymphocyte survival in rat popliteal lymph nodes. J. Immunol. *86*: 331–338 (1964).

16. MITCHISON, N.A.: Induction of paralysis in two zones of dosage. Proc. roy. Soc. B *161*: 275–295 (1964).

17. MITCHISON, N.A.: Antigen recognition responsible for the induction *in vitro* of the secondary response. Cold. Spr. Harb. Symp. quant. Biol. (in press).

18. MORRISON, S.L. and TERRES, G.: Enhanced immunologic sensitization of mice by the simultaneous injection of antigen and specific antiserum. II. Effect of varying the antigen-antibody ratio and the amount of immune complex injected. J. Immunol. *96*: 901–905 (1966).

19. MÖLLER, G.: Antibody-induced depression of the immune response. A study of the mechanism in various immunological systems. Transplant. Bull. *2*: 405–412 (1964).

20. MÖLLER, G. and WIGZELL, H.: Antibody-synthesis at the cellular level. Antibody-induced suppression of 19S and 7S antibody response. J. exp. Med. *121*: 969–989 (1965).

21. PAUL, W.E.; SISKIND, G.W. and BENACERRAF, B.: Specificity of cellular immune responses. Antigen concentration dependence of stimulation of DNA synthesis *in vitro* by specifically sensitized cells, as an expression of the binding characteristics of cellular antibody. J. exp. Med. *127*: 25–42 (1968).

22. PLOTZ, P.H. and TALAL, N.: Fractionation of spleenic antibody-forming cells on glass bead columns. J. Immunol. *99*: 1236–1242 (1967).

23. ROWLEY, D.A. and FITCH, F.W.: Homeostasis of antibody formation in the adult rat. J. exp. Med. *120*: 987–1005 (1964).

24. ROWLEY, D.A. and FITCH, F.W.: The mechanism of tolerance produced in rats to sheep erythrocytes. II. The plaque-forming cell and antibody response to multiple injections of antigen begun at birth. J. exp. Med. *121*: 683–695 (1965).

25. SAHIAR, K. and SCHWARTZ, R.S.: Inhibition of 19S antibody synthesis by 7S antibody. Science *146*: 67–69 (1964).

26. SISKIND, G.W.; DUNN, P. and WALKER, J.G.: Studies on the control of antibody synthesis. II. Effect of antigen dose and of suppression by passive antibody on the affinity of antibody synthesized. J. exp. Med. *127*: 55–66 (1968).

27. SMITH, R.T.: Immunological tolerance of non-living antigens. Advanc. Immunol., vol. 1, pp. 67–125 (Acad. Press, New York 1961).

28. SMITH, T.: Active immunity produced by so called balanced or neutral mixtures of diphteria toxin and antitoxin. J. exp. Med. *11*: 241–253 (1909).

29. STERNER, L.A. and EISEN, H.N.: Symposium on *in vitro* studies of the immune response. I. Variations in the immune response to a simple determinant. Bact. Rev. *30:* 383–405 (1966).
30. STERZL, J.; JILEK, M.; VESELY, J. and MANDEL, L.: Differentiation of immunologically competent cells. In Genetic variations in somatic cells. (Czechoslovak Acad. Sci., Prague 1966.)
31. SUTHERLAND, G.B. and CAMPBELL, D.H.: The use of antigen-coated glass as a specific adsorbent for antibody. J. Immunol. *80:* 294–298 (1958).
32. TALMAGE, D.W.: The primary equilibrium between antigen and antibody. Ann. N.Y. Acad. Sci. *70:* 82–86 (1955).
33. TAO, T.W. and UHR, J.W.: Capacity of pepsin-digested antibody to inhibit antibody formation. Nature (Lond.) *212:* 208–209 (1966).
34. TORRIGIANI, G. and ROITT, I.M.: The enhancement of 19S antibody production by particulate antigen. J. exp. Med. *122:* 81–98 (1965).
35. UHR, J.W. and BAUMANN, J.B.: Antibody formation. I. The suppression of antibody formation by passively administered antibody. J. exp. Med. *113:* 935–958 (1961).
36. UHR, J.W. and BAUMANN, J.B.: Antibody formation. II. The specific anamnestic response. J. exp. Med. *113:* 959–972 (1961).
37. URSO, P. and MAKINODAN, T.: The roles of cellular division and maturation in the formation of precipitating antibodies. J. Immunol. *90:* 897–907 (1963).
38. WALKER, J.G. and SISKIND, G.W.: Studies on the control of antibody synthesis. Effect of antibody affinity upon its ability to suppress antibody formation. Immunology (Lond.) *14:* 21–28 (1968).
39. WIGZELL, H.: The rise and fall of 19S immunological memory against sheep red cells in the mouse. Ann. Med. exp. Fenn. *44:* 209–215 (1966).
40. WIGZELL, H.: Antibody synthesis at the cellular level. Antibody-induced suppression of 7S antibody synthesis. J. exp. Med. *124:* 953–969 (1966).
41. WIGZELL, H.; MÖLLER, G. and ANDERSSON, B.: Studies at the cellular level of the 19S immune response. Acta path. microbiol. scand. *66:* 530–540 (1966).
42. WIGZELL, H.: Studies on some factors regulating antibody synthesis (Thesis, Stockholm 1967).

Author's address: Dr. H. WIGZELL, Department of Tumor Biology, Karolinska Institute, *10701 Stockholm 60* (Sweden).

Antibiotica et Chemotherapia, vol. 15, pp. 98–109 (Karger, Basel/New York 1969)

Immunological Tolerance and Inhibition by Hapten

J. L. Boak, E. Kölsch and N. A. Mitchison

National Institute for Medical Research, London and Department of Surgery,
St. Mary's Hospital London

The subject of this paper is the factors which control the induction of tolerance. In terms of the reaction of the antigen-sensitive cell, the problem can be posed in the following terms: what are the factors which determine whether an encounter between antigen and the cell leads to induction of tolerance or immunity? The outcome of the encounter can at present be judged only from the subsequent overall behaviour of the cell population—spontaneous antibody synthesis and heightened reactivity to antigen boost on the one hand, reduced reactivity towards antigen in adjuvant or to other forms of challenge on the other. Ultimately we would like to know what occurs in the sensitive cell immediately after the encounter with antigen that leads to tolerance, but this is a matter on which we are still ignorant. The available evidence favours the view that induction of tolerance depends on the selective destruction of antigen-sensitive cells endowed with a limited range of reactivities [3]. The means by which this destruction is brought about is still a subject of speculation.

A good case can be made for the hypothesis that direct exposure of lymphocytes to antigen leads to tolerance, whereas exposure via a macrophage leads to immunity. In considering the evidence it would be prudent to bear in mind the following three major reservations: (1) The greater part of the evidence in favour of this hypothesis has been obtained with foreign serum protein antigens, and a limited range of other proteins of fairly low molecular weight. Although they vary greatly among one another in immunogenic capacity they can all be regarded as weak antigens. Very different results are obtained when larger proteins, or proteins with naturally-occurring opsonins are employed. (2) The application of the hypothesis to transplantation antigens is doubtful. The discovery of a transplantation dose-effect akin to low-zone tolerance [1] has encouraged the belief that findings made with protein antigens can be transposed to transplantation, but much further work is required before the transposition can be taken for granted. (3) Exceptions have already been found to the direct access/macrophage hypothesis. In the secondary response lymphocytes can be stimulated directly, as will be mentioned, and flagellin may well induce tolerance when presented via macrophages. With these reservations in mind then, let us consider the evidence in favour of the hypothesis that has been obtained with the weak antigens.

1. *An Additional Step Required for Immunisation*

A range of weak antigens has been subjected to a standard test of tolerance-inducing capacity, in which repeated injections are given to irradiated mice and the results assessed by later challenging the mice with antigen in adjuvant [12]. A more limited range of antigens, particularly BSA, has been subjected to similar tests under other circumstances in which the propensity of the host to make antibody is reduced: these include neonatal life, the period of recovery from paralysis ("maintenance"), and normal adult life (for BSA only, although comparable dosage requirements have been recorded for BGG in slightly different tests [4, 12]. In every case the threshold concentration of antigen required for induction of tolerance is in the region of 10^{-8} molar. Thresholds in the same region have also been obtained in rats, rabbits, and guinea pigs [21]. The threshold concentration required for immunisation, on the other hand, varies greatly from one antigen to another within the range tested [4]. The constancy of low-zone induction threshold suggests that agents which facilitate tolerance induction, such as radiation, and others which inhibit, such as tubercle bacilli [5] or endotoxin [9], act on a step in the immune response which does not operate during the induction of tolerance. In more general terms, immunisation requires an additional step which is not needed in tolerance induction.

2. *Presentation of Antigen by Macrophages*

Antigen which has been taken up by macrophages is more potent than the free form in inducing primary immunisation; in the case of BSA the discrepancy is very large (of the order of one thousand-fold)

[13]. Other possible explanations of the finding have been largely eliminated, and the finding now stands as the principal evidence in favour of the view that immunisation proceeds via a macrophage-uptake step. The evidence need not be cited in detail; some parallel recent findings obtained with haemocyanins are discussed in another contribution to this symposium [10].

Two points in the biology of the handling of antigen by macrophages have prepared the ground for a more detailed analysis of intracellular events. These are as follows:

a) Radiation sensitivity. Irradiation of the macrophage donor at a suitable time before injection of antigen impedes the immunogenic activity of the cells. This finding was originally made with a Shigella antigen [8], and has been confined and extended with BSA [13]. Certain discrepancies with the Shigella study cannot, however, be entirely disregarded. With BSA there is an appreciable lag-period before the effects of radiation appear, and radiation applied *in vitro* is not effective; this is not the case with Shigella, for reasons which are not clear.

b) Persistence of antigen. Most of the BSA which is first taken up by peritoneal macrophages is then rapidly broken down, so that during the first 24 hours after injection the quantity of macrophage-bound antigen declines steeply, approximately in parallel with the decline in extracellular concentration. The immunogenic capacity of the macrophage-bound BSA remains approximately constant throughout this period, per unit weight, so that the net immunogenic capacity of the cells falls. There is some evidence of short-term retention of immunogenic capacity in the cells, based on the lack of activity of allogeneic cells [13], and also of much longer term retention over a period of months [14]. The evidence for retention of haemocyanin in an immunogenic form is more direct [10] and there is little or no indication of a comparable early loss of immunogenic activity.

3. The Intracellular Distribution of Antigen

Applying the "pulse and chase" technique to the study of phagocytosis of antigen by macrophages it was possible to demonstrate that coagulated BSA (cBSA) is retained in a subcellular storage compartment, from which it can be neither washed nor diluted out by material phagocytosed subsequently. This could explain the retention of antigen over months [14].

The cBSA found in the storage compartment accounts for 10% of the antigen taken up by the phagocytic cells. The residual 90% is found in lysosomes and phagolysosomes where it is degraded within 2 to 4 h and excreted as TCA non-precipitable material.

The intracellular distribution of antigen in macrophages was further studied by isopycnic centrifugation of macrophage homogenates in sucrose gradients. The subcellular particles of the storage compartment band at the same density as the nuclear fraction, and their nature has still to be determined. They can be separated from the lysosomal particles of the turnover compartment, which have a main-band density of 1.15 or 1.19, depending on the previous history of the macrophages. Figure 1 shows an experiment in which macrophages were exposed to I^{125} cBSA for 70 min in tissue culture, and were subsequently exposed to I^{131} cBSA for 5 or 20 min.

Irradiated macrophages have less antigen in the storage compartment than normal macrophages. So far it is not known whether

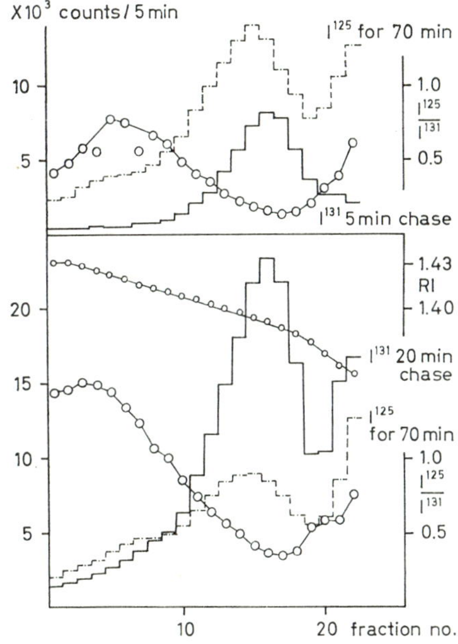

Fig. 1. 'Pulse and chase' in tissue culture. Isopycnic centrifugation of macrophage homogenates in a Spinco SW25 at 25000 rpm for 18 h. Bottom fraction of the centrifuge tube in fraction No. 1. Fractions were counted in a Packard Autogamma spectrometer and the ratio of I^{125}cBSA/I^{131}cBSA for each fraction was determined (0 —— 0). RI is the Refraction Index of the fractions (o —— o).

transport into the storage compartment or retention there is impaired. The defect in the storage compartment might well provide the basis of the impaired immunogenic activity of irradiated macrophages.

4. Direct Exposure of Lymphocytes

Exposure of lymphocytes to antigen *in vitro* does not induce tolerance repeatably, but brief exposure *in vivo* provides a substitute method. If cells are exposed *in vivo* to sufficiently high concentrations of antigens they will not respond to immunisation when transferred into an immunologically inert host. The effect of 100 mg BSA or HSA in a mouse can be detected by this method in peripheral leukocytes (mostly lymphocytes) within 2 h [15]. The interpretation of this observation is not entirely straightforward, and lower doses require longer periods of exposure to be effective [15, 23]. Nevertheless, it does indicate that direct exposure of lymphocytes to antigen can lead to the induction of tolerance. In passing it is worth noting that this provides an argument against the hypothesis that lymphocytes receive a "message" from macrophages during immunisation: once it has been established that lymphocytes can recognise antigen in the context of tolerance induction, simplicity dictates that recognition does not occur in any other cell in any other context.

In addition to the three lines of evidence just referred to, the direct access/macrophage hypothesis receives support from the well-known experiment on antigens which have been freed of aggregated matter by centrifugation [4] or *in vivo* passage [7]. It is not our intention to detract in any way from the importance of these experiments, but one discrepancy ought to be mentioned. BSA which has been passaged *in vivo* can still be taken up by mouse peritoneal macrophages and apparently enter their immunogenic pool on equal terms with non-passaged material [13]; and as might therefore be expected, passaged BSA is no less immunogenic in mice than non-passaged [7, 16]. The property of immunogenicity on the part of antigens cannot therefore be simply equated with susceptibility to phagocytosis.

5. Other Protein Antigens

A table is shown (table I) in which the properties of protein antigens are compared over a wide range of immunogenic capacity. The proteins are arranged in order of the size of the single dose required

Table I. The antigen-concentrating hierarchy

	Immunity			Paralysis		
	Threshold for 1° response/g. body weight	Potency of macrophage-bound antigen relative to free form	Inhibition of macrophage effect by radiation	Paralysis thresholds		*In vitro* paralysis
				Low-zone	High-zone	
BSA, HSA [3]	10^1 μg	$\times 10^3$	yes	10^{-1} μg	10^3 μg	no
Lysozyme, OA [3]	10^{-2} μg	$\times 10^1$–10^2	—	10^{-1} μg	10^3 μg	—
MSH [5]	10^{-3} μg	$\times 10^1$	no	—	—	—
KLH [6]	$<10^{-3}$ μg	< 1	—	—	—	—
Flagellin [2]	10^{-7} μg	—	—	10^{-7} μg	10^{-3} μg	yes
E. coli lipopolysaccharide [1]	—	—	—	—	—	yes

to procure primary immunity. The relative size of the macrophage effects begins to make sense when the proteins are ordered in this way.

The least immunogenic proteins, i.e. those for which the largest dose is required, exhibit the largest macrophage effect; as the requisite dose falls, so does the size of the macrophage effect. The size of the macrophage effect is presumably determined to some extent by the amount of macrophage uptake: if the uptake is high, less of the antigen is wasted when the free form is injected, and the discrepancy from the macrophage-bound form will be correspondingly less. A negative effect of the type encountered with KLH, i.e. a lesser immunogenic capacity on the part of the macrophage-bound form, might be explained in this way if it is assumed that uptake after injection of the free form is highly efficient, and takes place in macrophages which are more favourably placed for transmitting stimulation to lymphocytes than is the case with transferred macrophages. The size of the macrophage effect obtainable with cBSA can be predicted, on the basis of this explanation, from a comparison of the uptake and immunogenic capacity with those of normal BSA, and the prediction is borne out by experiment [13]. So far as the haemocyanins are concerned, however, it remains equally possible that macrophage-presentation plays a minor and possibly redundant role in immunisation, and that the proteins can stimulate lymphocytes directly without the intervention of a co-operative cell.

A partial explanation of the lack of radiation effect with MSH can be advanced. Cells from irradiated donors are evidently incapable of performing some operation that normal cells are capable of, perhaps involving the transfer of antigen into a heavy compartment of the type suggested by the double isotope experiments. This operation may be required for weak antigens such as BSA, but for antigens better endowed with intrinsic immunogenic activity the operation may be redundant. So far, proteins of highly different immunogenic capacity have not been compared after uptake by the same population of macrophages; this is an experiment that should certainly be performed with populations obtained from irradiated donors.

In the second part of table I data relevant to the induction of tolerance are summarised. Here the big surprise is ultra-low-zone induction by flagellin. The number of molecules administered in this dosage is so small that it has been inferred that the molecules are locked into some site, presumably by naturally-occurring opsonins, in such a manner that lymphocytes circulate past them and in doing so receive tolerance-inducing stimulation [20]. Autoradiographic and other studies indicate that the site where the localisation is likely to occur is on dendritic macrophages. We are left then with a picture, for antigens of this type, which is the exact reverse of that appertaining to BSA: exposure of lymphocytes via macrophages leads to tolerance, while direct exposure immunises!

It is tempting to speculate that the failure of BSA to induce tolerance *in vitro* can also be attributed to the lack of an antigen-concentrating mechanism. Whatever the final answer turns out to be, one thing is already clear. The concentrations of lipopolysaccharide [2] and flagellin [20] required to induce tolerance during brief exposure of lymphocytes are much smaller than that required for BSA or HSA [15].

6. *Specificity of Tolerance: Evidence of Cell-Cell Co-operation*

The "termination" of tolerance by immunisation with cross-reactive antigens is a phenomenon that has long required explanation. It occurs in one form which has been systematically studied by WEIGLE, in which tolerance of a protein is terminated to cross-immunisation either with another native protein or with the original protein conjugated with hapten. It occurs also in the reverse form, in which tolerance of one hapten-conjugate is terminated by cross-immunisation with the same hapten conjugated to a second carrier. There is some doubt whether termination in the first form occurs at all, strictly speaking, since the antibody that is elicited has only slight affinity for the antigen that was tolerated [19]. Nevertheless, secondary responses have been elicited with the antigen that was originally tolerated, after termination; furthermore, the affinity objection has not so far been found to apply in studies of termination in the second form [22].

Figure 2 illustrates an experiment which probably exemplifies termination in the second form. If the experiment is interpreted in this way, dextran is the tolerated antigen and the dextrin-protein conjugate represents the cross-reactive antigen. The experiment is shown only for the connoisseurs—it will be partially incomprehensible because it draws on unpublished work, carried out in collaboration with K. HIMMELSPACH.

We believe that a mechanism which accounts at least in part for termination operates as follows: immunisation occurs initially against

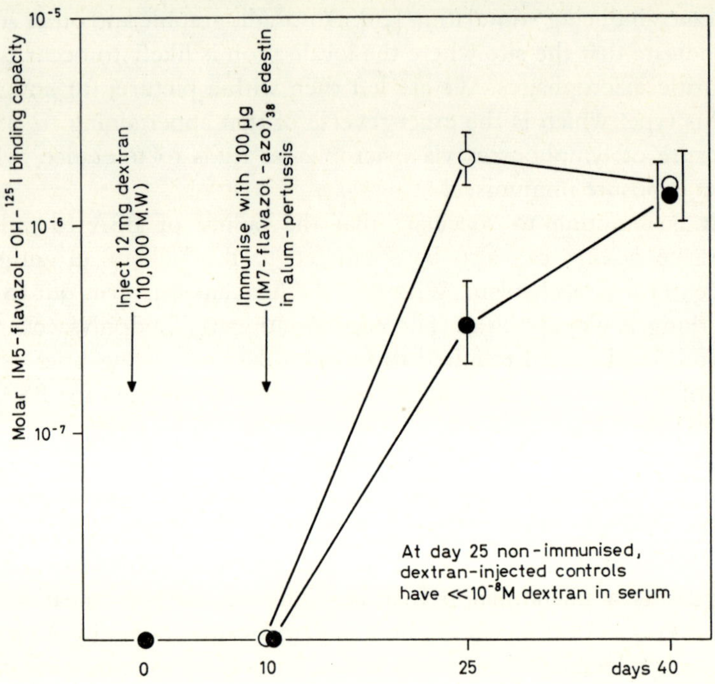

Fig. 2. Inhibition of the anti-dextrin response by prior injection of dextran in mice immunised with a dextrin-edestin conjugate. Groups of six mice showing mean and standard deviation of binding capacity for a radioactive hapten containing the dextrin group. Binding capacity measured by salt precipitation of serum immunoglobulin (K. HIMMELS-PACH and N. A. MITCHISON – unpublished data).

those determinants on the cross-reactive molecule which are new, i.e. which were not present on the tolerated molecule. Co-operative antibody is then produced, which has the property of acting as an antigen-concentrating device. This raises the local concentration of antigen in the neighbourhood of other lymphocytes, which then initiate a reaction against other determinants on the molecule. It is these secondary antibodies which make the state of tolerance appear to have been terminated. The essential feature of this hypothesis is the co-operating antibody which is directed against certain determinants and enhance the reaction against others on the same molecule; the main weakness is that this antibody has not yet been isolated, although very promising results have been obtained in another system [11]. The hypothesis is illustrated in figure 3.

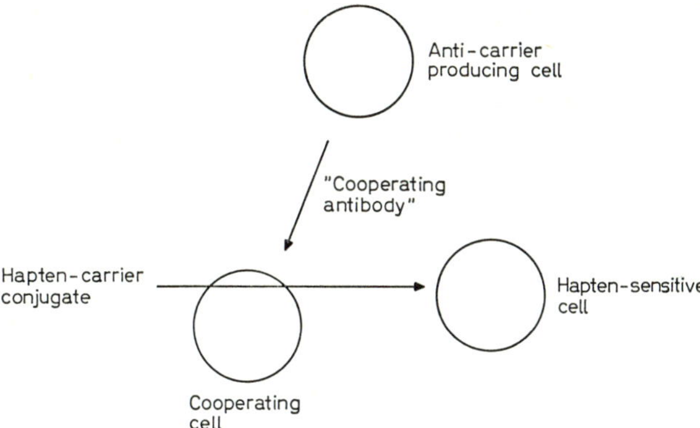

Fig. 3. A proposed mechanism for the carrier effect involving co-operating antibody. Note that the existence of a co-operating cell distinct from the hapten-sensitive cell is in doubt.

The evidence in favour of this hypothesis has recently been reviewed [17]. Our finding in the adoptive secondary response is that the sensitivity to NIP-BSA of cells primed with NIP-OA or NIP-CGG (antihapten response) can be enhanced by performing the stimulation (in irradiated syngeneic recipients) in the presence of cells primed with BSA (anti-carrier cells). The study is still incomplete, but other provisional findings can be summarised as follows:

a) Heat killed anti-carrier cells are ineffective.

b) Passive administration of anti-carrier antiserum is ineffective; for this reason co-operative antibody is envisaged as a type of antibody restricted in respect of either class or affinity.

c) The co-operating antibody may be directed against hapten sites. Thus the anti-NIP response can be enhanced by stimulating in the presence of NIP-DNP-conjugate + DNP-primed cells.

d) The anti-hapten response is proportional to the amount of anti-carrier antibody produced, and this in turn is proportional to the number of lymphocytes transferred from carrier-primed donors. The anti-hapten response bears no proportional relationship to the number of macrophages transferred from the carrier-primed donors.

e) Irradiation of the carrier-primed cells can, if performed at a suitable time and in suitable dose, reduce the anti-carrier response out of proportion to its co-operative effect on the anti-hapten response. This represents an exception to (d).

f) Co-operation can be detected *in vitro* to at least a minor extent.

7. The Site of Co-operation: A Footnote

It would fit with the immunogenic properties of macrophage-bound protein if the site of action of co-operative antibody proved to be the macrophage, and the properties of cytophilic antibody are in accordance with this expectation. Recent experiments, however, indicate that thoracic duct lymphocytes from primed donors can be stimulated efficiently by incubation *in vitro* with NIP-OA. This finding contradicts a previous report [18], and at present requires further investigation. In the light of this new evidence the co-operative cell which is postulated in figure 3 should be regarded sceptically.

References

1. Bainbridge, D.R. and Gowland, G.: Detection of homograft sensitivity in mice by the elimination of chromium-51 labelled lymph node cells. Ann. N.Y. Acad. Sci. *129*: 257–273 (1966).
2. Britton, S. and Möller, G.: Immunity and tolerance to a lipopolysaccharide antigen. Mendel Memorial Symposium 213–218 (Czechoslovak Academy of Science, Prague 1965).
3. Dresser, D.W. and Mitchison, N.A.: The mechanism of immunological paralysis. Adv. Immunol. *8*: 129–181 (Academic Press, New York 1968).
4. Dresser, D.W.: Specific inhibition of antibody production. II. Paralysis induced in mice by small quantities of protein antigen. Immunology *5*: 378–388 (1962).
5. Dresser, D.W.: Effectiveness of lipid and lipidophilic substances as adjuvants. Nature (Lond.) *191*: 1169 (1961).
6. Feldman, M.: (in present symposium).
7. Frei, P.C.; Benacerraf, B. and Thorbecke, G.J.: Phagocytosis of the antigen, a crucial step in the induction of the primary response. Proc. nat. Acad. Sci., Wash. *53*: 20–23 (1965).
8. Gallily, R. and Feldman, M.: (in present symposium).
9. Golub, E.S. and Weigle, W.O.: Studies on the induction of immunologic unresponsiveness. I. Effects of endotoxin and phytohemagglutinin. J. Immunol. *98*: 1241–1247 (1967).
10. Humphrey, J.H.: (in present symposium).
11. Jerne, N.K.: Summary: Waiting for the end. Cold Spr. Harb. Symp. quant. Biol. *32*: 591–603 (1967).
12. Mitchison, N.A.: The dosage requirements for immunological paralysis by soluble proteins. Immunology *15*: 509–530 (1968).
13. Mitchison, N.A.: The immunogenic capacity of antigen taken up by peritoneal exudate cells. Immunology *16*: 1–14 (1968).
14. Mitchison, N.A.: Recovery from immunological paralysis in relation to age and residual antigen. Immunology *9*: 129–138 (1965).
15. Mitchison, N.A.: Immunological paralysis induced by brief exposure of cells to protein antigens. Immunology *15*: 531–547 (1968).
16. Mitchison, N.A.: Induction of immunological paralysis in two zones of dosage. Proc. roy. Soc. B *161*: 275–292 (1964).

17. MITCHISON, N.A.: Recognition of antigen. Int. Soc. Cell. Biol. Symp. *7:* 29–42 (1968).
18. MITCHISON, N.A.: Antigen recognition responsible for the induction *in vitro* of the secondary response. Cold Spr. Harb. Symp. quant. Biol. *32:* 431–439 (1967).
19. PAUL, W.E.; SISKIND, G.W. and BENACERRAF, B.: A study of the 'termination' of tolerance to BSA with DNP-BSA in rabbits: relative affinities of the antibodies for the immunizing and the paralysing antigens. Immunology *13:* 147–157 (1967).
20. SHELLAM, G.R. and NOSSAL, G.J.V.: Mechanism of induction of immunological tolerance. IV. The effects of ultra-low doses of flagellin. Immunology *14:* 273–284 (1968).
21. THORBECKE, G.J. and BENACERRAF, B.: Tolerance in adult rabbits by repeated non-immunogenic doses of bovine serum albumin. Immunology *13:* 141–145 (1967); also references cited in (1) p. 138.
22. Unpublished data.
23. WEIGLE, W.O. and GOLUB, E.S.: Kinetics of the establishment of immunological unresponsiveness to serum protein antigens. Cold Spr. Harb. Symp. quant. Biol. *32:* 555–558 (1967).

References Included in Table I

1. BRITTON, S. and MÖLLER, G.: See ref. 17 in main list.
2. DIENER, E. and ARMSTRONG, W.D.: Induction of antibody formation and tolerance *in vitro* to a purified protein antigen. Lancet *ii:* 1281–1285 (1967).
3. MITCHISON, N.A.: See refs. 3, 8 and 12 in main list.
4. NOSSAL, G.J.V.; AUSTIN, C.M. and ADA, G.L.: Antigens in immunity. VII. Analysis of immunological memory. Immunology *9:* 333–348 (1965).
   See also ref. 16 in main list.
5. UNANUE, E.R. and ASKONAS, B.A. The immune response of mice to antigen in macrophages. Immunology *15:* 287–296 (1968).
6. UNANUE, E.R. and ASKONAS, B.A.: Two functions of macrophages and their role in the immune response. J. Reticuloendothelial Soc. *4:* 440 (1967).

Authors' addresses: Dr. J. L. BOAK and Dr. E. KÖLSCH, Department of Surgery, St. Mary's Hospital, *London, W. 2* and Dr. N. A. MITCHISON, National Institute for Medical Research, Mill Hill, *London, N.W. 7* (England).

Antibiotica et Chemotherapia, vol. 15, pp. 110–116 (Karger, Basel/New York 1969)

Immunosuppression by Antigen?

A. L. DE WECK and J. R. FREY

Division of Allergy and Clinical Immunology, Inselspital, Bern and
Medical Research Department, Hoffmann-La Roche Ltd., Basle

We are going to hear a great deal these days about unspecific immunosuppression by all possible means, drugs, anti-lymphocyte serum, irradiation, ribonuclease and so on. This is, if I may say so, "immunosuppression across the board": it has its limits, and its dangers which I do not need to recall here. On the other hand, specific immunosuppression is an ideal, which theoretically at least would fullfil the needs as well in transplantation as in therapy of autoimmune and allergic diseases. A great deal of work has been spent on the induction of specific immunological tolerance in virgin newborn or adult animals. Less seems to have been done, in comparison, with the endeavour to suppress specifically an immune response already established or being established. And nevertheless, for all practical purposes, it is this situation which we have to cope with when we treat a patient suffering from an immunological disease or starting to reject a foreign transplant.

I will raise only one question in operational terms: is it possible to achieve long-lasting unresponsiveness in already sensitized individuals or animals and this with antigen alone? The answer is a qualified yes and refers to delayed-type hypersensitivity only for the time being.

Attempts to achieve specific and permanent desensitization in delayed hypersensitivity reactions have been numerous and have met mostly with only moderate success or with no success at all (table I). There have been some occasional claims of long-lasting desensitization, e.g. in contact dermatitis. However, the results, especially in man, have never been that striking, reproducible or spectacular that a technique of specific desensitization may have gained recognition

Table I. Desensitization in delayed-type hypersensitivity; establishment of unresponsiveness in sensitized animals

Authors	Animal	Antigen	Manifestation	Desensitizing procedure	Duration of unresponsiveness
Bauer, 1909	man	tuberculin	delayed id. reaction	repeated injections of large doses of tuberculin in various schedules	variable
Fernbach, 1932	guinea pig	tuberculin			
Oliveira, 1958 and many others	guinea pig	tuberculin			
Kligman, 1958	man	Rhus	contact dermatitis	repeated im. injections or per os in various schedules	variable decrease in skin reactivity
Park, 1944	man	sulfonamide			
Morris-Owen, 1956	man	penicillin			
Jadassohn et al., 1959	guinea pig	DNCB	contact dermatitis	repeated (40–100) epicutaneous applications	several weeks (up to 28 weeks)
Rajka, 1960	guinea pig				
Lowney, 1964	guinea pig				
Schulz, 1965	guinea pig				
Frey, de Weck et al., 1962	guinea pig	DNCB	contact dermatitis	iv. injection DNBSO$_3$, DNP-amino acids or proteins	48–96 h
Uhr, Pappenheimer, 1958	guinea pig	Ag-Ab complexes	Jones-Mote	ip. injection of Ag	2–10 days
Gell, Benacerraf, 1962	guinea pig	Pic-proteins	delayed id. reaction contact to PicCl	iv. injection of Pic-protein	transient
Leskowitz, Jones, 1963	guinea pig	ABA-pTyr	delayed id. reaction	iv. injection of ABA-hapten and ABA-proteins	1–2 days up to 11 days
Crowle, 1963	mice	OVA, BSA	delayed id. reaction	massive ip. injection	"biphasic"
Frey, de Weck et al., 1964	guinea pig	NEO	delayed id. reaction	"double shot" iv. + id.	up to 80 weeks
Polak, Turk, 1967	guinea pig	Cr	contact dematitis	"double shot" iv. + epic.	up to 6 months
Waldorf et al., 1967	man	Nitrogen mustard	contact dermatitis	"double shot" iv. + epic.	up to 9 months

For references, see reference 2.
iv = intravenous – ip = intraperitoneal – id = intradermal – epic = epicutaneous – DNCB = 2,4-dinitrochlorobenzene – DNBSO$_3$ = 2,4-dinitrobenzenesulfonic acid – PicCl = picryl chloride – OVA = ovalbumin – BSA = bovine serum albumin – NEO = neoarsphenamine – Cr = potassium bichromate – ABA = p-azobenzenearsonate – pTyr = polytyrosine

and acceptance. Four years ago, we struck on a rather peculiar phenomenon in experiments on delayed-type hypersensitivity to Neoarsphenamine. Guinea pigs highly sensitized to Neoarsphenamine could be rendered completely and permanently unresponsive, provided that an intravenous and an intradermal injection of the antigen were administered in short succession (fig. 1).

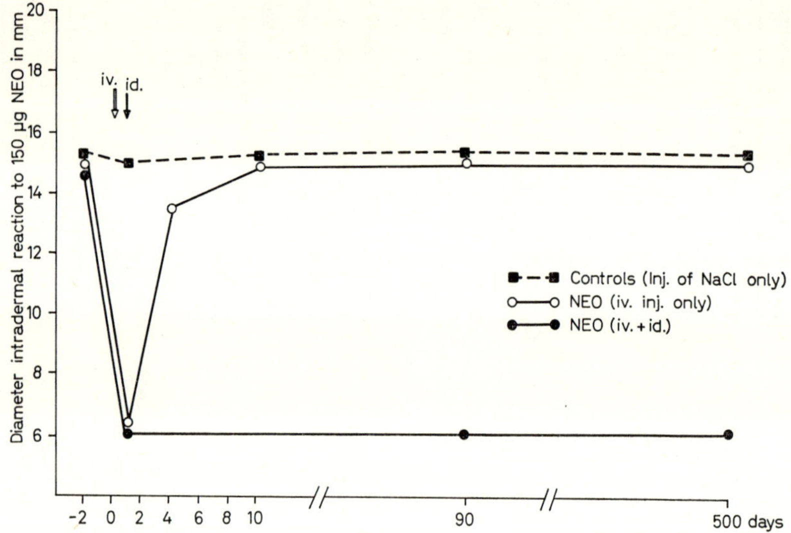

Fig. 1. Desensitization to Neoarsphenamine in guinea pigs by "double shot" procedure (60 mg/kg intravenously and 150 μg intradermally within six hours). For experimental details, see ref. 2.

These experiments have been in large part published [1, 2] and I will only point here to our main conclusions:

1. The unresponsiveness achieved by such a procedure is of very long duration, in fact lasts in many animals for their life time (up to 80 and more weeks).

2. The unresponsiveness is due merely to the conjunction of one single intravenous injection followed within 6 to 48 h by an intradermal injection of a minute dose of antigen (150 μg). It is enouni- of this "double shot" to achieve complete desensitization. If the agh mals are not tested at all for three months after the desensitizing "double shot", they are still unresponsive. This shows that the long lasting unresponsiveness is due only to these two injections and is

not eventually maintained by further doses of antigen administered by repeated testing.

The intravenous dose is critical: below a treshold of 30 mg/kg, the desensitizing effect is not manifest. The intradermal injection is critical, it cannot be replaced by another intravenous injection for example. The interval between both injections is critical, if it is longer than 48 hours, the animals show only a temporary desensitizing effect (or inhibition) like after any intravenous injection of antigen in a delayed hypersensitive animal [3]. The phenomenon is immunologically specific, as a concomittant sensitivity to another unrelated sensitizer, e.g. 2.4-dinitrochlorobenzene (DNCB) is not affected.

Having made this observation and established these rules for Neoarsphenamine, we then of course tried to reproduce the phenomenon with the classical contact and delayed-type hypersensitivity to 2.4-dinitrochlorobenzene (DNCB). For the last three years, we have used many conceivable ways and schedules to administer DNCB, 2.4-dinitrobenzenesulfonic acid ($DNBSO_3$), DNP-amino acids or DNP-protein conjugates in already sensitized guinea pigs. The experimental details of these rather disappointing attempts will eventually be published elsewhere. We have only succeeded at best in prolonging somewhat the temporary unresponsive state which normally follows for two to four days an intravenous injection of antigen. By prolongation, we mean two to three weeks of unresponsiveness or markedly diminished responsiveness, but the guinea pigs almost always became again fully responsive in the end.

Having reached a state of complete frustration, we have recently come across two observations. One is from Dr. John Turk and concerns the contact dermatitis of the guinea pig to chromium. Following our model, Dr. Turk and Dr. Polak have injected potassium bichromate intravenously into sensitized guinea pigs and have also applied potassium bichromate on the skin within 24 h [4, 5]. In so doing they obtained a complete desensitization which lasted for at least six months. The same rules as we had defined with Neoarsphenamine seemed to apply to potassium bichromate. If the epicutaneous application was postponed for four days of more, the animals became responsive again. The intravenous dose was also critical, as below a treshold of 20 mg/kg, the desensitizing effect remained only temporary.

An apparently very similar phenomenon has recently been observed in man by the group of van Scott in Bethesda [6]. Some patients with mycosis fungoides were treated with nitrogen mustard in topical applications and several of such patients became contact sensitive to nitrogen mustard. They were given intravenous injections of nitrogen mustard over a few hours period, followed by skin tests at various intervals (table II). Strikingly enough three patients showed a complete desensitization at eight weeks. In two of them tested again later, the effect was still present at five and nine months. Three other patients showed a definite partial desensitization, whereas two had reacted to the intravenous injection of nitrogen mustard by a generalized dermatitis, apparently similar to the dermatitis we have described in guinea pigs sensitized to DNCB or Neoarsphenamine and intravenously injected with the corresponding antigen [3]. The effect was specific, as a concomittant sensitization to DNCB was unaffected. Interestingly, the permanently and completely desensitized patients appear to have been those who had been tested two days after the intravenous injection [7]. The other patients had been tested only seven days after the intravenous injection.

So that our state of frustration has now somehow transformed again in a state of excitement. It seems to us that we are now justified in assuming that we deal here with a general biological phenomenon, at least in operational terms. Obviously this phenomenon does not apply to all antigens, e.g. it does not seem to apply to DNCB. We could be tempted to state it applies mostly to antigens which are not rapidly metabolized and eliminated, as is obviously the case for potassium bichromate and Neoarsphenamine. It is much too late today or too early, as far as the evidence is concerned, to speculate about the ways in which this state of long-lasting unresponsiveness is brought about. Does the intravenous injection "knock off" all committed lymphocytes, making temporarily again of the sensitized guinea pig a virgin animal? And is it then enough for an intradermal injection to induce low-dose tolerance? Is it required that the antigen remains fixed in the skin to maintain the unresponsive state? And do we deal here with true tolerance or merely with a masking of the reactivity by some kind of "threadmill" mechanism?

In any case, the preliminary conclusion should be that it is possible in some cases and with some antigens by a relatively simple combination of intravenous and intradermal antigen injections to achieve long-lasting unresponsiveness in delayed-type hypersensitivity in guinea pigs. Theoretical and eventual practical implications in man will have to await further developments.

Table II. Specific desensitization in contact dermatitis to nitrogen mustard (NH_2) in patients with mycosis fungoides

Procedure	R.H.	L.D.	O.K.	L.L.	W.M.	G.L.	A.W.	A.L.
1. Reference patch test to:								
Nitrogen mustard	++	++	++	++++	++++	++	+++	++
DNCB[2]	++	++	+++	+++	++		++	++
2. Intravenous injection of nitrogen mustard (1.11–6.11 mg)								
3. Patch-test 2–7 days after i.v. injection								
Patch-test to nitrogen mustard	0	0	0	+	+	+	+++[1]	++[1]
Patch-test to DNCB	++	++	+++	+++	++		++	++
4. Patch-test 8 weeks after i.v. injection nitrogen mustard	0	0	0	+++	+	+	+++	++
5. Patch-test 5 or 9 months after i.v. injection nitrogen mustard	0	0						

[1] Patients showing a morbilliform exanthema 5 h and 4 days after the intravenous injection.
[2] After prior experimental sensitization to DNCB.
Condensed from Waldorf, D.S.; Haynes, H.A. and van Scott, E.J.: Ann. Int. Med. *67*: 282 (1967).

Summary

Guinea pigs hypersensitive to Neoarsphenamine or to potassium bichromate may be rendered specifically unresponsive for prolonged periods of time (up to 18 months) by a simple "double shot" (intravenous and intradermal) of antigen, administered at intervals not exceeding two days. A similar phenomenon appears to have been observed in a few patients with contact sensitivity to nitrogen mustard.

References

1. FREY, J.R.; DE WECK, A.L. and GELEICK, H.: Immunological tolerance induced in animals previously sensitized to simple chemical compounds. Science *144*: 853 (1964).
2. FREY, J.R.; DE WECK, A.L. and GELEICK, H.: Sensitization, immunological tolerance and desensitization of guinea pigs to Neoarsphenamine. IV. Desensitization to Neoarsphenamine. Int. Arch. Allergy *30*: 521 (1966).
3. DE WECK, A.L.; FREY, J.R. and GELEICK, H.: Specific inhibition of contact dermatitis to dinitrochlorobenzene in guinea pigs by injection of haptens and protein conjugates. Int. Arch. Allergy *24*: 63 (1964).
4. POLAK, L. and TURK, J.L.: Studies on the effect of systemic administration of sensitizers in guinea pigs with contact sensitivity to inorganic metal compounds. I. The induction of immunological unresponsiveness in already sensitized animals. Clin. exp. Immunol. *3*: 207 (1968).
5. POLAK, L. and TURK, J.L.: Situdes on the effect of systemic administration of sensitizers in guinea pigs with contact sensitivity to inorganic metal compounds. II. The flareup of previous test sites of contact sensitivity and the development of a generalized rash. Clin. exp. Immunol. *3*: 215 (1968).
6. WALDORF, D.S.; HAYNES, H.A. and VAN SCOTT, E.J.: Cutaneous hypersensitivity and desensitization to mechloirethamne in patients with mycosis fungoides lymphoma. Amer. Int. Med. *67*: 282 (1967).
7. WALDORF, D.S.: Personal communication.

Authors' addresses: P.D. Dr. A.L. DE WECK, Division of Allergy and Clinical Immunology, Inselspital, *3000 Bern* and Dr. J.R. FREY, Medical Research Department, Hoffmann-La Roche Ltd., *4000 Basle* (Switzerland).

Antibiotica et Chemotherapia, vol. 15, pp. 117–121 (Karger, Basel/New York 1969)

Specific Anti-Thymocytes Antibodies Activities

P. Grabar

Institut Pasteur, Paris

During the past years, we have studied with several different collaborators constituents of rat tissues and particularly the reticulo-endothelial system, using immunochemical methods.

We firstly analyzed the spleen [2], then the bone-marrow [1] and recently the thymus [3, 5]. It was possible to detect some constituents which are common to various tissues and some which are specific for a given organ or tissue.

I. *In studies on thymus* performed with Miss Buffe and Tadje-bakche [3] rabbit antisera have been used. In order to render them specific for thymus constituents, they have been absorbed with blood (serum and hemolysate) and with extracts of liver, spleen, bone-marrow, etc... These sera served then for the detection and definition of soluble thymus constituents in gel diffusion and particularly in immuno-electrophoretic analysis (I.E.A.). It has been shown that among the soluble components of the thymus, at least two are thymus specific, because they could not be detected in extracts of other organs and certainly not in bone-marrow and spleen.

Analogous results have been published by Tallberg [6]. These two thymus specific constituents migrate in the zone of the serum alpha-globulins and their mobilities are nearly the same.

Using immunofluorescence technics, and the same absorbed immunesera, it could be observed that these soluble components are situated in the peripheral part of the thymocytes (the tests have been made with suspensions of these cells). But absorption of these sera with the soluble extract of thymus did not suppress completely fluorescence, which seems then to persist only on the membranes of these cells. This observation led us to envisage the possibility of some insoluble antigens which would be also specific for thymocytes. In order to control this possibility the cytotoxic activity of the immunsera on thymocytes has been investigated.

The immunesera have been again conveniently absorbed with extracts of other tissues. As controls, normal rabbit sera have been utilized but, as they normally possesses a certain cytotoxic activity on rat cells, they have been also absorbed with the same amounts of other tissues as the immunsera. The cytotoxic activity of the immune and of the normal sera on suspensions of thymocytes and of spleen cells has been evaluated by counting dead cells. A very rapid and important cytotoxic activity on thymocytes was observed with the immunesera, whereas the action on spleen cells was faint and nearly the same with the immune- and normal sera.

The inhibition of the cytotoxic activity of the immunesera could be obtained when the sera were absorbed by the insoluble fraction of thymocyte homogenates, whereas the addition of soluble components was without action. These observations prove that the thymocytes differ from the lymphocytes of the spleen and of the bone-marrow cells.

II. *Studies on the cytotoxicity of anti-thymus immunesera* were resumed several months ago in collaboration with BACHVAROFF and Miss COURCON, in order to discover which of the cell components is involved and also to study the *in vivo* activity of the corresponding antibody.

Series of new rabbit antisera have been prepared; some were obtained as previously by injection either of total homogenates or of the soluble extracts of rat thymuses; but some others were prepared by injecting rabbits with sub-cellular fractions of thymocytes, obtained by fractional centrifugation.

In previous studies, the aim was to obtain potent precipitating antibodies and therefore we were obliged to immunize our rabbits for many months. But, in recent studies it was observed that immunesera possessing a convenient cytotoxic activity can be obtained much more rapidly than those containing a high precipitating titer.

The immunesera obtained, as well as the normal rabbit sera which were used as controls, have been absorbed as previously with serum, hemolysate and lyophilysates of several other tissues (liver, spleen, lymph nodes).

When the immunesera are added to suspensions of thymocytes in the absence of complement, the cells are agglutinated and, in presence of complement (i.e. fresh guinea pig serum), they were killed. This cytotoxic action has been evaluated by counting the cells which are coloured by eosin.

In order to find out which of the thymocytes components are involved in the cytotoxic activity of the specific immunesera, sub-cellular fractions have been used for testing the inhibition of this activity. With the new series of immunesera, the results were even more clear-cut than in the previous experiments. It was observed that any fraction which contains membrane structure such as cell membranes, membranes of the endoplasmic reticulum, or mitochondria, except purified nuclei, are active in neutralization of the cytotoxic effect in the order as above. The cell sap and the ribosomal fraction did not absorb the cytotoxic antibodies. The specificity of the absorption was verified using analogous sub-cellular fractions from spleen and liver cells (see table I).

A partial absorption of the cytotoxicity was observed when sub-cellular fractions of lymph node cells were used.

Using specific sera against thymus microsome or mitochondria, we attempted to render the serum specific for the thymocytes only. The original serum had a cytotoxic titer higher for these than for lymph node cells.

Table I. Cytotoxicity of anti-thymus antibody and its absorption with subcellular fractions (per cent of dead cells)[1]

Dilutions of the serum	1/2	1/4	1/8	1/16	1/32	1/64	1/128
Absorptions							
Initial serum[2]	100	100	100	100	99	97	90
1 ml serum absorbed with:							
40 mg thymus cell-sap	100	100	99	97	95	93	87
40 mg purified thymus nuclei	100	100	100	98	97	92	90
10 mg thymus ribosomes	100	100	100	97	94	92	85
10 mg thymus microsomes	10	10	10	10	10	10	10
10 mg thymus mitochondria	15	10	10	10	10	10	10
1 mg thymus cell-membranes	15	10	10	10	10	10	10
2 mg thymus endoplasmic reticulum membranes	15	10	10	10	10	10	10
2 mg liver cell-membranes	100	100	98	96	93	90	87
10 mg lymph node microsomes	98	95	87	82	77	71	65
10 mg spleen microsomes	100	98	93	88	81	76	71

[1] 0.1 ml of a 10^{10} thymocytes suspension + 0.1 serum (or its dilution) + 0.05 ml of a 1/4 dilution of fresh guinea pig serum. After 1 h incubation at 37° C, the dead cells were counted using eosin dye exclusion test.

[2] Previously absorbed only with normal rat serum and red blood cells.

By absorbing the original serum progressively with microsomes or mitochondria from lymph node cells, the cytotoxicity for them was substantially decreased while the titer against thymocytes was only slightly lowered (see table II). Despite the large quantities of material used for absorption, a certain cytotoxicity against the lymph node cells remained. It is conceivable that a small proportion of these cells contain the same antigen (or antigens) as the thymocytes.

Some preliminary experiments in which the cell membranes have been treated with urea or methyl cellosolve, seem to indicate that the proteins thus extracted are capable of neutralizing the cytotoxic antibodies, but only partially, as compared with the original membranes or reconstituted membranes.

Experiments on the *in vivo* activity of the anti-thymus antibodies have been performed on new born rats (strains I.C. and WAG).

The immunsera, rendered thymus specific by absorption as in the other experiments, have been administered to these rats by peritoneal injections (roughly on the basis of 0.07 ml per gram of body weight) daily for 10 to 15 days. Analogous control animals received the same amounts of the same immuneserum but absorbed also with the thymus.

These experiments must be considered as only preliminary because the number of treated animals was not large enough and because their mortality was high, probably due to an infection. But some results may be mentioned, as they were constantly observed: After 10 days

Table II. Comparison of the cytotoxicity (per cent of dead cells) of the anti-thymus-microsomal serum on thymocytes and lymph node cells[1]

Lymph node microsomes used for absorption of the serum (mg/ml)[2]	Cells	Dilutions of the serum							
		1/2	1/4	1/8	1/16	1/32	1/64	1/128	1/256
2	Thymus	100	100	100	100	98	98	97–95	90
	Lymph node	100	98	95	90	88	75	60–70	50–60
4	Thymus	100	100	100	99	97	95	95–90	75
	Lymph node	95	93	85	75–80	55–60	30–40	25–30	25–30
8	Thymus	100	100	95	92	90	87	85	65
	Lymph node	50	43	35–40	28–32	25–30	25–30	25–30	25–30

[1] 0.1 ml of a 10^{10} cells/ml suspension + 0.1 ml serum (or its dilution) + 0.05 ml of a 1/4 dilution of fresh guinea pig serum. After 1 h incubation at 37°C, the dead cells were counted using eosin dye exclusion test.

[2] The serum was previously absorbed with normal rat serum, red blood cells and microsomes of spleen and liver.

of treatment (the first autopsy) in the rats treated with the immune-serum, the thymuses nearly disappear completely, the spleens are much smaller than in the controls and lymph nodes could hardly be found.

Dr. A. Aschkenasy has kindly examined some slides of these organs. The microscopic image showed some important modifications, such as a diminution of the perifollicular zone of Malpighian corpuscules in the spleen. The small resting part of the thymus has also an abnormal appearance.

The *in vivo* action of the immune sera on the spleens seems at first sight to contradict the absence of cytotoxic action of the same sera in *in vitro* experiments on suspensions of lymph node cells. But, if one admits that certain cells in the spleen originate from the thymus [see for example ref. 4] this could be the case for the perifollicular cells. Their absence in treated animals may be due either to their destruction in the thymus prior to their migration, or to their destruction in the spleen.

We hope that our experiments in progress will furnish more complete and more precise data, but from the results already obtained, we may conclude that thymocytes possess specific components which distinguish them from other lymphocytes and that our immunesera contain antibodies for these components among which at least one is part of the cell membranes. These antibodies specifically agglutinate thymocytes and, in presence of complement, are cytotoxic for these cells. Injected into young rats, they provoke involution of their thymuses and modifications in their spleens.

References

1. Beernink, K.D.; Courcon, J. and Grabar, P.: Immunochemical studies on bone marrow of the rat. Immunology *9:* 377–389 (1965).
2. Grabar, P.; Pisi, E.; Courcon, J. et Lespinats, G.: Analyse immunochimique des constituants solubles de la rate de rat. Ann. Inst. Pasteur *107:* 749–763 (1964).
3. Grabar, P.; Tadjebakche, H. et Buffe, D.: Activités spécifiques d'anticorps anti-thymus du rat. Ann. Inst. Pasteur *114:* 159–172 (1968).
4. Parrot, D.M.V.; de Sousa, M. and East, J.: Thymus dependent areas in the lymphoid organs of neo-nataly thymectomized mice. J. exp. Med. *123:* 191–203 (1966).
5. Salerno, A.; Courcon, J. et Grabar, P.: Analyse immunochimique des constituants solubles du thymus de rat normal. Ann. Inst. Pasteur *112:* 38–53 (1967).
6. Tallberg, T.; Kosunen, T.U.; Rioslahti, E. and Ehnholm: Detection of an organ specific protein in the human thymus. Ann. Med. exp. biol. Fenn. *44:* 221–226 (1966).

Author's address: Prof. Dr. P. Grabar, Institut Pasteur, *Paris 15e* (France).

Antibiotica et Chemotherapia, vol. 15, pp. 122–134 (Karger, Basel/New York 1969)

Effect of Growth Hormone and Anti-Growth Hormone Serum on the Lymphatic Tissue and the Immune Response

W. Pierpaoli[1] and E. Sorkin[2]

Schweizerisches Forschungsinstitut, Medizinische Abteilung, Davos-Platz

Introduction

Hormones can probably interfere at several levels with the development of the immunological capacity. One point of interference is in the recruitment of antigen-reactive cells which are dependent on the activity of the thymus and of the bursa of Fabricius [23] while corticosteroids can produce thymus atrophy and wasting disease [19]. Parallel to these effects, involution of lymphatic organs and the thymus by adrenal cortical hormones and the action of these hormones on lymphocytes have been extensively studied by Dougherty *et al.* [3]. Attention has also been drawn to the possible significance of one or several hypothetical thymus hormones for the development of the immunological capacity [10]. Another type of interference by steroid hormones at the efferent level of the immune response might concern the reaction of normal and sensitized cells.

The significance of hormones as control mechanisms in protein synthesis is well exemplified by the metamorphosis in amphibians induced by thyroxin. Such a study would seem at first rather remote from one on the immune response. However, expression of immunological capacity is almost certainly connected with synthetic processes which are under hormonal control. Recent findings indicated that the control by growth promoting and developmental hormones is exerted at the DNA and ribosomal and transfer RNA synthesis level [6, 20,

[1] Research fellow of the National Research Council, Rome.
[2] This work was supported by the Schweizerischen Nationalfonds zur Förderung der wissenschaftlichen Forschung (No. 4518).

21]. In fact we must ask whether formation of antigen-sensitive cells from stem cells and transformation of lymphocytes into antibody-producing plasma cells is dependent on one or several hormones so that the "message" of antigen into antibody proteins can be transcribed. Thyroxin and somatotropic hormone come to mind. Both these hormones which have been shown to be essential for protein synthesis are likely to be involved in the immunological maturation including the antibody-producing mechanisms.

It is the purpose of the present communication to investigate the significance of growth hormone for the immunological capacity. Ideally, animals with a naturally lowered somatotropic hormone level or with a deficiency in somatotropic hormone would be most suitable for such an investigation. Such animals do exist [2]. Experiments with so-called dwarf mice which are somatotropic hormone-deficient and have been shown to be immunological cripples will be reported elsewhere.

Thymus-Hypophysis Relationship

The high mitotic index of thymocytes and the cellular turnover in the thymus [8] suggested to us that these processes might be under hormonal control [13, 14]. Similar to other target organs such as the thyroid, gonads and adrenal cortex which are directed by specific hypophyseal hormones, the thymus could be under hypophyseal control. Characteristic cellular changes have been observed in the hypophysis after removal of such target glands. Accordingly, neonatal thymectomy should result in changes in the hypophysis. When mice were neonatally thymectomized, modifications were indeed observed in the acidophilic cells, which produce somatotropic hormone [14].

Another line of evidence for the relationship between the hypophysis, possibly the somatotropic hormone, and the thymus was sought by injecting anti-hypophysis serum [13]. Such a treatment might conceivably result in changes in the thymus and other target glands of the pituitary gland. Indeed a single injection of anti-hypophysis serum into mice produced body growth inhibition, thymus atrophy and a wasting syndrome. The fact that such a syndrome could only be produced in young mice suggested that the relationship between the pituitary gland and the thymus might be critical in the neonatal or perinatal age when the processes of immunological maturation are thymus-dependent. Figure 1 demonstrates growth patterns of various groups of young male mice [1] untreated, [2] wasting after

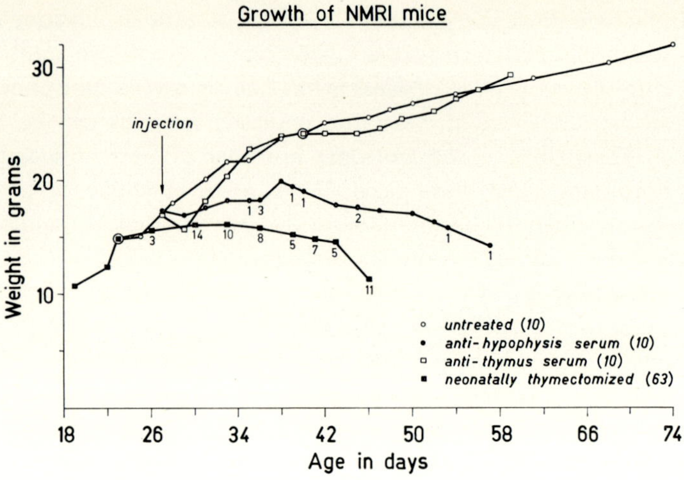

Fig. 1. Comparison of growth of NMRI male mice after a single intraperitoneal injection of rabbit anti-mouse hypophysis serum, anti-thymus serum or after neonatal thymectomy. The numbers in the curves indicate the wasted mice dying on the various days after thymectomy or anti-hypophysis serum treatment. ○, untreated (10); ●, anti-hypophysis serum (10); □, anti-thymus serum (10); ■, neonatally thymectomized (63). (From: PIERPAOLI, W. and SORKIN, E.: Nature *215:* 834–837, 1967).

treatment with anti-hypophysis serum, [3] treated with anti-thymus serum and [4] wasting after neonatal thymectomy. Untreated control animals and those treated with a single injection of anti-thymus serum behaved similarly except for the passing initial reduction in weight after the injection of the immune serum. Wasting animals injected with anti-hypophysis serum showed a growth pattern similar to the neonatally thymectomized mice. It must be emphasized that the mice were injected with the anti-hypophysis serum at approximately the age when they would develop the wasting syndrome if neonatally thymectomized.

Parallel to the induction of the wasting disease and changes in the thymus, anti-hypophysis serum produced also striking changes in the total number of peripheral blood leucocytes as is shown in figure 2. Variations in body growth, thymus volume and cellularity are accompanied by similar changes in total peripheral leucocyte counts. Thus the recovery of body growth and thymus volume was regularly accompanied by an increase in peripheral leucocyte counts. Figure 3 shows the thymus and the spleen of a mouse of the experiment indicated in figure 2. This mouse was killed during the wasting phase after one injection of anti-hypophysis serum.

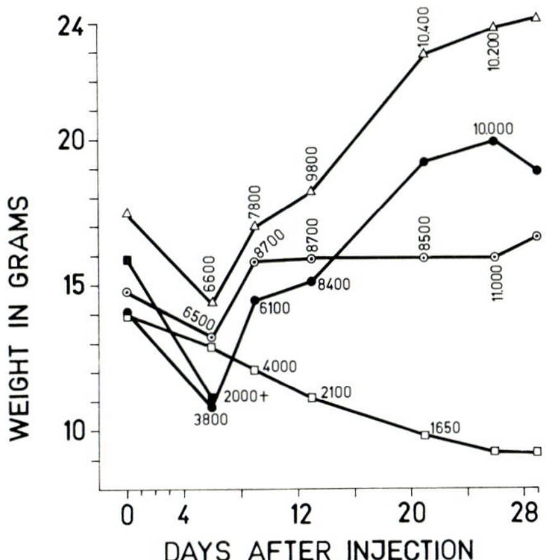

Fig. 2. Parallelism between body growth inhibition and total peripheral blood leucocyte counts in C57/B1 mice after a single intraperitoneal injection of rabbit anti-mouse pituitary serum.

Antisomatotropic Hormone Serum and Wasting Disease

So far the experiments concerned the effects of neonatal thymectomy and anti-hypophysis serum. These results suggested to us that somatotropic hormone might be responsible at-least in part for the observed findings. But also other hormones, especially thyroxin had to be considered. Anti-somatotropic hormone serum was therefore prepared by repeated injections in rabbits. Technical details are reported elsewhere [16]. For immunization the somatotropic hormone (STH) preparation (Rabentype bovine growth hormone, Nutritional Biochemicals Co., Cleveland, Ohio, USA) was incorporated in Freund's complete adjuvant. The hormone preparation was practically free of other anterior pituitary hormones. Anti-somatotropic hormone antisera have been prepared earlier by several groups of workers [5, 1, 17, 4, 9] who also showed that such antisera possess anti-growth activity in hypophysectomized animals which were restored with somatotropic hormone [1]. Anti-thyrotropic hormone serum was also prepared in a way similar to anti-somatotropic hormone serum.

The following questions were investigated: (1) Can anti-somatotropic hormone serum reproduce the effects of anti-hypophysis serum on the thymus? (2) If so, what are these effects: a) in young two or three weeks old animals and b) in adult animals. (3) Can the effect

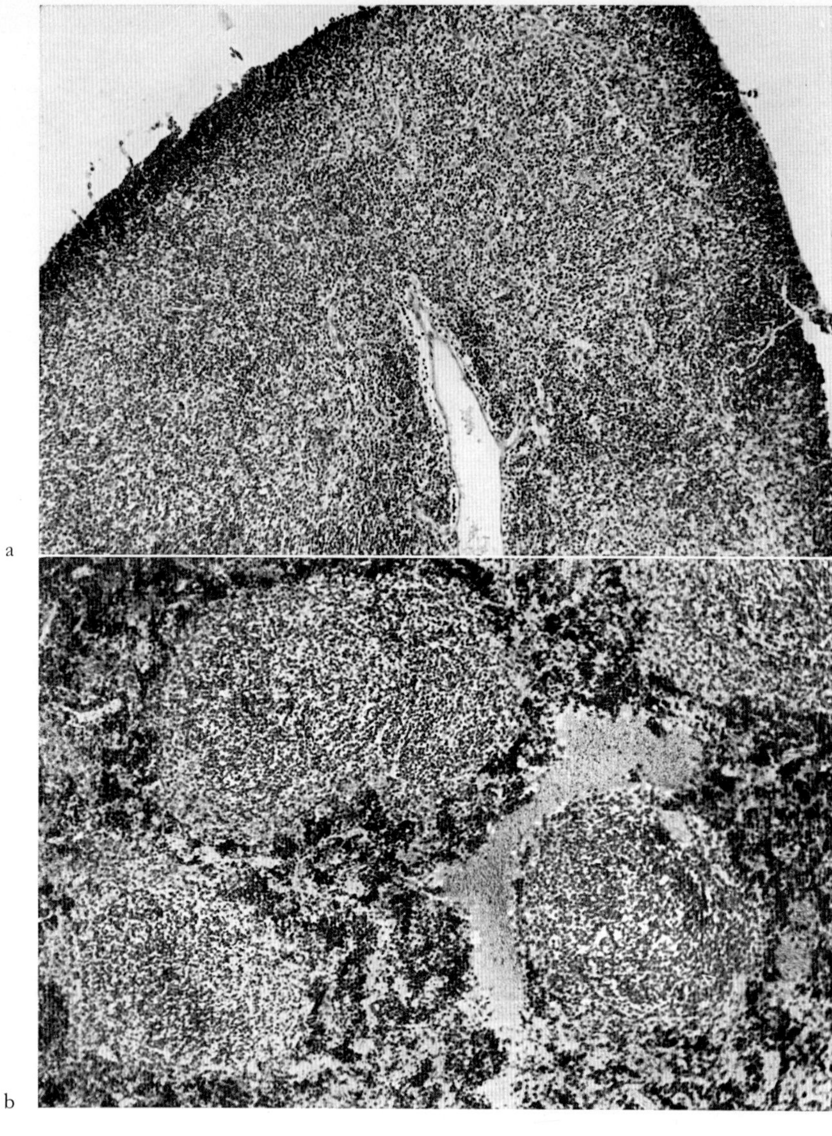

Fig. 3. Thymus (a) and spleen (b) of a C57/B1 mouse (see also fig. 2) killed six days after a single intraperitoneal injection of rabbit anti-mouse hypophysis serum. Note in the thymus complete involution of the cortex and loss of thymocytes. The spleen shows absence of perifollicular mantles around the lymphoid follicles and extreme poverty or absence of lymphocytes in the red pulp. Haematoxylin and eosin, × 70.

of anti-somatotropic hormone treated animals be reversed by somato-tropic hormone? (4) Is thyroxin also dependent on somatotropic hor-mone as far as the effects on the lymphatic tissue and the immune response are concerned? (5) Has anti-somatotropic hormone serum an effect on the immune response?

Daily injections (up to seven) of anti-somatotropic hormone globulins into two weeks old Charles River mice produced a wasting syndrome as seen in animals after treatment with anti-hypophysis serum or after neonatal thymectomy. Anti-somatotropic hormone treatment produces inhibition of body growth, thymus atrophy and affects strongly the reaction of the spleen to inoculation with hetero-logous globulins. The action of anti-somatotropic hormone globulins on spleen and thymus could be reversed by simultaneous injection of somatotropic hormone.

Experiments with groups of three-week-old normal male Charles River mice gave essentially the same results as those with the two weeks old mice. The effect of anti-somatotropic hormone serum on the spleen was even more pronounced. Mice injected with the same quantities of normal rabbit serum globulins (NRS globulins) showed normal body growth and splenic enlargement. Detailed results on these experiments will be reported elsewhere [16].

These results answered several of the posed questions: anti-somatotropic hormone serum can reproduce the effects of anti-hypo-physis serum, that is, thymus atrophy and a wasting syndrome, and these effects can be reversed by somatotropic hormone.

We would like now to discuss the results using five to eight weeks old adult mice treated with anti-somatotropic hormone or NRS glo-bulins for six consecutive days. The adult animals treated with anti-somatotropic hormone globulins showed a variable inhibition of body growth. In contrast to the younger animals, anti-somatotropic hor-mone treated adult mice never showed a wasting syndrome. This is of interest in connection with the interpretation of the pathogenesis of the wasting disease after neonatal thymectomy or after anti-hypo-physeal serum treatment. However, in these adult mice the spleen reaction to the injected foreign proteins was clearly inhibited by anti-somatotropic hormone globulins (fig. 4). This effect was completely reversed by simultaneous administration of somatotropic hormone. Somatotropic hormone alone induces spleen enlargement. This could be partially due to the antigenicity of the somatotropic hormone prep-aration, which is of bovine origin.

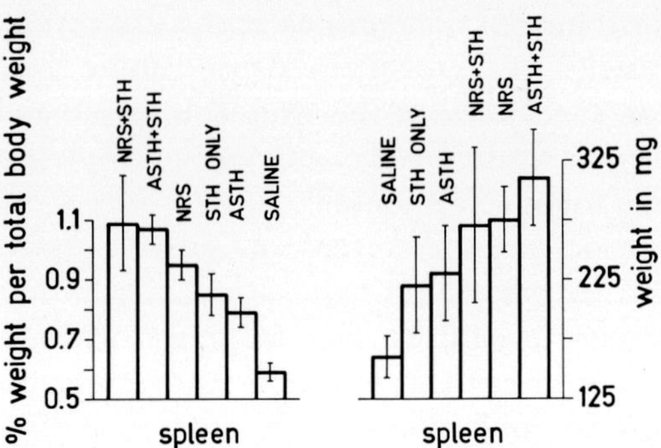

Fig. 4. Effect of daily injections of rabbit anti-somatotropic hormone (ASTH) and normal rabbit serum (NRS) globulins alone or together with somatotropic hormone (STH), of STH alone or of saline on spleen weight in relation to body weight in adult male Charles River mice. The mice received daily injections for six consecutive days and were killed on the seventh day after beginning of treatment. Note reconstitution of ASTH-treated mice with STH.

Somatotropic Hormone and Cellular Dynamics of Lymphoid Tissue

We like now to pass on to the microscopic findings in the spleen of adult mice treated with anti-somatotropic hormone and NRS globulins alone or together with somatotropic hormone and to those in mice treated with somatotropic hormone only and untreated controls

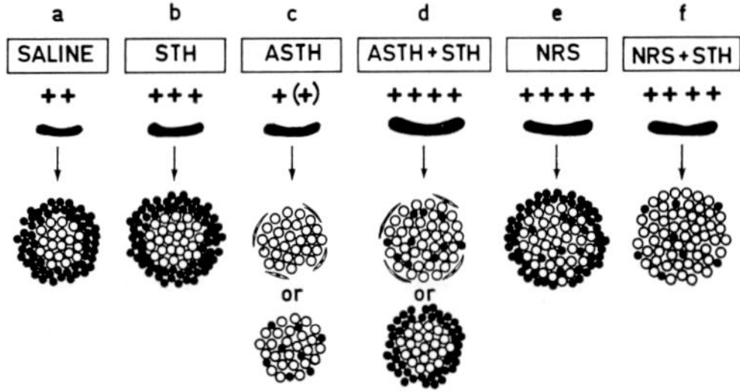

Fig. 5. Same mice and treatment as in figure 4. This schematic representation shows the effect of various agents on spleen size and on the number and cellular composition in splenic germinal centers of adult mice. Treatment with STH alone (b) produces spleen enlargement and an increase in number of germinal follicles and in perifollicular lymphoid cells. Injection of ASTH globulins (c) strongly affects spleen size, number, size and cell composition of germinal centers (compare with [e] NRS-treated mice). The germinal follicles of ASTH-treated mice are very few, scanty and show extreme poverty or complete absence of lymphoid cells. These effects of ASTH globulins are reversed by simultaneous injection of STH (d).

Figure 5 shows a schematic representation of the modifications seen in number, size and cell population of splenic germinal centers of the variously treated mice. In the somatotropic hormone treated mice the spleen is enlarged, the number of germinal follicles is increased and their perifollicular mantles are richer in lymphoid cells. The anti-somatotropic hormone treated mice show a decreased spleen volume, the number of germinal follicles is strongly reduced and their perifollicular lymphoid cells are reduced in number or absent. Thymus-dependent areas [12] are completely devoid of lymphoid cells. This effect can be reversed by somatotropic hormone. In mice treated with NRS globulins the spleen is enlarged and the number and size of germinal centers is increased. A comparison of this group with the anti-somatotropic hormone injected animals, which received the same quantity of protein, shows especially striking differences. In conclusion, the cell population of the perifollicular zones of the germinal centers is influenced and modified by somatotropic hormone or anti-somatotropic hormone in that its reproductive activity seems to be somatotropic hormone dependent. Since the anti-somatotropic hormone effect can be reversed by somatotropic hormone, this clearly indicates that somatotropic hormone regulates cellular dynamics of lymphoid cells and probably also the immunological capacity.

We turn now to the question of how far the well known interdependence of growth hormone and thyroxin is expressed in effects on the lymphatic tissue. This was studied by injecting young male mice with anti-thyrotropic hormone antibody and by treating some

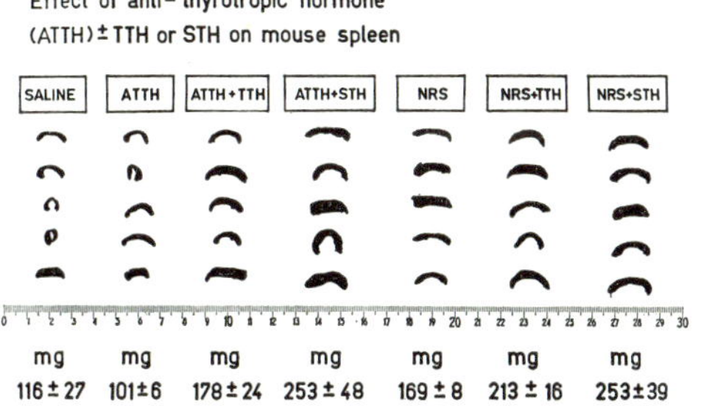

Fig. 6. Effect on young male Charles River mice of injections with rabbit anti-thyrotropic hormone globulins (ATTH) alone or together with thyrotropic hormone (TTH) or somatotropic hormone (STH), for six consecutive days. The inhibition of the spleen cellular reaction and weight in ATTH-treated mice is reversed by simultaneous administration of TTH or STH. Controls were injected with the same quantity of NRS globulins.

groups of these animals with somatotropic or thyrotropic hormone. As shown in figure 6, the spleens of anti-thyrotropic hormone treated mice are very small as compared with those of mice treated with NRS globulins. This effect of anti-thyrotropic hormone globulins can be completely reversed and in fact overcompensated for, not only by giving thyrotropic hormone but surprisingly, also by somatotropic hormone; the thymuses of these animals do not seem to be affected by the anti-thyrotropic hormone activity and no wasting disease was observed, although there was complete inhibition of body growth.

Immunosuppression by Antisomatotropic Hormone

These striking effects of somatotropic hormone on the lymphatic tissue and its importance in protein synthesis in general indicated that interference with somatotropic hormone might result in immuno-supression. Figure 7 shows that rabbit anti-somatotropic hormone

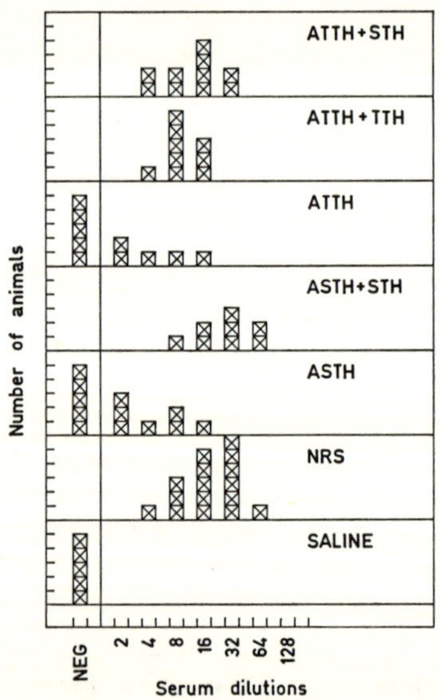

Fig. 7. Effect of injections of rabbit ASTH or ATTH globulins alone or together with STH or TTH on the production of precipitating antibody in individual young male Charles River mice. The globulins were injected intraperitoneally for six consecutive days and the mice were killed on the seventh day. The control mice received the same quantity of NRS globulins. The precipitin test was performed using normal rabbit serum globulins as antigen.

globulins besides being antigenic for the mouse have a built-in immunosuppressive action (anti-somatotropic hormone activity). In fact anti-STH globulins strongly inhibit the formation of precipitating antibody to substances present in these globulin preparations, whereas normal rabbit serum globulins give strong precipitating sera. Inhibition of antibody formation is reversed by somatotropic hormone or thyrotropic hormone and this is parallel to the effects of these hormones on spleen volume (see fig. 6).

Discussion

We would like now to attempt to interpret the meaning of our results in connection with the development of the immunological capacity and wasting disease. Although hormones such as corticosteroids and other steroids are known to depress immunological reactivity, it is astonishing to see that the effects of some other hormones have been largely ignored. The results with somatotropic hormone, at-least as far as the thymus and the peripheral lymphatic organs are concerned, are however so striking that an important role must be assumed for this hormone. We will first consider the wasting disease and death of animals after neonatal thymectomy. These events have been interpreted to be a consequence of bacterial or viral infections in these immunologically deficient animals. We feel that this interpretation in the light of our findings with anti-hypophysis or anti-somatotropic hormone serum may be both correct and wrong. It would seem to us that the primary course of the wasting syndrome, at least as far as our experiments are concerned, is dependent on the induction of a deficiency of somatotropic hormone and other hormones resulting in an inhibition of thymus mitotic activity. In the thymus of young animals this hormone-dependent activity might be essential for a normal development of the immune system and even for body growth [15]. These processes are of lesser importance in the adults in which no wasting disease can be induced by thymectomy nor by anti-somatotropic hormone serum.

We pass now to a short discussion of the action of somatotropic hormone on cells. The levels at which this hormone acts is largely unknown but it is likely that it interferes at several cellular and molecular levels [18, 7, 22, 20]. As shown in figure 8, which is based on MILLER's and other authors findings [11], one site of action for somatotropic

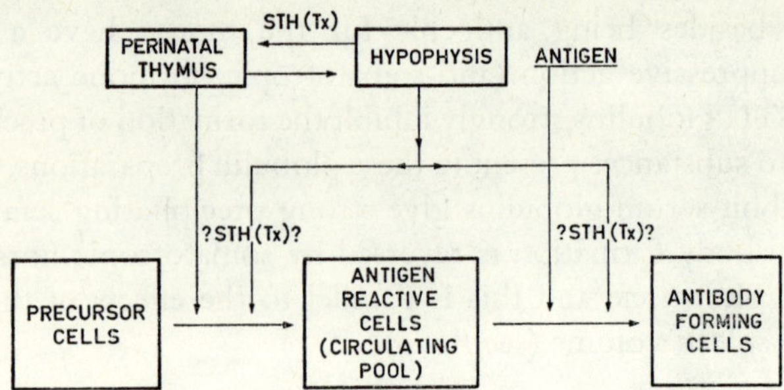

Fig. 8. Scheme showing the possible role of hormones on thymus growth and function and on direct or thymus-mediated differentiation and maturation of antibody-producing cells. STH = somatotropic hormone; Tx = thyroxin.

hormone is almost certainly the thymus as was shown above. In fact, we can ask the somewhat heretical question whether it is the somatotropic hormone and perhaps in addition thyroxin which are the long disputed hormonal factors in the thymus responsible for the differentiation of precursor cells into antigen-reactive cells. Proof for the presence of somatotropic hormone in the thymus is therefore needed. Alternatively growth hormone might act directly on thymocytes or through a specific thymus hormone synthesized by the thymus epithelial cells. It is also possible that somatotropic hormone alone or together with thyroxin is the lymphopoietic factor in the thymus. Experimentation in tissue culture will be needed to establish these points.

Besides the action on the thymus, it appears likely that somatotropic hormone also acts directly on the antigen-sensitive cells. It is known that somatotropic hormone has an important influence on protein synthesis and by implication presumably on antibody synthesis. As was pointed out by TATA [20], growth-promoting and developmental hormones do not directly control cell division or initial differentiation, but help the already differentiated but immature cell to complete its functional specialization or to regulate its size. Accordingly as a working hypothesis we should like to suggest that growth-promoting and developmental hormones including somatotropic hormone and thyroxin might also act on antigen-sensitive cells either before or after contact with the antigen thereby converting them into antibody producing plasma cells. It is still unknown whether antigen-sensitive cells are dependent on somatotropic hormone for their further differentiation after contact with the antigen or if somatotropic hormone is responsible for the maturative step which renders immunocytes sensitive to the action of the antigen.

Finally, we would like to mention that interference with the action of somatotropic hormone should result in immunosuppression. Since we have demonstrated that lymphoid tissue is much more sensitive than other tissue to somatotropic hormone deficiency, such a temporary inhibition might not necessarily be unphysiological.

Summary

A relationship between the function of the thymus and the hypophysis was previously described and has been now further analyzed. Neonatal thymectomy in mice produces changes in the somatotropic hormone-producing-cells of the anterior pituitary gland. Anti-pituitary serum globulins produce thymus atrophy and a wasting syndrome in young male mice. The role of somatotropic hormone in these events was studied. Somatotropic hormone strongly influences the thymus and peripheral lymphatic tissue. Evidence was obtained for atrophy of the thymus and the spleen and for the induction of a wasting syndrome following treatment of mice with anti-somatotropic hormone globulins. The effect exerted by anti-somatotropic hormone is directed against the rapidly reproducing cells in the perifollicular zones of the Malpighian corpuscles and in the thymus-dependent areas of the spleen and in the thymus cortex. Interference with the activity of somatotropic hormone or of hormones which are interdependent with it, like thyroxin, results in immunosuppression.

These findings suggest a twofold role of somatotropic hormone for the development of the immunological capacity. The one at the level of the thymus and peripheral lymphatic tissue has been experimentally demonstrated. The other concerns the possible role of somatotropic hormone in the mechanisms controlling maturation and differentiation of antigen-reactive cells to antibody-producing cells. These points need experimental verification.

References

1. ANIGSTEIN, L.; RENNELS, E. G. and ANIGSTEIN, D. M.: Inhibitory effects of antirat pituitary serum (APS) on hypophysectomized rats injected with pituitary hormones. Acta endocrin., Kbh. *35:* 139–160 (1960).

2. BARONI, C.: Thymus, peripheral lymphoid tissues and immunological responsiveness of the pituitary dwarf mouse. Experientia *23:* 282–283 (1967).

3. DOUGHERTY, T. F.; BERLINER, M. L.; SCHNEEBELI, G. L. and BERLINER, D. L.: Hormonal control of lymphatic structure and function. Ann. N.Y. Acad. Sci. *113:* 825–843 (1964).

4. GRUMBACH, M. M. and KAPLAN, S. L.: Immunochemical studies on human growth hormone: a consideration of the human growth hormone-anti-human growth hormone system and its application to the assay of growth hormone. Ciba Foundation Colloquia on Endocrinology, vol. 14, pp. 63–102 (Churchill, London 1962).

5. HAYASHIDA, T. and LI, C. H.: Immunological investigation of human pituitary growth hormone. Science *128:* 1276–1277 (1958).

6. KIDSON, C.: Cortisol in the regulation of RNA and protein synthesis. Nature (Lond.) *213:* 779–782 (1967).

7. KORNER, A.: Regulation of the rate of synthesis of messenger ribonucleic acid by growth hormone. Biochem. J. *92:* 449–456 (1964).

8. METCALF, D.: Functional interactions between the thymus and other organs. In DEFENDI and METCALF's The thymus, pp. 53–73 (Wistar Institute Press, Philadelphia 1964).

9. McGARRY, E.E.; BECK, J.C.; AMBE, L. and NAYAK, R.: Some studies with antisera to growth hormone, ACTH, and TSH. Recent Progr. Hormone Res. *20:* 1–23 (1964).

10. MILLER, J.F.A.P. and OSOBA, D.: Current concepts of the immunological function of the thymus. Physiol. Rev. *47:* 437–520 (1967).

11. MILLER, J.F.A.P. and MITCHELL, G.F.: The thymus and the precursors of antigen reactive cells. Nature (Lond.) *216:* 659–663 (1967).

12. PARROTT, D.M.V.; DE SOUSA, M.A.B. and EAST, J.: Thymus-dependent areas in the lymphoid organs of neonatally thymectomized mice. J. exp. Med. *123:* 191–203 (1966).

13. PIERPAOLI, W. and SORKIN, E.: Relationship between thymus and hypophysis. Nature (Lond.) *215:* 834–837 (1967).

14. PIERPAOLI, W. and SORKIN, E.: Cellular modifications in the hypophysis of neonatally thymectomized mice. Brit. J. exp. Path. *48:* 627–631 (1967).

15. PIERPAOLI, W. and SORKIN, E.: Effect of gonadectomy on the peripheral lymphatic tissue of neonatally thymectomized mice. Brit. J. exp. Path. *49:* 288–293 (1968).

16. PIERPAOLI, W. and SORKIN, E.: Hormones and immunologic capacity. I. Effect of heterologous anti-growth hormone (ASTH) antiserum on thymus and peripheral lymphatic tissue in mice. Induction of a wasting syndrome. J. Immunol. (in press 1968).

17. READ, C.H.; EASH, S.A. and NAJJAR, S.: Experiences with the haemagglutination method of human growth hormone assay. Ciba Foundation Colloquia on Endocrinology, vol. 14, pp. 45–61 (Churchill, London 1962).

18. RIGGS, T.R.: Hormones and the transport of nutrients across cell membranes. In LITWACK and KRITCHEVSKY's Action of hormones on molecular processes, pp. 1–57 (Wiley and Sons, New York 1964).

19. SCHLESINGER, M. and MARK, R.: Wasting disease induced in young mice by administration of cortisol acetate. Science *143:* 965–966 (1963).

20. TATA, J.R.: Growth and developmental hormones as tools for the study of biosynthetic control mechanisms. In Developmental and metabolic control mechanisms and neoplasia, pp. 335–356 (The Williams and Wilkins Co., Baltimore 1965).

21. TATA, J.R.: Thyroid hormones and the formation and distribution of ribosomes. Acta endocrin., Kbh. Suppl. *124:* 141–152 (1967).

22. TOMKINS, G.M. and THOMPSON, E.B.: Hormonal control of protein synthesis at the translational level. In Wirkungsmechanismen der Hormone, pp. 107–120 (Springer, Berlin 1967).

23. WARNER, N.L. and BURNET, F.M.: The influence of testosterone treatment on the development of the bursa of Fabricius in the chick embryo. Austr. J. Biol. Sci. *14:* 580–587 (1961).

Authors' address: Dr. W. PIERPAOLI and Prof. Dr. E. SORKIN, Schweiz. Forschungsinstitut, Medizinische Abteilung, *7270 Davos-Platz* (Switzerland).

Antibiotica et Chemotherapia, vol. 15, pp. 135–154 (Karger, Basel/New York 1969)

Studies on Differentiation of Immunocompetent Cells Using Immunological Inhibition

J. ŠTERZL

Department of Immunology, Institute of Microbiology, Czech. Acad. Sci., Prague

Introduction

Immune inhibition has been established using various methods. This procedure can be used not only for practical purposes, when suppression of immune response is required, but also for studies on the differentiation of immunocompetent cells.

According to different authors and experiments, the state of immune inhibition can result from various mechanisms. There is evidence that the inhibition follows immediately on contact with a critical dose of an antigen. This may be either due to blocking of receptor sites on a cell sensitive to antigen, or due to allergic death of the cells [BURNET, 1959]. The antigen can affect not only the cell, which was contacted for the first time, i.e. the immunocompetent cell, but such immediate inhibition can be evoked also in presensitized cells, prepared for secondary reaction [MICHIE and HOWARD, 1962; MITCHISON, 1966].

However, there are types of inhibition preceeded by active immune response. After the second dose of antigen, both possibilities—immunological inhibition or secondary reaction—may be expected.

In this paper I would like to present data demonstrating that these two alternative situations (inhibition or secondary response) are dependent on active proliferation or on restriction of proliferation of the cells stimulated by the antigen.

1. Cellular Dynamics after Immunization

At first, let us consider the fact that the preparation of secondary response results from the increased number of cells capable of reacting with an antigen.

If newborn colostrum-free piglets are reared under sterile conditions for one to two months after birth and if possible "natural" stimulation with cross-reacting antigens is minimized using synthetic diet, no antibody-forming cells against sheep red blood cells (SRBC) are detected (table I) in their lymphatic organs. If a sufficient quantity of an antigen (beyond a critical level) is administered to animals, the number of antibody-forming cells initially appearing was found to be about $100/10^8$ lymphoid cells, which means that the maximum number of immunocompetent cells (capable of reacting after the first antigenic stimulus) is $1–10/10^6$ lymphoid cells.

Table I. Number of antibody forming cells/10^8 lymphoid cells in sterile and conventional piglets before and on various days after immunization

Age of piglets in days (when tested or immunized)	Sterile animals			Conventional piglets
	Before immunization	Hours after immunization with 4×10^{10} SRBC i.p.		Before immunization
		48 hrs	72 hrs	
1	0; 0; 0; 0	0; 0; 0; 0	0; 0; 37; 50	0
5	0; 0; 0	0	6; 53	0
12	0	0	35; 270	9
16	0; 0	0	16	20
18	0; 0; 0; 0	—	—	—
26	0; 0; 0; 0; 0; 0	0; 4	3; 48	—
35	0; 0	3	358	—
55	0; 0	—	172	—

Even if sterile newborns are injected immediately after birth with non-specific stimuli (lipopolysaccharide, phytohaemagglutinin, adjuvants), which increase proliferating activity of lymphoid cells, the immunocompetent cells do not react to this stimulation: in piglets stimulated nonspecifically immediately after birth and immunized at the age 1 month, a similar number of antibody producing cells (per 10^8 lymphoid cells) has been found as in animals immunized immediately after birth (table II). Thus proliferation of immunocompetent cells is started only with a specific antigen.

Table II. Influence of non-specific stimulation in newborn sterile piglets on the numbers of antibody producing cells

Non-specific stimulation after birth	Numbers of Ab-producing cells in 10^8 lymphoid cells	Dose of SRBC in 3-week-old piglets
Phytohemagglutinin 5 ml i.c. (Difco M)	25, 620	4×10^{10}
Freund's adjuvant 15 ml s.c.	147, 270, 643	4×10^{10}
Endotoxin 10 μg/kg i.c.	257, 76	4×10^{10}
Controls (0)	95, 358, 318, 719, 776	4×10^{10}
Freund's adjuvant 5 ml s.c.	0, 0	2×10^8
Specific primary stimulus 10^9 SRBC	416 (19S), 3600 (7S)	2×10^8
Controls (0)	0, 0	2×10^8

In the true primary reaction it has been shown that the more antigen introduced, the greater number of cells capable of reacting with an antigen (immunocompetent cells) differentiate into antibody producing cells. Using increasing amounts of sheep red blood cell (SRBC) antigen increasing numbers of antibody forming cells were detected (table III). If the single dose of SRBC (10^9) is administered immediately after birth followed by revactination four weeks later, the quantity of antigen needed is by two to three orders lesser. We concluded that the number of the cells of 19S type is 100 times higher and the number of the cells forming antibodies of 7S type 1000 times

Table III. Relation between the quantity of the antigen and the number of Ab-producing cells in primary and secondary reactions

The dose of SRBC injected i.p.	Primary response in newborn piglets (7 days after antigen injection)	Secondary response of 1-month-old piglets primary stimulated after birth with 10^9 SRBC	
		Ab-producing cells detected 5 days after Ag injection	
		by complement only (19S)	by anti IgG serum and complement (7S)
2×10^6	0	4	56
2×10^7	0	48	640
2×10^8	1	416	3 600
2×10^9	22	800	8 000
2×10^{10}	162	1 040	20 000
2×10^{11}	1 861	3 030	30 060

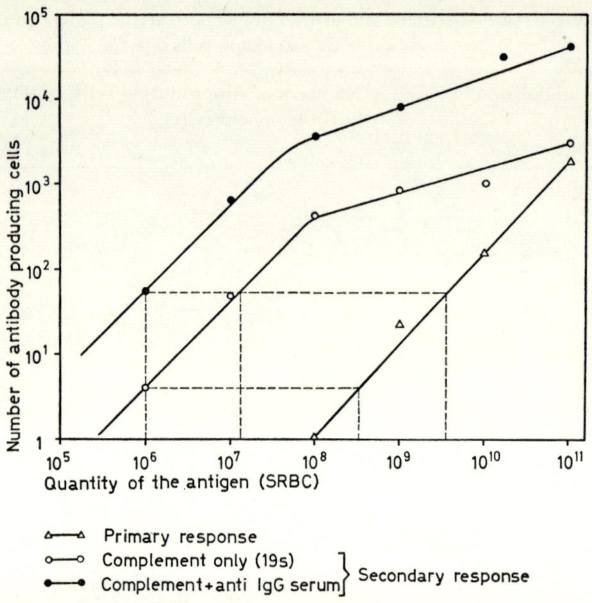

Fig. 1. Quantity of the antigen inducing the same number of antibody producing cells during the primary and secondary response.

higher when compared with the primary response (fig. 1) [Šterzl and Jílek, 1967]. Therefore this experiment shows, as the experiments with transfer of cells [Makinodan and Albright, 1963), that the preparation of secondary reaction is based on the proliferation of immunologically activated cells.

The cells undergoing proliferation and preparing secondary response represent a differentiation step on the way to antibody-forming cells. A secondary response may be prepared without completed primary response, without detection of antibody-forming cells (table IV). Low doses of an antigen stimulated cells to proliferate without transformation of activated cells into antibody-forming cells. This shows that there is a clear dissociation between the proliferating cell, i.e. the cell preparing secondary response (Y-cells) and the cell already producing antibodies (Z-cell). Experiments with transfer of cells [Trnka and Šterzl, 1960] confirmed that for the change of activated cell into the antibody-forming cell a further contact with an antigen is required, similarly as in experiments with cells brought into contact with low doses of an antigen in diffusion chambers [Šterzl, 1967].

Table IV. Secondary response in animals "primed" with low doses of antigen without detection of primary response (Number of Ab-forming cells/10^8 lymphoid cells)

Primary stimulus	Primary Ab-response	Secondary response in primed animals:		Nonprimed controls:	
		19S	7S	19S	7S
Sterile piglets with 10^9 SRBC	0	2×10^8 SRBC (secondary dose)			
		2 173	14 160	0	0
Newborn rabbits with 0.01 ml of SRBC fluid antigen	0	2×10^9 SRBC (secondary dose)			
		6 797	4 700	423	166
Mice (8 weeks old) with 10^6 SRBC	23	10^8 SRBC (secondary dose)			
		14 700	66 000	4 470	3 260

2. The Effect of Metabolic Inhibitors

In studies using metabolic inhibitors it is necessary to differentiate their influence on synthesis of nucleic acids during induction of antibody formation from their action on proliferation of cells engaged in antibody response. As has already been shown, when antigen is administered to an organism, mitotic divisions of cells activated with the antigen as well as the cells already forming antibodies form an indivisible part of the immune reaction. Therefore any intervention into mitotic activity of cells results in inhibition either of primary or of secondary reactions.

In order to dissociate the effect of inhibitors on the intracellular process of induction from their effect on the process of proliferation, an experimental system has been used, in which proliferation activity is highly restricted: transfer of isolated spleen cells mixed with an antigen *in vitro* to a non-inbred allogeneic recipient, a young rabbit. The cells are transfered either free in the peritoneum or closed in a diffusion chamber. The cells of allogeneic donor survive in the recipient only a few days and cytological analysis of the cell population does not show proliferation of the cells transferred [HOLUB, 1962].

This experimental model proved that only simultaneous administration of metabolic inhibitors (6-mercaptopurine) together with the transfer of cells mixed with the antigen, leads to complete inhibition of antibody response (fig. 2). If 6-MP is administered 24, 48 or 72 h after the transfer of cells mixed with the antigen, its effect is gradually lowered; when the administration of 6-MP starts 72 h after the transfer of cells, values of antibody response are almoste qual to

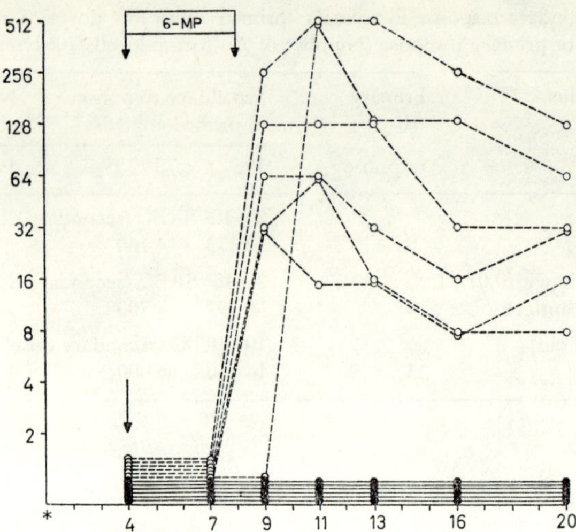

Fig. 2. The effect of 6-MP (0.5 mg/100 gm of body weight for five days) on antibody formation by transferred cells (50×10^6) mixed with *Br. suis* antigen *in vitro* when 6-MP is administered starting on the day of cell transfer (solid line). Controls (dashed line) are recipients receiving the cells only.

controls (fig. 3). When cells already producing antibodies are transferred and 6-MP is applied simultaneously, no inhibition is shown (fig. 4). On the basis of the results obtained it has been concluded that 6-MP affects the process of induction, because the onset of proliferation starts (in vivo system) 72–96 h after the administration of the antigen. However, at this time no effect of inhibitors has been observed [Šterzl, 1960].

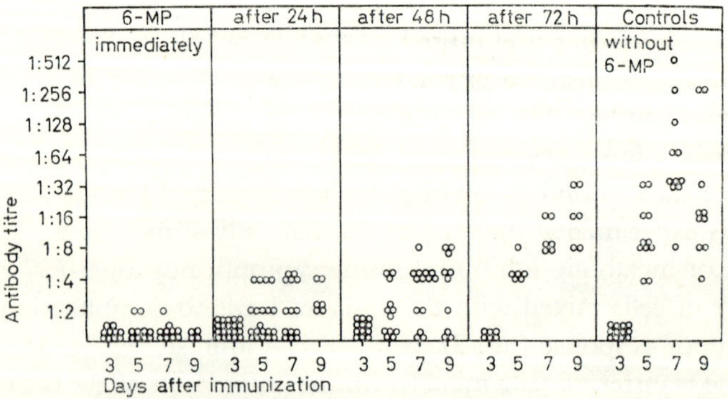

Fig. 3. Inhibition of antibody formation by 6-MP (0.5 mg/100 gm body weight administered at various intervals after transfer of spleen cells (50×10^6) into newborn rabbits.

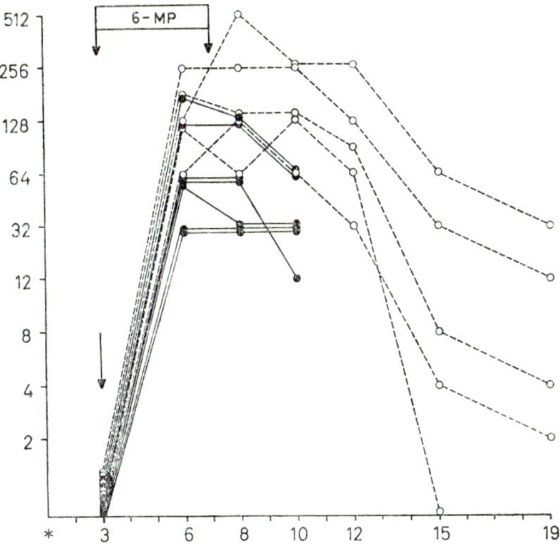

Fig. 4. Transfer of spleen cells (50×10^6) from immunized donors to recipient, newborn rabbits. 6-MP administration (0.5 mg/100 gm for five days) was started on the day of transfer (solid line). Controls not treated with 6-MP (dashed line).

We tried to obtain further informations about the role of proliferation in the onset of antibody formation using the same model, with other types of metabolic inhibitors. 6-Azathymine, 5-fluorouracil, alkylating agents and derivates of folic such as aminopterin have been used, which affect mainly the synthesis of desoxyribonucleic acid. Also agents affecting inhibition of mitotic division—colchicine and actinomycin C—were applied. As shown in table V. toxicity of these drugs was found to be higher than their effect on antibody formation. Only purine antagonists, especially 6-MP and 6-thioguanine and their derivates, exerted higher inhibitory effect on antibody formation in comparison with their toxicity. On the basis of the results we conclude that in the model, in which the cells do not proliferate, we can demonstrate the effect of those inhibitors only, which interfere with the induction of antibody response, as 6-MP and 6-TG. As soon as the process of induction has been realized, antibody production proper is not blocked by these inhibitors. Also application of inhibitors of DNA synthesis has no effect in this system, which indicate that the cells differentiating into antibody-forming cells, need not necessarily go through mitotic division [ŠTERZL, 1961]. This conclusion is supported by our experiments with incorporation of ^{14}C thymidine; incorporation into earliest appearing antibody-forming cells was de-

Table V. Action of metabolic inhibitors on antibody formation

Type of inhibitors	Compound	Dose (mgm/100 gm) body-weight)	a) Inhibition of antibody formation	b) Toxicity
Pyrimidine antagonists	5-fluorouracil	2.0	0	+
		1.0	0	0
	5-bromouracil	5.0	0	0
		2.0	0	0
	6-azauracil	1.0	0	0
		0.5	0	0
	6-azauridine	50.0	0	+
		5.0	0	0
	6-azathymine	2.0	0	0
		1.0	0	0
Purine antagonists	6-mercaptopurine	1.0	+	+
		0.5	+	0
		0.05	±	0
	Buthiopurine	8.0	+	+
		4.0	+	0
		2.0	±	0
		1.0	±	0
	6-thioguanine	0.1	+	+
		0.05	+	0
		0.02	+	0
		0.01	0	0
	6-thioguanosine	0.5	+	+
		0.1	+	0
Folic acid antagonist	Aminopterine	0.15	0	+
		0.05	0	0
		0.025	0	0
		0.01	0	0
Inhibitors of mitotic division	Colchicine	0.2	0	+
		0.05	0	0
	Actinomycin C	0.002	0	+
		0.001	0	0
Polyfunctional alkylating agents	TS-160 (trichlorethylamine)	0.5	—	+
		0.2	0	0
		0.1	0	0
	Endoxan (Cytoxan)	5.0	0	+
		2.5	0	+
		2.0	0	+

a) Antibody formation was estimated in newborn rabbits to which spleen cells isolated from nonimmunized adult rabbits and mixed with *Brucella suis* antigen *in vitro* were transferred.

tected only in 25 % of cells using plaque technique [ŠTERZL *et al.*, 1965].

As stated in the first chapter, if an experimental animal is immunized, proliferation of cells occurs. The cells, which have not been stimulated by further dose of antigen, remain as a reserve for secondary response. Therefore, in most of experiments, the inhibitors administered even after the antigenic stimulus (also inhibitors without any effect in our non-proliferating system, e.g. aminopterin), affect antibody formation. I would like to present one of our experiments on the effect of 6-MP, administered during primary reaction, on the secondary response: Three groups of mice were injected with 6-MP in three doses, each of 50 mg per 1 kg. In animals injected with 6-MP immediately after administration of the antigen, primary antibody response was completely inhibited, however the secondary response was almost as high as in control animals (fig. 5). If 6-MP is administered during both primary and secondary reactions or secondary only the onset of secondary reaction is inhibited. From this experiment it may be concluded that although the expression of capability to form antibodies has been inhibited, the proliferating activity induced by administration of the antigen has not been demaged by shortterm action of this inhibitor. The results indicate that the induction of antibody formation is comprised at two phases; first one, in which the cell is stimulated by the antigen to proliferation and the second phase, i.e. specific induction of proteosynthesis, which is common for both primary and secondary reactions and which is sensitive to 6-MP (fig. 6) [ŠTERZL, 1962].

In the previous experiment, only three doses of the antigen were administered at the beginning of immunization. Later, we followed the influence of 6-MP administered to young rabbits in seven doses, on the seven days following the administration of red blood cell antigen. Intensity of antibody response was followed in secondary reaction three weeks after the first dose of antigen. Secondary response in animals, in which antigen and 6-MP was given during the primary reaction, was almost completely inhibited in comparison with

---

Agglutinating antibodies were estimated at 3, 5, 7 and 9 days after transfer and were statistically evaluated using the Wilcox test. In comparison to controls, the effect of antimetabolites in 20 experimental animals per group were classified as complete inhibition (+), inhibition in 50 % of the animals (±), and no significant inhibition (—).

b) Toxic effects in more than 50 % of experimental animals were classified as +, and no significant toxic effects as 0.

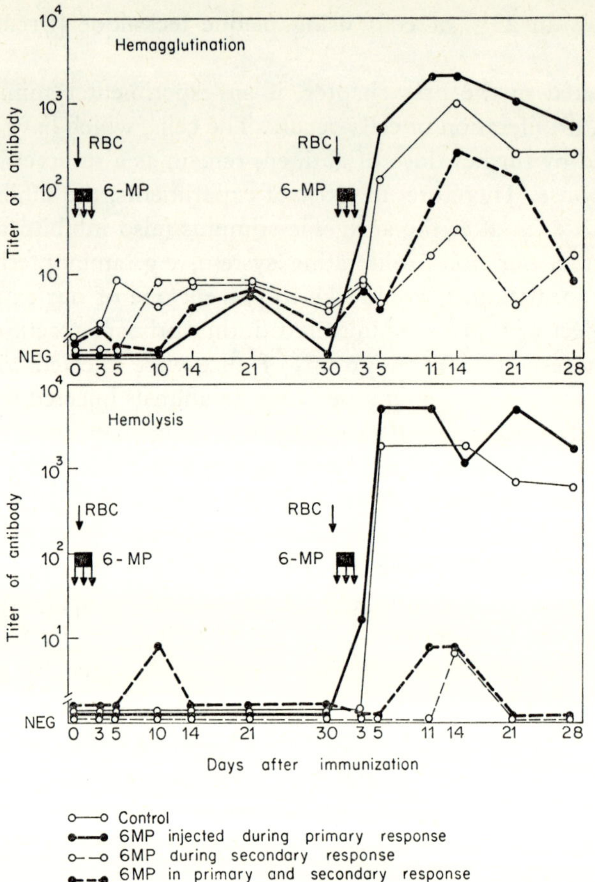

Fig. 5. The effect of 6-MP on the primary and secondary reaction of antibody formation. Mice immunized and revaccinated intravenously with 0.5 ml of 0.01 % suspension of sheep red blood cells (SRBC); 6-MP injected subcutaneously on three successive days in amounts of 50 mg/kg body weight.

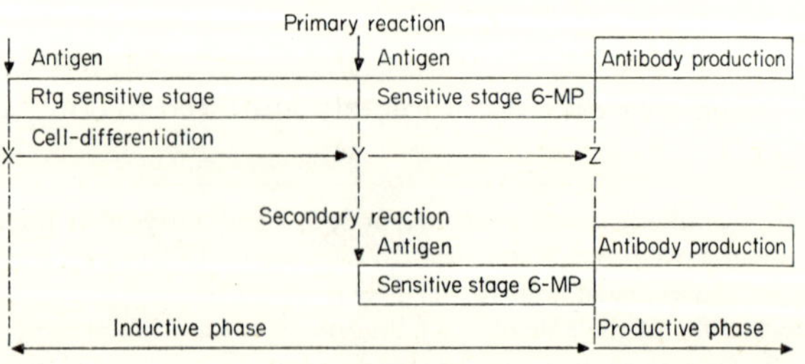

Fig. 6.

Table VI. Influence of 6-mercaptopurine injected with primary stimulus on the secondary response produced three weeks later

Primary stimuli after birth			
7 doses 2.5×10^{10} SRBC during 7 days		7 doses 2.5×10^{10} SRBC and 7 doses 6-MP (3 mg/kg) during 7 days	
Complement only (19S)	With anti-IgG serum (7S)	Complement only (19S)	With anti-IgG serum (7S)
2 140	9 120	40	80
8 080	10 000	36	80
1 872	6 736	24	56
		12	20

Number of antibody forming cells estimated per 10^8 spleen lymphoid cells by plaque technique 5 days after secondary stimulus (2.5×10^8 SRBC).

controls (table VI). These experiments indicate that 6-MP, given in series of successive days after antigen administration, also inhibits the proliferation of cells activated by the antigen, which prepare the secondary response.

3. The Dose of Antigen and the Establishment of Immunological Inhibition

Our interest in the effect of the dose of antigen was mainly stimulated by results published in 1957 [ŠTERZL and TRNKA, 1957]. Young rabbits, injected with bacterial antigen, in a dose sufficient for evocation of immune response in adult animals (S. para B suspension, 10^8 microbes per ml) started to form antibodies after only few weeks of delay (table VII). When a 50% lethal dose (4×10^9 microbes per ml) was injected, the onset of antibody formation was substantially accelerated; in some animals, antibodies were detected already on the fourth day after immunization. However with this large quantity, immediate inhibition of antibody formation was never observed. The group injected with normal dose of the antigen (10^8) as primary stimulus, showed higher antibody formation than controls. On the contrary, in the group immunized with high dose of the antigen immediately after birth (4×10^9) which rapidly formed antibodies in primary response, statistically significantly lower antibody response after revaccination was observed (table VIII).

Table VII. Primary response of newborn rabbits to the different doses of antigen S. paratyphi B.

5-day-old rabbits, 10^8 i.p.	5-day-old rabbits, 10^8 i.c.	0–1-day-old rabbits, 2×10^9 i.p.		5-day-old rabbits, 2×10^9 i.c.	5-day-old rabbits, 4–6×10^9 i.p.	
29	21	14	24	14	9	23
29	21	14	24	17	10	23
>29	21	14	24	17	10	23
>29	>21	14	24	19	11	23
>29	22	14	31	19	13	23
>29	29	14	31	21	14	26
>29	29	17	45	22	14	
>35	36	17	45	29	14	
38	>36	17	45	29	14	
38	>36	24	59		15	
38	36	24	>59		15	
>38	50	24	>59		15	
	50	24	>59		15	
	50	24	>59		15	
		24			23	
M>29	29<M<36	M=24		M=19	M=15	

Table VIII. Secondary response in groups of rabbits injected at birth with different dosages of S. paratyphi B. antigen

1–5-day-old rabbits, 4–6×10^9 i.p.	0–1-day-old rabbits, 2×10^9 i.p.	5-day-old rabbits, 10^8+spleen cells i.p.		Controls
8	32	16	256	32
8	32	16	256	32
8	32	16	256	32
8	32	64	512	64
16	64	64	512	64
16	64	64	512	64
16	64	128	512	64
16	64	128	512	64
32	128	128	512	128
32	128	128	1024	128
32	128	128	1024	128
32	256	128	1024	128
32	256	128	1024	256
	256	256	2048	256
	512	256	2048	256
		256	2048	512
		256	2048	512
		256		
M=16	M=64	M=256		M=128

We repeated these experiments, using sheep erythrocytes as antigen. Antibody formation was estimated by the number of antibody-forming cells detected by plaque technique. Newborn rabbits and newborn sterile piglets were injected after birth with increasing doses of the antigen (table IX, table X). In both types of experiments we have found that in primary response the increasing dose of antigen results in increasing numbers of cells detected as antibody-forming cells. All groups immunized with different doses immediately after

Table IX. Antibody formation in young rabbits immunized after birth with different doses of sheep red blood cells (SRBC) and revaccinated three weeks after the primary immunization

Dose of SRBC in primary immunization	Average number of plaque-forming cells per 10^8 lymphoid cells		
	8 days after primary stimulus	5 days after secondary stimulus with 2×10^9 SRBC	
	developed by complement	by complement only	by anti-γ-G + complement
0	0	2 585	732
1 ml 0.01 % SRBC (2×10^6 cells)	0	2 735	532
1 ml 0.1 % SRBC (2×10^7)	3	14 070	102 433
1 ml 1 % SRBC (2×10^8)	9	1 788	7 810
1 ml 10 % SRBC (2×10^9)	35	978	1 445
1 ml conc. SRBC (2×10^{10})	46	66	166

Table X. Antibody formation in sterile piglets immunized after birth with different doses of sheep red blood cells (SRBC) and revaccinated three weeks after the primary immunization

Dose of SRBC in primary immunization	Average number of plaque-forming cells per 10^8 lymphoid cells		
	10 days after primary stimulus	5 days after secondary stimulus with 2×10^8 SRBC	
	developed by complement	by complement only	by anti-γ-G + complement
0	0	0	0
10 ml 0.01 % SRBC (2×10^7 cells)	0	0	0
10 ml 0.1 % SRBC (2×10^8)	0	0	0
10 ml 1 % SRBC (2×10^9)	22	2 640	21 600
10 ml 10 % SRBC (2×10^{10})	89	1 180	1 660
10 ml conc. SRBC (2×10^{11})	389	0	800

birth were reinjected with the same dose of the antigen. Estimating hemolytic antibodies of 19S and 7S type by plaque technique it was demonstrated that the group of animals, immunized with minimum critical dose of the antigen, showed highest secondary response. If a subminimum quantity is administered, then animals reared under conventional conditions show only an slight increase of ab-forming cells, caused by the immunization with cross-reacting antigens in the environment (table IX). On the contrary, in groups with increasing doses in primary reaction, a gradual lowering of the number of cells during the secondary reaction was found. In the secondary reaction, maximum dose given in primary leads to the response, which may be characterized as the real inhibition of antibody formation.

The results, therefore, indicate that a certain type of immunological inhibition does not result from a direct inhibition of the capability of cells to react immunologically, but that the inhibition preceeds immune response, which is exhausted because the proliferation of activated cells is limited.

In order to support such an idea, it was necessary to use different antigens, eventually clasical models of the onset of the inhibition. Dr. TLASKALOVÁ and Dr. MEDLÍN [1967] repeated experiments with the effect of various doses of bacterial antigen on the secondary response and they proved that if a high quantity of bacterial or lipopolysaccharide antigen is administered to animals tested, the number of Ab-producing cells in secondary response is significantly inhibited in comparison to controls (fig. 7).

In an other set of experiments, Dr. MEDLÍN used a model of immunological paralysis by injecting pneumococcal polysaccharide. In the first dose, 10–100 gamma one mouse was injected, i.e. a dose, which does not result into detectable antibody response in the serum. However, shortly after the administration of this dose, specific antibody-forming cells were detected in the spleen in significant numbers ($500–1000/10^8$), but later disappeared. After the immunogenic dose, the cells appeared in greater number, but later on.

These results were supported by experiments of SISKIND *et al.* [1968]. Injecting 50 mg of DNP antigen into rabbits they observed a rapid antibody response, which results in depression of immune response. On the contrary, if the animals are immunized with 0,5 mg of the antigen, which results in slight primary antibody response, the authors found a vigorous secondary response upon boosting at 50 days. They concluded that "a single hit or binding by a few antigen mole-

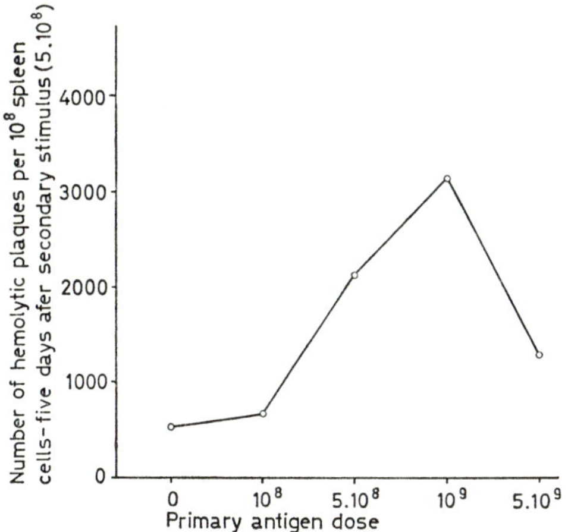

Fig. 7. The secondary response of young rabbits primed with different doses of S. paratyphi B on the 15th day of life.

cules might result in proliferation without differentiation to antibody
secretion. A large dose of antigen would thus favor differentiation
of cells for antibody production, resulting in the rapid appearance of
high antibody titers, but would tend to deplete the pool of proliferating cells and thus later limit the extend of the immune response.
Lower doses of antigen, which would result in less immediate diver-
sion of cells for antibody synthesis, would favour a more sustained
and ultimately a greater immune response.''

Regulatory influence of the quantity of the antigen on the process
of immune reaction may be followed not only by administration of
different doses during the immunization, but also by lowering of the
quantity of antigen, using antiserum to the antigen used. Series of
papers proved that antiserum injected simultaneously with the antigen
or shortly after it can inhibit the onset of antibody response. In our
experiments, we have fully verified these findings.

We assume (fig. 6) that in the induction of antibody formation, a
proliferative period exists during which only a further antigenic stimulus evokes the specific differentiation. Therefore we were interested
in whether the administration of the antiserum in various phases after
antigenic stimulus, would remove the remaining antigen and so inhibit the completion of the primary antibody response or whether this
would limit the onset of the secondary response. It has been demonstrated that the dose of antiserum, which completely inhibits antibody

formation, results in the elimination of the secondary response. This is an analogy of experiments mentioned above, in which the quantity of antigen did not reach the values necessary for the critical concentration on the surface or inside the immunocompetent cells (table III). If the quantity of antiserum given is lowered, then the onset of antibody response is not detected in the usual time sequence, i.e. fourth day after antigen administration. A slight antibody response has been detected about the 15th day (also cells of 7S type are detected). In these individuals, a second dose leads to a typical secondary response, with a majority of 7S antibodies (table XI). An interesting situation may be observed, if the inhibitory quantity of the antiserum is given 24 h after the administration of an antigen: four days after the antigen injection the intensity of primary response is significantly lowered. Later, 15 and 30 days after immunization number of ab-forming cells is comparable to non immunized individuals. In the secondary response significant increase in the number of cells has been detected, but only in cells forming antibodies of 19S type. Cells detectable in numbers higher by one order using anti IgG serum i.e. the group of cells forming antibodies of 7S type, are not present at all. If the antiserum against SRBC is given later, 72 or 96 h after the antigen injection, the secondary reaction is normal, even at the significant inhibition of the primary response.

Table. XI. The effect of antiserum given simultaneously with antigen

Dose of antigen	Dilution of anti-serum	Antibodies detected					After revaccination with 10^8 SRBC	
		4th day	15th day compl.	anti-IgG	30th day compl.	anti-IgG	4th day compl.	anti-IgG
10^{10}	1:10	403	—	—	—	—	—	—
SRBC	1:100	960	—	—	—	—	4.500	510.000
	1:1000	13.503	108	4.063	—	—	4.800	348.500
	0	61.353	58	3.803	—	—	16.675	175.000
10^9	1:10	5	943	3.436	5	173	41.500	460.000
SRBC	1:100	2.029	2.685	23.530	33	183	100.500	1,913.000
	1:1000	10.910	615	17.470	—	—	—	—
	0	48.000	1.130	6.000	—	—	30.400	1,120.000
10^8	1:10	21	46	—	—	—	8.650	7.000
SRBC	1:100	182	353	3.660	3	390	60.900	384.000
	1:1000	3.262	865	16.630	30	80	94.000	1,518.000
	0	42.480	1.224	19.748	106	52	835.000	2,533.000

These results introduce the problem of mutual relations of cells forming 19 and 7S antibodies. Some authors consider the origin of cells forming 19 and 7S antibody from two separate independent lines. If a large quantity of the antigen is injected, antibodies of 7S type appear early. Hypothetically for the induction of cells forming 7S antibodies, much more antigen is required than for the induction of cells forming 19S antibodies. However, there are facts against this opinion: firstly, the cells forming 7S antibodies have greater affinity for the antigen, i.e. they are able to bind the antigen even if present in the organism in minimum quantity only. If the organism is injected with a small quantity of antigen, cells forming antibodies of 19S type appear first; the cells forming antibodies of 7S type appear only later on, i.e. at the time, when the quantity of antigen in the organism has been considerably lowered. Therefore, we favor the second alternative hypothesis, that there is a common immunocompetent cell which differentiate into precursors for 19S and 7S types during the proliferation of the cells activated by the antigen. This is supported by the fact that all procedures which influence the proliferation activity regulate the onset of the cells forming 19 and 7S types: a small dose of antigen induces only 19S type, while the same dose in Freund's adjuvant leads to the appereance also of cells forming 7S antibodies. Inhibition of proliferation by X-irradiation or by 6-MP prevents the appearance of antibodies of 7S type. This hypothesis is supported by the above mentioned experiments with antiserum to the antigen used, which indicate that antibodies of 19S and 7S type are not induced simultaneously: 24 h after antigen injection, the onset of antibody-forming

Table XII. The effect of antiserum (1:10) given in various time intervals after administration of 10^8 SRBC

Serum given	Antibodies detected					After revaccination with 10^8 SRBC	
	4th day	15th day		30th day		4th day	
		compl.	anti-IgG	compl.	anti-IgG	compl.	anti-IgG
simultaneously	21	46	0	—	—	8.650	7.200
24 hrs after antigen	1.880	57	132	26	261	329.000	304.000
48 hrs after antigen	2.550	40	50	61	26	705.000	700.600
72 hrs after antigen	10.350	180	60	48	6	327.000	1,360.000
96 hrs after antigen	88.000	733	1.098	21	7	680.000	1,460.000
0	42.480	1.224	19.748	106	52	835.000	2,533.000

cells was not completely inhibited in primary and secondary response, but these cells were only of 19S type. The reduction of the quantity of the antigen after 24 h prevented the shift between the precursors of 19 to 7S. Similar example of the sequential gene expression in the same line of cells produces the change in the synthesis of fetal to adult hemoglobin.

Conclusions

On the basis of studies with immunosuppressive drugs and different doses of antigens, a possible picture of differentiation of immuno-competent cells may be discussed.

We advance the idea that the fate of cells activated by antigen (i.e. the cells endowed with a proliferative potential) is of central importance: stimulation or limitation of their proliferative activity (affected either by function of drugs or by quality and quantity of antigen) leads either to secondary response or to immunological inhibition.

From our data, some working conclusions may be drawn: Immunocompetent cells (X) are resting (not actively proliferating) cells and are activated only after a contact with specific antigen.

The cell activated by the antigen (Y) has proliferating activity; its appearance is only the first step in the induction of antibody-formation.

Further contact with the antigen shifts the activated cell in the differentiation sequence to the antibody-forming cell (Z); at this stage, specific nucleic acid is formed and this phase of induction is sensitive to 6-MP.

According to the quantity and quality of the antigen injected, different results are observed, which can be interpreted as follows (fig. 8):

If a sufficient amount of antigen is present during the whole process of induction, antibody-forming cells are detected and are differentiated without intensive mitotic divisions (forming antibodies of 19S type) (fig. 8/1 b). Small dose of antigen injected as a true primary stimulus (in sterile newborns fed with non-antigenic diet) leads to the activation of immunocompetent cells, to the proliferative state only (1 a).

We assume that limited proliferation of precursor cells (five to seven generations) provides the basis for formation of antibodies of

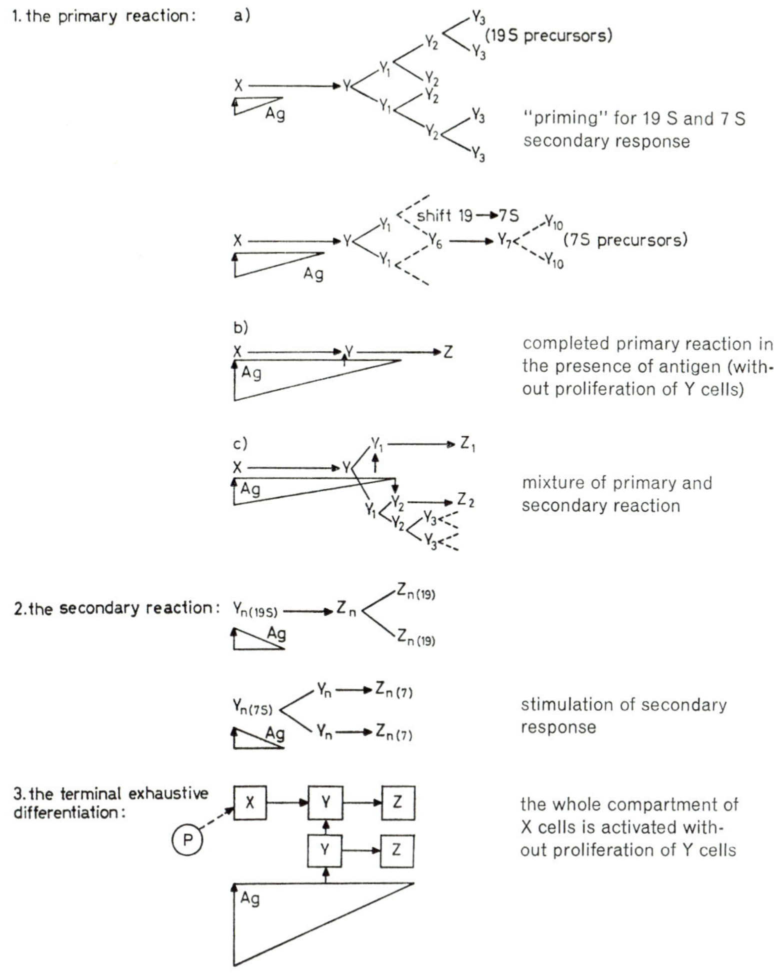

Fig. 8. Unitarian concept of immune reactions based on the model of immunocompetent cell differentiation.

19S type. The proliferation may be limited either by antigen dosage (very large or very small quantities of antigen) or by external inhibitors (6-MP, X irradiation etc.). If the proliferation of activated cells continues, "genetic shift" may occur, i.e. the activation of gene region controlling gamma-chain synthesis.

Our results lead to the conclusion that immunological inhibition may result from induction of antibody formation under conditions in which the proliferation of activated cells is restricted. After primary stimulus with the large dose of antigen all immunocompetent cells are activated and differentiated into antibody-forming cells, about 1–10 per 10^6 lymphoid cells. Antibody-forming cells live two to three days; subsequent doses of the antigen will react only with a small number of immunocompetent cells (fig. 8/3). In adult individuals already purposely or naturally stimulated (with large stock of Y-cells) only repeated doses of antigen may be effective to complete the process of terminal exhaustive differentiation of immunologically reacting cells.

References

BURNET, F.M.: The clonal selection theory of acquired immunity (Cambridge Univ. Press, London 1959).

HOLUB, M.: Potentialities of the small lymphocyte as revealed by homotransplantation and autotransplantation experiments in diffusion chambers. Ann. N.Y. Acad. Sci. *99*: 477–486 (1962).

MAKINODAN, T. and ALBRIGHT, J.F.: In: Immunopathology, p. 99 (Eds.) P. GRABAR and P.A. MIESCHER (Schwabe and Co., Basel 1963).

MICHIE, D. and HOWARD, J.G.: Transplantation tolerance and immunilogical immaturity. Ann. N.Y. Acad. Sci. *99*: 670–678 (1962).

MITCHINSON, N.A.: Immunological paralysis as a problem of cellular differentiation; Ontogeny of immunity, pp. 135–140 (Eds.) R.T. SMITH; R.A. GOOD and P.A. MIESCHER (University of Florida Press, 1967).

SISKIND, G.W.; DUNN, P. and WALKER, J.G.: Studies on the control of antibody synthesis. II. Effect of antigen dose and of suppression by passive antibody on the affinity of antibody synthesized. J. exp. Med. *127*: 55–66 (1967).

ŠTERZL, J. and TRNKA, Z.: Effect of very large doses of bacterial antigen on antibody production in newborn rabbits. Nature *179*: 918–919 (1957).

ŠTERZL, J.: Inhibition of the inductive phase of antibody formation by 6-mercaptopurine studied by the transfer of isolated cells. Nature *185*: 256–257 (1960).

ŠTERZL, J.: Effect of some metabolic inhibitors on antibody formation. Nature *189*: 1022–1023 (1961).

ŠTERZL, J.: Allergology, pp. 269–281 (Ed.) E.A. BROWN (Pergamon Press, N.Y. 1962).

ŠTERZL, J.; VESELÝ, J.; JÍLEK, M. and MANDEL, L.: Molecular and cellular basis of antibody formation. pp. 463–475 (Publish. House Czech. Acad. Sci., Prague 1965).

ŠTERZL, J.: Factors determining the differentiation pathway of immunocompetent cells. Cold Spring Harbor Symp. Qant. Biol. *32*: 493–506 (1967).

ŠTERZL, J. and JÍLEK, M.: Number of antibody-forming cells in primary and secondary reactions after administration of antigen. Nature *216*: 1233–1236 (1967).

TLASKALOVÁ, H.; MEDLÍN, J. and ŠTERZL, J.: Pathophysiology of fetal and neonatal development. Symp. Jena (1967). Bull. mikrobiol. soc., Prague (in press).

TRNKA, Z. and ŠTERZL, J.: Mechanisms of antibody formation, pp. 190–194 (Eds.) M. HOLUB and L. JAROŠKOVÁ (Publish. House Czech. Acad. Sci., Prague 1960).

Author's address: Dr. J. ŠTERZL, Czechoslovak Academy of Science, Institute of Microbiology, Department of Immunology, *Prague 4* (Czechoslovakia).

Antibiotica et Chemotherapia, vol. 15, pp. 155–176 (Karger, Basel/New York 1969)

Immunosuppressive Agents:
The Design of Selective Therapeutic Schedules

M. C. BERENBAUM

Department of Immunology, Institute of Child Health,
University of London, London

The problem of the clinical use of immunosuppressive agents is largely the problem of specificity, that is, how to act against the cells with the undesired property without causing unacceptable damage to other cells that may be of vital importance. There are two types of specificity here. An immunologically specific treatment would have little or no effect on immunologically competent cells except those with the undesired immunological activity. A tissue-specific treatment would damage immunologically competent cells generally, but have little or no effect on other tissues, e.g., bone marrow. We may therefore have treatments that are immunologically specific but not tissue specific (i.e. they damage a particular set of immunologically active cells more than other cells of the same sort, but they also damage other vulnerable tissues), treatments that are tissue-specific but not immunologically specific (i.e. they damage immunologically active cells in general, more than other vulnerable tissues), and treatments that are both immunologically and tissue-specific.

Immunological Specificity

Specificity of this type is obtainable by (a) induction of immune tolerance, with massive doses of antigen; (b) induction of tolerance with rather smaller amounts of antigen in animals treated with immunosuppressive agents; (c) exploitation of the time-dependent effects of immunosuppressive agents.

Discussion of the first two manoeuvres would lead too far from the main subject matter of this review, but the use of time-dependence is sufficiently relevant to merit brief discussion. It is known that radiation, busulphan and anti-lymphocyte serum suppress antibody production most effectively if they are given before the antigen but have little or no effect if given afterwards. Most antimetabolites, alkylating agents and alkaloids behave in the contrary way, being relatively ineffective if given before the antigen and strongly immunosuppressive if given afterwards [TALIAFERRO and TALIAFERRO, 1954; GENGOZIAN and MAKINODAN, 1958; BERENBAUM, 1961, 1962, 1967b, 1967c; FRISCH et al., 1962; MERRITT and JOHNSON, 1963; BROWN, 1964; RIETHMÜLLER et al., 1967].

It follows that, if two antigens are given on two different occasions, it should be possible to suppress the response to one without affecting the response to the other by giving an immunosuppressive agent between the two injections of antigen. This expectation was confirmed by experiments in which thioguanine, cyclophosphamide or methotrexate were given to mice between injections of sheep and human red cells. The response was inhibited only to the antigen that was given before the drug [FRISCH and DAVIES, 1962; 1966; SANTOS and OWENS, 1963].

In man also, given three antigens in series, a 5-day course of 6-mercaptopurine or methotrexate markedly inhibits the response to an antigen given on the second day of the course, slightly inhibits the response to one given a day after the end of the course, and has no effect on the response to an antigen given 3 days after the course is completed [HERSH et al., 1966]. Some degree of specific immunological depression can therefore be achieved by appropriate timing of administration of immunosuppressive agents if the timing of exposure to antigen is known.

Tissue Specificity

There are three general approaches to the problem of ensuring that immunosuppressive agents damage immunologically competent cells more than other tissues.

a) Study of factors underlying differential cell susceptibility. It is a commonplace that toxic agents are generally selective, damaging some tissues more than others. The factors responsible for such selectivity embrace practically every physical and chemical property of the drugs and the cells that they affect. The relevant factors include cell permeability to different agents, the binding constants of these agents to various enzymes, the amounts of these enzymes in various cells and the ability of the cell to synthesize them, the effect of varying intracellular conditions (e. g., pH) on the activity of different agents, the rates of breakdown or detoxication of agents by various cell types, cell dependence on particular metabolic paths, ability to repair damage of various types and so on. It need hardly be said that our knowledge of such factors in regard to human cells is scanty indeed; it is virtually non-existent in regard to immunologically competent cells. There can be no doubt that the intensive study of this field will enable the selection or design of more effective and less toxic immunosuppressive agents.

b) Use of drug combinations. The use of pairs or groups of immunosuppressive agents to achieve potentiation of the immunosuppressive effect without corresponding potentiation of toxicity has not been explored in any systematic fashion. The use of other, non-immunosuppressive drugs to produce the same effect by enhancing the activity or modifying the disposal of immunosuppressive agents is also a relatively neglected field [see, e. g., ELION *et al.*, 1963a, b; McCONNELL and ZUKOSKI, 1963]. Some encouraging results have been obtained by using, with immunosuppressive agents, drugs that protect other vulnerable tissues from their toxic effects [BERENBAUM, 1967a].

c) Modifications of therapeutic schedule. The principles underlying the methods described above for achieving specificity in immunosuppression are clear enough, even if some of them might be difficult to put into practice at present. It may not be so evident that a certain degree of specificity may reside in the design of the therapeutic schedule, that is, in the size and frequency of the doses of the agent. The main purpose of this review is to show that this is so, at least in theory, and that, under certain circumstances, variation in these parameters might profoundly alter the effects of an agent on different tissues. It will be necessary first to establish what is the main cellular effect of standard immunosuppressives, after which the relation of the dose regimen to this effect can be examined.

Modes of Action of Immunosuppressive Agents

The immune response is a complex sequence of events that can be divided broadly into (1) uptake of antigen; (2) transfer of modified antigen or other informational macromolecules from ingesting cells to effector cells; (3) proliferation of effector cells and (4) differentiation and definitive function of effector cells. Conceivably, immunosuppression could be brought about by interference with any of these steps but there is evidence that the third step, cell proliferation, is particularly vulnerable to most of the immunosuppressive agents used at present. More particularly, the evidence suggests that these agents act in the main by causing so-called reproductive cell death.

a) Many immunosuppressive agents are also anti-neoplastic. Skipper and his colleagues, who have elaborated methods for studying the kinetics of neoplastic cells in mice treated with these agents, have shown that they cause a rapid fall in the number of reproductively competent cells but the cells that survive continue to multiply at the normal rate [Skipper *et al.*, 1964, 1965; Pittillo *et al.*, 1965; Wilcox *et al.*, 1965]. In other words, the reduction of a neoplastic cell population is not brought about by an overall slowing of proliferation, nor by induction of a lag in cell division, but by a rapid destruction of the reproductive ability of part of the cell population. Cells that are not affected in this way appear to suffer little permanent damage. It is relevant, therefore, that the doses of these agents that are immunosuppressive are in the same range as the doses that are effective in inhibiting tumours (figs. 13, 14). Although these agents have many other actions that could conceivably be responsible for their immunosuppressive effects (e. g. destruction of small lymphocytes, temporary delaying of mitosis, etc.), these are not generally produced in the same dose range as that required for immunosuppression. For instance, lymphocyte destruction is caused by nitrogen mustard at doselevels considerably less than those required for immunosuppression, whereas such agents as thioguanine would require doses well above the immunosuppressive level to produce this effect to any material degree.

b) Certain antimetabolites and alkaloids, e.g., 5-fluorouracil, methotrexate, 6-mercaptopurine, vincaleukoblastine, etc., are more effective in impairing cell reproductive integrity when the cells are rapidly proliferating than when they are resting [Schabel *et al.*, 1965; Pittillo *et al.*, 1965; Madoc-Jones *et al.*, 1966; Madoc-Jones and Bruce, 1967]. Similarly, it has been shown that these and similar agents are most effective in suppressing immune responses when given some one to four days after the antigen, i.e., at the time when immunologically competent cells are multiplying most rapidly [Berenbaum, 1961, 1962; Merritt and Johnson, 1963; Santos and Owens, 1964; Frisch and Davies, 1962]. In the case of 6-thioguanine it has been shown, by counting antibody-forming cells, that these are practically unaffected by administration of the drug one or six days before the antigen, are rapidly reduced in numbers by the drug given up to four days after the antigen (with a maximum effect on day $+2$) and are again relatively resistant to the agent 8 or 20 days after immunization [BERENBAUM, 1967b]. In other words, agents that impair cell reproductive integrity to the greatest extent when the cells are rapidly multiplying but have little effect on this function when the cells are resting, also impair immune responses most effectively when immunologically competent cells are multiplying rapidly and have little effect when these cells are resting.

c) In contrast to the antimetabolites, radiation causes reproductive lesions whether the cells are proliferating or not [GLINOS and NORTH, 1963]. Cells that are not multiplying at the time of irradiation store the lesion and show damage when they attempt to divide. Therefore, if radiation acted on immunologically competent cells by damaging the reproductive apparatus, we would expect that its immunosuppressive activity would not depend greatly on whether the immunologically competent cells were proliferating or not at the time of irradiation. In other words, it should be immunosuppressive whether given before or after the antigen. Now it is certainly true that radiation is immunosuppressive if given before the antigen, i.e. at a time when immunologically competent cells are not proliferating rapidly [TALIAFERRO and TALIAFERRO, 1954, 1964; TALIAFERRO et al., 1952; GENGOZIAN and MAKINODAN, 1958]. It is more difficult to show that it is also immunosuppressive if given after the antigen. This difficulty is largely due to certain experimental artefacts that have been discussed elsewhere and it has been shown that, when antibody-forming cells are counted, the immune response is radiosensitive at all stages [BERENBAUM, 1966a, 1967b].

d) Radiation-induced damage to cell reproductive integrity is persistent. Cells that are irradiated in the resting state store the damage for weeks or months [ALBERT and BUCHER, 1960; WEINBREN et al., 1960; LEONG et al., 1961]. If radiation acted on immunologically competent cells by impairing their reproductive integrity, we would accordingly expect such impairment to last for weeks or months. This expectation is borne out in practice. The effects of single doses of radiation in the immunosuppressive range (200–700r) last for several weeks, although they diminish slowly during that time [TALIAFERRO and TALIAFERRO, 1954, 1964; TALIAFERRO, TALIAFERRO and JANSSEN, 1952; GENGOZIAN and MAKINODAN, 1958]. The slow recovery after irradiation is probably due to replacement of the defective cell population by proliferation of undamaged cells. The work of NETTESHEIM *et al.*, [1967] showed that spleen cells from irradiated donors could not mount a secondary response even 18 months after radiation doses of 400r or more. Also relevant is the finding by NOWELL [1965a] that, in irradiated patients, immunologically competent small lymphocytes (i.e. those stimulated to divide by exposure to tuberculin) still carried chromosomal abnormalities six months after irradiation.

These lines of evidence may be summed up as follows. Agents that inhibit tumour growth by impairing cell reproductive integrity also suppress immune responses, and the doses for the two effects are in the same range. Agents that impair reproductive integrity most when cells are rapidly proliferating also impair immune responses most when immunologically competent cells are rapidly proliferating. Radiation, which impairs reproductive integrity whether the cells are multiplying or not, also impairs immune responses whether immunologically competent cells are multiplying or not. Radiation-induced impairment of reproductive integrity is persistent and so is radiation-induced immunosuppression. The evidence therefore points to the conclusion that the main mode of action of the immunosuppressive agents discussed so far is to impair the reproductive integrity of immunologically competent cells.

Of course, this is not the only mode of action. Some highly effective agents, e.g. anti-lymphocyte serum and the corticosteroids, produce a bewildering array of effects of possible immunological significance and it is not possible to say yet what the crucial actions of these agents are.

Now, if commonly used immunosuppressives, such as 6-mercaptopurine, azathioprine, actinomycin, irradiation, and cyclophosphamide, act mainly by impairing cell reproductive integrity, any attempt to use these agents rationally must be based on an understanding of the relation between the size and frequency of doses and the extent of reproductive impairment that results. In other words, we have to consider the relationship between dose-response curves and the design of therapeutic schedules.

Dose-Response Curves

Two main types of dose-response curve have been described for agents that act by impairing cell reproductive integrity; they are, respectively, the exponential type and hyperbolic type. There is a third type which will not be discussed here because it has so far been shown only by one class of agents, the vinca alkaloids, which are not commonly used as immunosuppressives [VALERIOTE *et al.*, 1966].

a) Exponential dose-response curves. An exponential curve is produced when a constant linear increment in dose causes a constant logarithmic decrease in cell survival. This may be expressed by the equation

$$\log. S = -aD \tag{1}$$

where S is the surviving fraction of the cell population, D the dose and a a constant. A plot of log. S against D therefore gives a straight line with a slope of $-a$ (fig. 1, a). More conventionally, the exponential relationship is expressed as

$$S = e^{-aD} \tag{2}$$

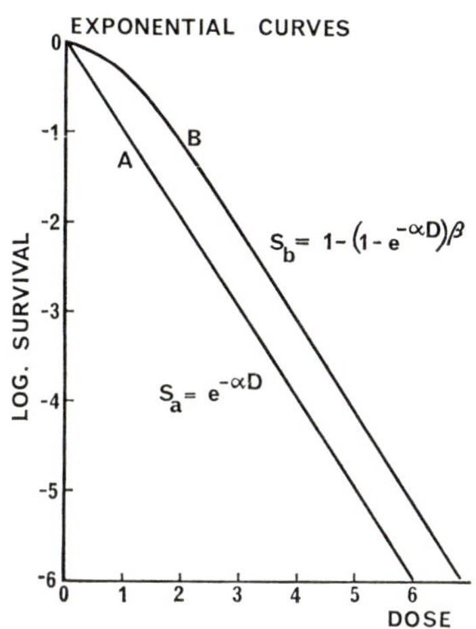

Fig. 1. Exponential dose-response curves.
A – simple exponential curve. B – exponential curve with shoulder.

This relationship may be explained by target theory if it is supposed that (1) reproductive integrity is governed by a single structure in each cell which is inactivated by reaction with a single molecule of drug or a single ionization produced by radiation, and (2) these reactions are independent of each other. A useful analogy is the destruction of a number of eggs by randomly thrown objects [WILCOX, 1966]. The relation between the proportion broken and the number of objects thrown is an exponential one.

Most exponential curves found experimentally are more complex than that shown in figure 1, A, in that they show a shoulder at low doses (fig. 1, B). This type of curve is approximated by the equation

$$S = 1 - (1 - e^{-\alpha D})^\beta \qquad (3)$$

It may be accounted for by supposing the existence of several targets requiring inactivation in each cell, or by mechanisms that repair damage to the reproductive apparatus, or by both.

Exponential dose-response curves are given *in vivo* by ionizing radiation and alkylating agents (figs. 2–5). There is a certain therapeutic attractiveness in agents that cause logarithmic decreases in cell survival for linear increments in dose. For instance, if one gave a series of leukaemic patients, containing an average of, say, 10^{11} leukaemic cells, a dose of agent that caused a 12-log fall in cell survival, there would remain an average of 0.1 leukaemic cell per patient. In other words, we would expect 9 out of 10 patients to have no leukaemic cells left; they would be cured. To use WILCOX's analogy, if enough objects are thrown at a pile of eggs, there is a reasonable chance of breaking them all.

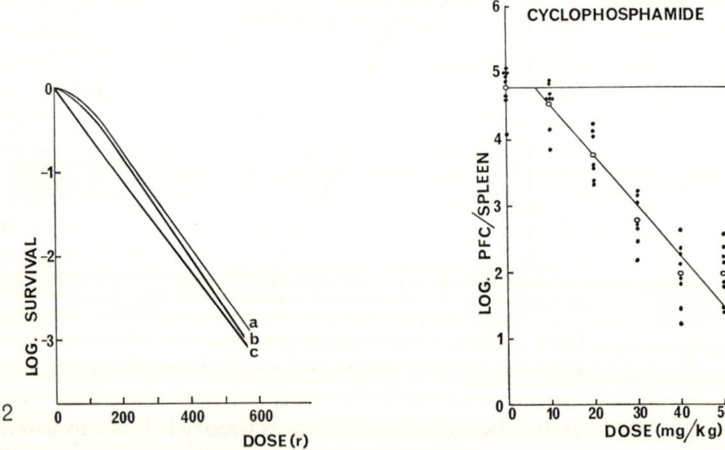

Fig. 2. Dose-response curves for effect of whole-body irradiation on immunologically competent cells. a – lymphocytes producing graft-versus-host reaction [SMITH and VOS, 1963]; b – haemagglutinin-forming cells [MAKINODAN *et al.*, 1962]; c – plaque-forming cells in mouse spleen [KENNEDY *et al.*, 1965].

Fig. 3. Dose-response curve for effect of cyclophosphamide on haemolysin-forming cells in mouse spleen. Animals given 0.2 ml 10 % formolised sheep red cells I.P. on day 0, and various doses of cyclophosphamide intraperitoneally on day 2. Numbers of plaque-forming cells per spleen counted on day 5. Individual counts ●, logarithmic means ○.

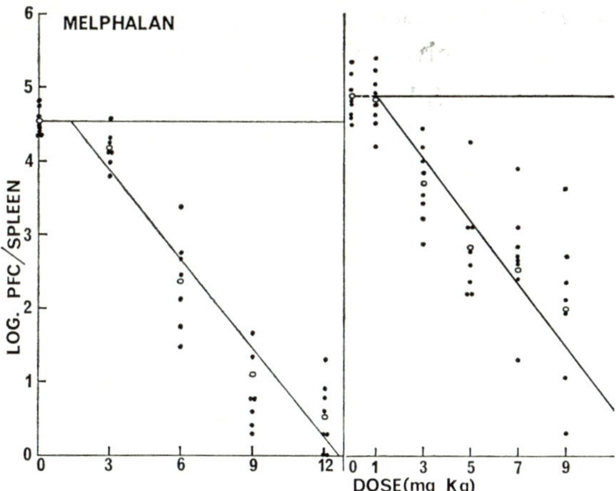

Fig. 4. Dose-response curve for effect of melphalan on haemolysin-forming cells in mouse spleen. Experimental details as in figure 2. Results of two experiments are shown.

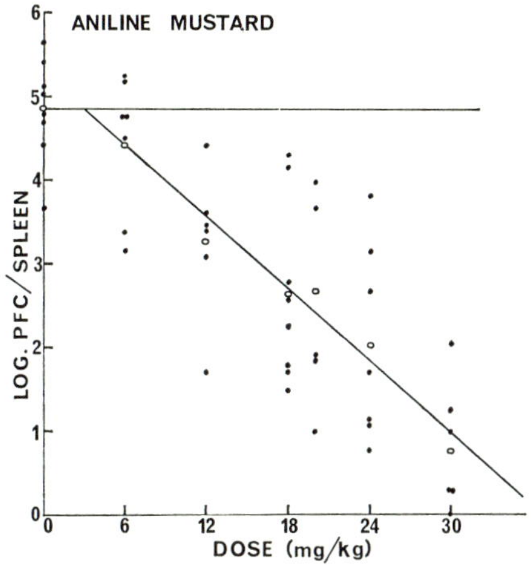

Fig. 5. Dose-response curve for effect of aniline mustard (C.B. 1074) on haemolysin-forming cells in mouse spleen. Experimental details as in figure 2.

It is not surprising, therefore, that data for survival of leukaemic cells in animals given commonly used antineoplastic drugs (alkylating agents and antimetabolites) have been treated as if they fitted exponential curves [SKIPPER *et al.*, 1964, 1965]. However, it has been shown that dose-response curves for antimetabolites are not exponential but hyperbolic [BERENBAUM, 1969a].

b) Hyperbolic dose-response curves. A hyperbolic dose-response curve, in its simplest form, is given when the product of the dose and the fraction of cells surviving is a constant, i.e.

$$SD = k$$
$$\therefore S = \frac{k}{D}$$

and

$$\log. S = \log. k - \log. D$$

If log. S is plotted against log. D, a straight line results, with an intercept log. k on the S = 1 axis and a slope of –1 (fig. 6, a). This intercept obviously represents the threshold dose, which we may term D_o, so that we may write

$$S = \frac{D_o}{D}$$

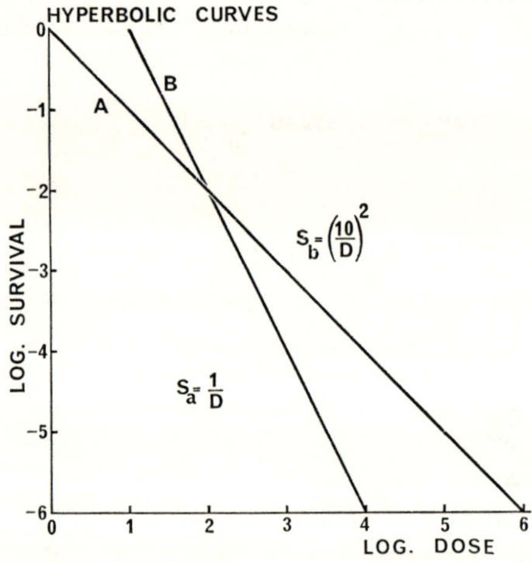

Fig. 6. Hyperbolic dose-response curves. For curve A, $D_o = 1$, $\gamma = 1$; for curve B, $D_o = 10$, $\gamma = 2$.

Some experimentally obtained hyperbolic dose-response curves have slopes steeper than –1, and the appropriate equation is

$$S = \left(\frac{D_o}{D}\right)^{\gamma} \tag{4}$$

where the slope is $-\gamma$ (fig. 6, b).

The biological explanation for hyperbolic dose-response curves is uncertain, but the following hypothesis may be put forward. Agents showing this type of curve act essentially by competition for sites on enzymes critical for cell reproduction. The not unreasonable assumption may be made that the reproductive integrity of a cell treated with an antimetabolite depends directly on the relative residual activity of the inhibited enzyme. This activity is indicated by the rate equation for competitive inhibition,

$$\frac{V_i}{V_m} = \frac{[M]}{[M] + \dfrac{K_m}{K_a} \cdot [A] + K_m}$$

where V_i is the rate of the inhibited reaction, V_m that of the un-inhibited reaction, [M] and [A] the concentrations of metabolite and antimetabolite respectively and K_m and K_a the dissociation constants for the enzyme-metabolite and enzyme-antimetabolite complexes. [M] can be regarded as reasonably constant for the purposes of this discussion. If [A] is high compared with [M], K_m and K_a, the equation approximates to

$$\frac{V_i}{V_m} \propto \frac{1}{[A]}$$

In other words, at high doses of antimetabolite, the proportion of enzyme molecules engaged in normal activity is approximately inversely proportional to the concentration, and therefore the dose, of antimetabolite.

If the above line of reasoning is correct, it follows that the ability of cells to reproduce will be inversely proportional to the dose of antimetabolite at high doses. At low doses, the relation between the proportion of unaffected enzyme molecules and dose is an asymptotic one. However, if it is assumed that a proportion of enzyme molecules are in excess of requirement for cell proliferation, doses of antimetabolite that block less than this amount will have no effect on cell reproductive integrity. In other words, the curve relating cell survival to dose will cut the $S = 1$ abscissa at a threshold dose and will closely resemble the curves shown in figure 6, a [for a fuller discussion see BERENBAUM, 1969a].

Some examples of hyperbolic dose-response curves given by immunosuppressive antimetabolites are shown in figures 7–9.

Therapeutic Implications of Dose-Response Curves

How can the information contained in the dose-response curve be used to design selective therapeutic regimens? We shall at present

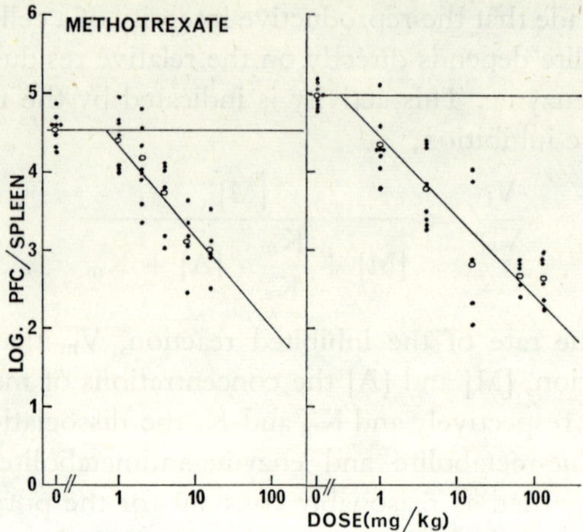

Fig. 7. Dose-response curves for effect of methotrexate on haemolysin-forming cells in mouse spleen. Experimental details as in figure 2. Results of two experiments are shown.

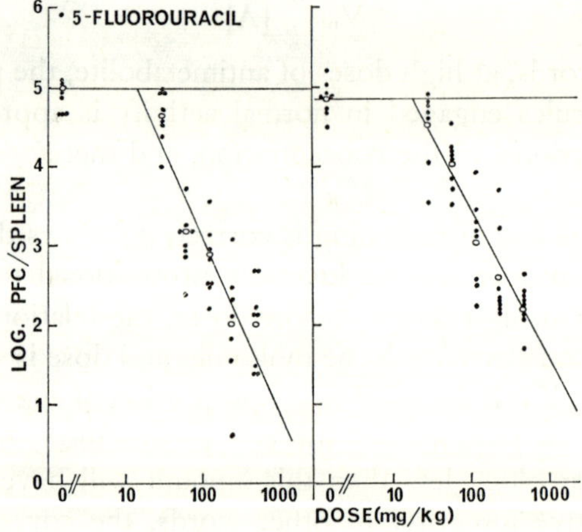

Fig. 8. Dose-response curves for effect of 5-fluorouracil on haemolysin-forming cells in mouse spleen. Experimental details as in figure 2. Results of two experiments are shown.

consider this problem only in an artificially simplified form, that is, in relation to homogeneous cell populations, multiplying asynchronously in the absence of homoeostatic mechanisms. Immunologically active cell populations are not homogeneous, their proliferation is partly synchronized, and they are strongly influenced by homoeostasis. Unfortunately, there is not enough quantitative information about any of these factors to allow us to take them into account with any

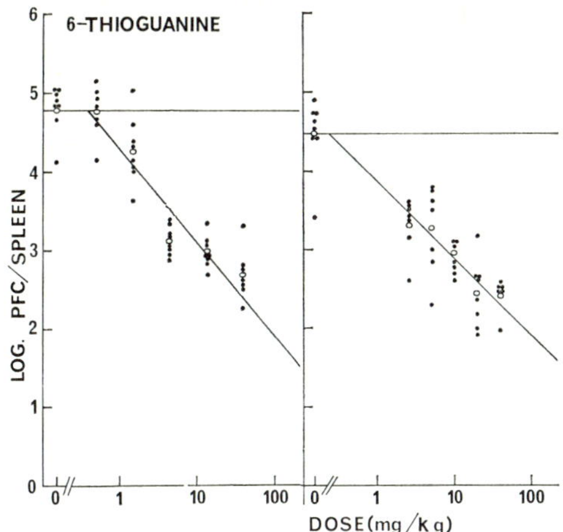

Fig. 9. Dose-response curves for effect of 6-thioguanine on haemolysin-forming cells in mouse spleen. Experimental details as in figure 2. Results of two experiments are shown.

confidence. However, what can be done mathematically with a simplified population has interesting clinical implications, and this may stimulate work aimed at providing a more complete quantitative account than has hitherto been available of the cellular kinetics of immune responses.

In our homogeneous population, multiplying asynchronously without homoeostasis, the increase in population with time is given by

$$N_t = N_o \cdot 2^{t/T_g}$$

where N_o and N_t are the numbers at time 0 and time t respectively and T_g is the cell doubling time. Suppose, now, that repeated doses of an immunosuppressive agent are given, the dose being D and the interval between doses t. If this dose reduces the size of the population to F (i.e. to a fraction less than one of the starting population) then the changes in size of the population with each dose are as shown in figure 10. The first dose reduces the population size to F. During the following interval t this grows to F. $2^{t/T_g}$. The second dose reduces this to F. F. $2^{t/T_g}$ and this grows during the next interval to F. F. $2^{t/T_g} \cdot 2^{t/T_g}$. Evidently, after n doses of size D at intervals of t, the population is

$$\left(F \cdot 2^{t/T_g}\right)^n \tag{5}$$

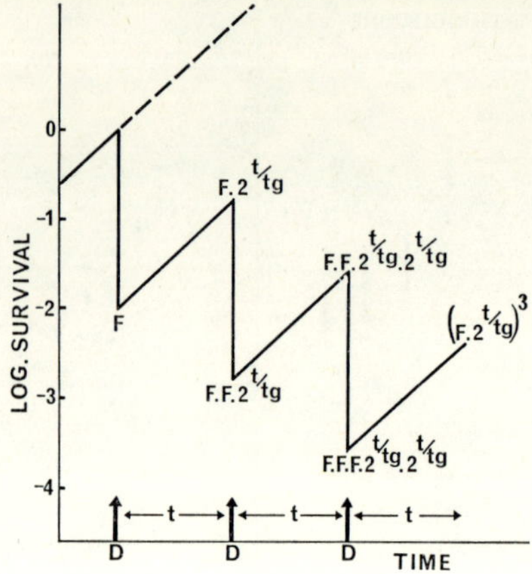

Fig. 10. Effect on a cell population multiplying with a doubling time T_g of repeated doses D at intervals t of an agent that impairs cell reproductive integrity. Each dose D reduces the reproductively competent population to a fraction F of its size before the dose is given (see text).

We can now substitute for F the expressions in equations (2), (3) and (4). For an agent giving a simple exponential dose-response curve, survival S after a regimen of n doses of D at intervals t is given by

$$S = \left[e^{-\alpha D} . 2^{t/T_g} \right]^n \tag{6}$$

For an agent giving an exponential dose-response curve with a shoulder it is

$$S = \left[1 - (1 - e^{-\alpha D})^{\beta} . 2^{t/T_g} \right]^n \tag{7}$$

For an agent with a hyperbolic dose-response it is

$$S = \left[\left(\frac{D_o}{D} \right)^{\gamma} . 2^{t/T_g} \right]^n \tag{8}$$

Although it is not directly relevant to the main theme, it is interesting to see that, when an agent shows a simple exponential curve, the outcome of treatment is independent of the regimen, provided the same total dose is given over the same total period. If, instead of giving n doses of D at intervals of t, we gave $\frac{n}{x}$ doses of Dx at intervals of tx, the final population would be given by

$$S = \left[e^{-\alpha Dx} . 2^{tx/T_g} \right]^{\frac{n}{x}}$$

$$= e^{-\alpha Dn} \cdot 2^{tn/T_g}$$

$$= e^{-\alpha \cdot \text{Total dose}} \cdot 2^{\left(\dfrac{\text{Total time}}{T_g}\right)}$$

This principle is illustrated in figure 11. In the case of an exponential curve with a shoulder, simple inspection of the curve shows that, if the total dose and time are fixed, the maximum effect is given by concentrating the total to be administered into a single dose, for this reduces to a minimum the loss of efficiency caused by the shoulder on the dose-response curve. The situation for agents giving hyperbolic dose-response curves is more complex. Obviously, doses below the threshold dose D_o are ineffective, and it can be shown that, if the total dosage and time are fixed, the most efficient regimen is one in which $D = e\,D_o$.

However, we are not concerned here with the most efficient way to design regimens with fixed overall dosage and time, but with the design of regimens of maximal selectivity of action. It will be noted that equations (6), (7) and (8) contain parameters of two sorts, viz., those that describe the cell population and its sensitivity to immunosuppressive agents (α, β, γ, D_o, T_g), and those that describe the

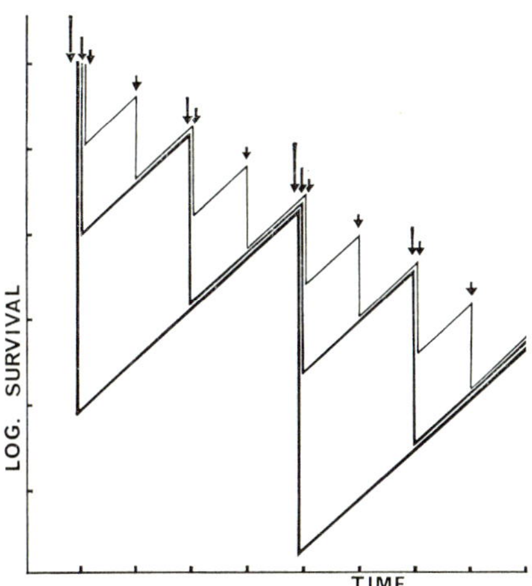

Fig. 11. Effect of different dose schedules on proliferating cell population with a simple exponential dose-response relation. The total dose administered over a given period is kept constant by maintaining a constant ratio between dose and the interval between doses. Note that, under these circumstances, the overall effect on the cell population is independent of manipulations in the dose schedule.

therapeutic regimens (D, t and n). In any therapeutic situation the first set of values is given, and the second can be varied at will. Equation (5) shows that the fate of a homogeneous, a synchronously multiplying population under a regimen of repeated doses of constant size and frequency is determined by the product of F and $2^{t/T_g}$. If this is less than 1, the population will progressively decrease in size under treatment; if it is greater than 1, it will grow in spite of treatment, although at a slower rate than normal. If, therefore, we have two cell populations A and B in the same individual, the differences between their drug-sensitivities and cell doubling times may allow us to design therapeutic regimens that will eliminate one population and allow the other to survive. If population A is to survive,

$$F_a \cdot 2^{t/T_{ga}} > 1 \tag{9}$$

and if population B is to be eliminated, then

$$1 > F_b \cdot 2^{t/T_{gb}} \tag{10}$$

Formulae (6), (7) and (8) can now be used to find the conditions for population A to survive and B to be eliminated with various types of dose-response curve. The most likely case is that in which both cell types show the same sort of dose-response curve to a given agent, the curves differing quantitatively but not qualitatively. There is, however, no difficulty in applying the method used below to cases, if any, where different cell populations give qualitatively different types of curve in response to the same agent.

    a) Simple exponential curve. For A to survive and B to die out, it is required, from equations (6), (9) and (10), that

$$e^{-\alpha_a D} \cdot 2^{t/T_{ga}} > 1 > e^{-\alpha_b D} \cdot 2^{t/T_{gb}}$$

and therefore that

$$\frac{t. \log_e 2}{T_{ga} \cdot \alpha_a} > D > \frac{t. \log_e 2}{T_{gb} \cdot \alpha_b} \tag{11}$$

It is clear that the outcome we wish can occur only if $T_{ga} \cdot \alpha_a > T_{gb} \cdot \alpha_b$, and that if this is so, A will survive to a greater extent than B under all regimens. In the converse circumstance, i.e. $T_{ga} \cdot \alpha_a < T_{gb} \cdot \alpha_b$, any regimen that eliminated B would eliminate A even more rapidly.

b) Exponential curve with shoulder. Here it is required that

$$\left[1-(1-e^{-a_aD})^{\beta_a}\right] \cdot 2^{t/T_{ga}} > 1 > \left[1-(1-e^{-a_bD})^{\beta_b}\right] \cdot 2^{t/T_{gb}}$$

for which it is necessary that

$$\frac{-\log_e\left[1-\left(1-2^{t/T_{ga}}\right)^{\frac{1}{\beta_a}}\right]}{a_a} > D > \frac{-\log_e\left[1-\left(1-2^{t/T_{gb}}\right)^{\frac{1}{\beta_b}}\right]}{a_b} \quad (12)$$

c) Hyperbolic curve. Here it is required that

$$\left(\frac{D_{oa}}{D}\right)^{\gamma_a} \cdot 2^{t/T_{ga}} > 1 > \left(\frac{D_{ob}}{D}\right)^{\gamma_b} \cdot 2^{t/T_{gb}}$$

for which it is necessary that

$$D_{oa} \cdot 2^{t/T_{ga}\gamma_a} > D > D_{ob} \cdot 2^{t/T_{gb}\gamma_b} \quad (13)$$

Let us consider a concrete example. Suppose, for a particular agent giving hyperbolic dose-response curves, the threshold dose D_{oa} for population A is 1 mg/kg and the slope of its dose-response curve is –1 (i.e. $\gamma_a = 1$). For population B in the same individual, let the threshold dose D_{ob} be 3 mg/kg and the slope of the curve –2 (i.e. $\gamma_b = 2$). Let us also suppose that the doubling time T_{ga} of population A is one day and that of population B, T_{gb}, two days.

To destroy population A without at the same time destroying population B, we require, from equation (13), that

$$3 \times 2^{t/4} > D > 2^{t}$$

For D to have a positive value here, t <2.113 days. If t is set at, say, 1.5 days, then

$$4.9 \text{ mg/kg} > D > 2.83 \text{ mg/kg}$$

In figure 12 (1), it can be seen that a regimen of this agent at a dosage of 3.3 mg/kg given every 1.5 days progressively reduces population A while population B continues to increase in numbers. In other words, the regimen has the desired selectivity.

Suppose the requirement that t <2.113 days is ignored and the therapeutic regimen altered so as to double the dose and the interval between doses. The total dosage given over the same period is, of course, unaffected by this alteration. Fix 12 (2) shows that this apparently trivial change in regimen completely reverses the effects on the

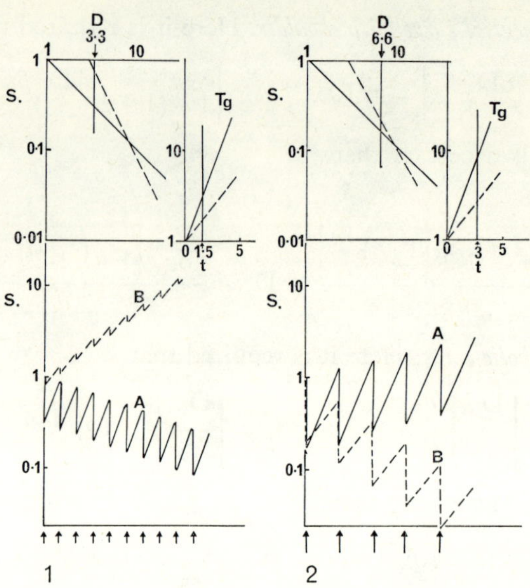

Fig. 12. Effect of two dose schedules on two proliferating cell populations with hyperbolic dose-response relations. For population A, $D_0 = 1$, $\gamma = 1$, $T_g = 1$; for population B, $D_0 = 3$, $\gamma = 2$, $T_g = 2$. – The top portion of the figure shows the dose-response curves and proliferative rates for these two populations and indicates the doses and intervals between doses selected for the two schedules. – Schedule 1 consists of doses of 3.3 mg/kg given every 1.5 days; schedule 2 consists of doses of 6.6 mg/kg every three days. The amount of drug administered over a given period is the same under both schedules, but, under schedule 1, population A decreases and population B increases whereas under schedule 2 the reverse is true.

Population A ——————, Population B ————————.

two cell populations—now population B is destroyed and population A continues to grow in spite of treatment. Such a reversal of effect can, of course, happen only in particular sets of circumstances. It underlines, however, the point of this discussion, for we have here an example of how the tissue specificity of an agent may be manipulated at will simply by adjusting the dose regimen.

The important reservations laid down at the outset, namely, that real cell populations are to varying extents inhomogeneous, may be partly synchronized and are subject to homoeostasis, inevitably complicate and blur the situation (the design of selective regimens when cell populations are homoeostatically regulated is discussed elsewhere) [Berenbaum, 1969b]. Nevertheless, as different cell types undoubtedly vary in their sensitivity to immunosuppressive agents (figs. 13, 14) and in their doubling times, it is apparent that the specificity of drug action may be greatly affected by the design of the therapeutic schedule.

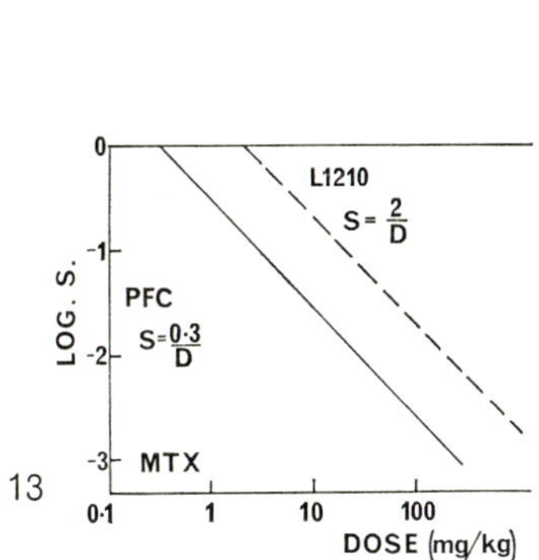

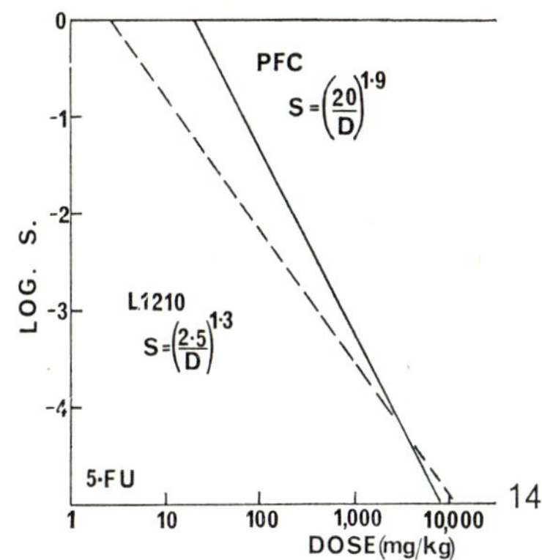

Fig. 13. Dose-response curves for haemolytic plaque-forming cells (PFC) and L 1210 leukaemia cells in mice treated with single doses of methotrexate. Data for PFC taken from figure 6; data for L 1210 cells from SKIPPER *et al.* [1965].

Fig. 14. Dose-response curves for haemolytic plaque-forming cells (PFC) and L 1210 leukaemia cells in mice treated with single doses of 5-fluorouracil. Data for PFC taken from figure 7; data for L 1210 cells from SKIPPER *et al.* [1965].

We hardly know enough yet to be able to use this approach clinically, although we do know that the design of the dose regimen may considerably affect therapeutic efficiency in the treatment of leukaemia [FREIREICH and FREI, 1964; SELAWRY and FREI, 1964; PIERCE *et al.*, 1966]. A great deal has yet to be learned about the characteristics of various cell types, including their generation rates and quantitative responses to immunosuppressive agents. With this knowledge it should be possible to make considerable advances in immunosuppressive therapy.

Acknowledgement

I am indebted for support to the Medical Research Council, the British Empire Cancer Campaign for Research and the Leukaemia Research Fund.

References

1. ALBERT, M.D.: X-irradiation induced mitotic abnormalities in mouse liver regenerating after carbon tetrachloride injury. I. Total-body irradiation. J. nat. Cancer Inst. *20:* 309–319 (1960).
2. BERENBAUM, M.C.: The action of antimitotic substances on the immune response. Proc. 10th Int. Congr. Cell. Biol.; Path. Biol. *9:* 963–966 (1961).

3. BERENBAUM, M.C.: The effect of cytotoxic agents on the production of antibody to T.A.B. vaccine in the mouse. Biochem. Pharmacol. *11:* 29–44 (1962).

4. BERENBAUM, M.C.: Radiosensitivity of immunologically activated cells. Nature (Lond.) *209:* 1313–1315 (1966a).

5. BERENBAUM, M.C.: Role of mitosis and mitotic inhibition in the immunosuppressive action of thioguanine. Nature (Lond.) *210:* 41–43 (1966b).

6. BERENBAUM, M.C.: Differential protection in the use of immunosuppressive agents. In: Int. Symp. Transplant. Tissues and Organs, Frankfurt, pp. 81–89 (Eds.) K.E. SEIFFERT and R. GEISSENDÖRFER (Georg Thieme, Stuttgart 1967a).

7. BERENBAUM, M.C.: Immunosuppressive agents and the cellular kinetics of the immune response. pp. 217–237. In: Immunity, Cancer and Chemotherapy (Ed.) E. MIHICH (Academic Press, New York 1967b).

8. BERENBAUM, M.C.: Time-dependent immunosuppressive effects of anti-thymocyte serum. Nature (Lond.) *215:* 1481–1482 (1967c).

9. BERENBAUM, M.C.: Dose-response curves for agents that impair cell reproductive integrity. I. A fundamental difference between dose-response curves for antimetabolites and those for radiation and alkylating agents (Brit. J.Cancer, in the press, 1969a).

10. BERENBAUM, M.C.: Dose response curves for agents that impair cell reproductive integrity. II. The relation between dose response curves and the design of selective therapeutic regimes in cancer chemotherapy (Brit. J. Cancer, in the press, 1969b).

11. BROWN, I.N.: Effect of actinomycin C on immune response *in vivo*. Nature (Lond.) *204:* 487–488 (1964).

12. ELION, G.B.; CALLAHAN, S.; NATHAN, H.; BIEBER, S.; RUNDLES, R.W. and HITCHINGS, G.W.: Potentiation and inhibition of drug degradation: 6-substituted purines and xanthine oxidase. Biochem. Pharmacol. *12:* 85–93 (1963a).

13. ELION, G.B.; CALLAHAN, S.; RUNDLES, R.W. and HITCHINGS, G.W.: Relation between metabolic fates and antitumor activities of thiopurines. Cancer Res. *23:* 1207–1217 (1963b).

14. FREIREICH, E.J. and FREI, E.: Recent advances in acute leukaemia. (Eds.) MOORE, C. and BROWN, E. Progr. Haemat. *4:* 187 (1964). (Grune & Stratton).

15. FRISCH, A.W. and DAVIES, G.H.: Inhibition of hemagglutinin formation by thioguanine: dose-time relationships. Proc. Soc. exp. Biol. Med. (N.Y.) *110:* 444–447 (1962).

16. FRISCH, A.W. and DAVIES, G.H.: Inhibition of hemagglutinin synthesis by Cytoxan: Specificity and drug-induced 'tolerance'. J. Lab. clin. Med. *68:* 103–112 (1966).

17. FRISCH, A.W.; DAVIES, G.H. and MILSTEIN, V.: The inhibition of hemagglutinin formation in mice by thioguanine. J. Immunol. *89:* 300–305 (1962).

18. GENGOZIAN, N. and MAKINODAN, T.: Relation of primary antigen injection to time of irradiation on antibody production in mice. J. Immunol. *80:* 189–197 (1958).

19. GLINOS, A.D. and NORTH, H.H.: Cellular growth and tissue radiosensitivity: Cell studies *in vitro* and general concepts. Trans. N.Y. Acad. Sci. *26:* 145–158 (1963).

20. HERSH, E.M.; CARBONE, P.P. and FREIREICH, E.J.: Recovery of immune responsiveness after drug suppression in man. J. Lab. clin. Med. *67:* 566–572 (1966).

21. KENNEDY, J.C.; TILL, J.E.; SIMINOVITCH, L. and McCULLOCH, E.A.: Radiosensitivity of the immune response to sheep red cells in the mouse, as measured by the hemolytic plaque method. J. Immunol. *94:* 715–722 (1965).

22. LEONG, G.F.; PESSOTTI, R.L. and KREBS, J.S.: Liver cell proliferation in X-irradiated rats after single and repetitive partial hepatectomy. J. nat. Cancer Inst. *27:* 131–143 (1961).

23. McCONNELL, D.V. and ZUKOSKI, C.F.: Effect of 6-MP and BW 56–158 on canine renal homografts. Fed. Proc. *22:* 501 (1963).

24. MADOC-JONES, H. and BRUCE, W.R.: Sensitivity of L cells in exponential and stationary phases to 5-fluorouracil. Nature (Lond.) *215:* 302–303 (1967).

25. Madoc-Jones, H.; Bruce, W.R.; Meeker, B.E. and Valeriote, F.A.: The sensitivity of proliferating and non-proliferating cells to 5-fluorouracil. Proc. Amer. Ass. Cancer Res. *7:* 46 (1966).

26. Makinodan, T.; Kastenbaum, M.A. and Peterson, W.J.: Radiosensitivity of spleen cells from normal and pre-immunized mice and its significance to intact animals. J. Immunol. *88:* 31–37 (1962).

27. Merritt, K. and Johnson, A.G.: Studies on the adjuvant action of bacterial endotoxins on antibody formation. V. The influence of endotoxin and 5-fluoro-2-deoxyuridine on the primary antibody response of the Balb mouse to a purified protein antigen. J. Immunol. *91:* 266–272 (1963).

28. Nettesheim, P.; Makinodan, T. and Williams, M.L.: Regenerative potential of immunocompetent cells. 1. Lack of recovery of secondary antibody-forming potential after X-radiation. J. Immunol. *99:* 150–157 (1967).

29. Nowell, P.C.: Unstable chromosome changes in tuberculin-stimulated leukocyte cultures from irradiated patients. Evidence for immunologically committed, long-lived lymphocytes in human blood. Blood *26:* 798–804 (1965).

30. Pierce, M.; Shore, N.; Sitarz, A.; Murphy, M.L.; Louis, J. and Severo, N.: Cyclophosphamide therapy in acute leukemia of childhood: Co-operative study conducted by members of Children's Cancer Cooperative Group A. Cancer, Philad. *19:* 1551–1560 (1966).

31. Pittillo, R.F.; Schabel, F.M. Jr.; Wilcox, W.S. and Skipper, H.E.: Experimental evaluation of potential anticancer agents. XVI. Basic study of effects of certain anticancer agents on kinetic behavior of model bacterial cell populations. Cancer Chemother. Reps. *47:* 1–26 (1965).

32. Riethmüller, G.; Rieber, P. and Riethmüller, D.: Effect of intact and of pepsin-digested anti-mouse-thymus-γG on antibody forming spleen cells and on the homograft reaction. Proc. 1st. Int. Congr. Transplant. Soc., Paris, p. 155 (1967).

33. Santos, G.W. and Owens, A.H. Jr.: Specific suppression of agglutinin response by methotrexate. Pharmacologist *5:* 272 (1963).

34. Santos, G.W. and Owens, A.H. Jr.: A comparison of the effects of selected cytotoxic agents on the primary agglutinin response in rats injected with sheep erythrocytes. Bull. Johns Hopk. Hosp. *114:* 384–401 (1964).

35. Schabel, F.M. Jr.; Skipper, H.E.; Trader, M.W. and Wilcox, W.S.: Experimental evaluation of potential anticancer agents. XIX. Sensitivity of nondividing leukemic cell populations to certain classes of drugs *in vivo*. Cancer Chemother. Reps. *48:* 17–30 (1965).

36. Selawry, O.S. and Frei, E.: Prolongation of remission in acute lymphocytic leukemia by alteration in dose schedule and route of administration of methotrexate. Clin. Res. *12:* 231 (1964).

37. Skipper, H.E.; Schabel, F.M. Jr. and Wilcox, W.S.: Experimental evaluation of potential anticancer agents. XIII. On the criteria and kinetics associated with 'curability' of experimental leukemia. Cancer Chemother. Reps. *35:* 1–111 (1964).

38. Skipper, H.E.; Schabel, F.M. Jr. and Wilcox, W.S.: Experimental evaluation of potential anticancer agents. XIV. Further study of certain basic concepts underlying chemotherapy of leukemia. Cancer Chemother. Reps. *45:* 5–28 (1965).

39. Smith, L.H. and Vos, O.: Radiation sensitivity of mouse lymph node cells relative to their proliferative capacity *in vivo*. Radiat. Res. *19:* 485–491 (1963).

40. Taliaferro, W.H. and Taliaferro, L.G.: Further studies on the radiosensitive stages in hemolysin formation. J. infect. Dis. *95:* 134–141 (1954).

41. Taliaferro, W.H. and Taliaferro, L.G.: The relation of radiation dosage to enhancement, depression, and recovery of the initial Forssman hemolysin response in rabbits. J. infect. Dis. *114:* 285–303 (1964).

42. TALIAFERRO, W.H.; TALIAFERRO, L.G. and JANSSEN, E.F.: The localization of X-ray injury to the initial phases of antibody response. J. infect. Dis. *91:* 105–124 (1952).
43. VALERIOTE, F.A.; BRUCE, W.R. and MEEKER, B.E.: A model for the action of vinblastine *in vivo*. Biophys. J. *6:* 145–152 (1966).
44. WEINBREN, K.; FITSCHEN, W. and COHEN, M.: The unmasking by regeneration of latent irradiation effects in the rat liver. Brit. J. Radiol. *33:* 419–425 (1960).
45. WILCOX, W.S.: The last surviving cancer cell: The chances of killing it. Cancer Chemother. Reps. *50:* 541–542 (1966).
46. WILCOX, W.S.; GRISWOLD, D.P. and LASTER, W.R. Jr.: Experimental evaluation of potential anticancer agents. XVII. Kinetics of growth and regression after treatment of certain solid tumors. Cancer Chemother. Reps. *47:* 27–39 (1965).

Author's address: Dr. M.C. BERENBAUM, Department of Experimental Pathology,
St. Mary's Hospital Medical School, *London, W. 2.* (England).

Antibiotica et Chemotherapia, vol. 15, pp. 177–181 (Karger, Basel/New York 1969)

Immunosuppressive Effect of a New Antibiotic: Ovalicin

S. Lazary and H. Stähelin

Biological and Medical Research Division, Sandoz Ltd., Basle

Ovalicin was isolated in our chemical laboratories from culture filtrates of *Pseudeurotium ovalis*. During investigations of the biological properties of ovalicin we found this substance to be able to inhibit several immunological reactions in laboratory animals. In the following we will describe the effect of ovalicin on the immune response to sheep red cells in mice, studied by measurement of hemagglutinin titres [Nathan *et al.*, 1961], and at the cellular level by determination of the number of primary hemolysin forming spleen cells with Jerne's method [Jerne and Nordin, 1963]. Further, we investigated the effect of the drug on the symptoms of experimental allergic encephalomyelitis (EAE) in rats.

Materials and Methods

Animals. Mice: Albino and (albino $\times$ DBA/2) F_1 mice, two to three months of age of both sexes. Rats: two months old male Wistar rats.

Antigens, immunisation. 0.5 ml of a 10% suspension of washed sheep red blood cells in saline was administered intravenously to each mouse.

For EAE, the antigen was whole rat spinal cord, emulsified in a modified Freund's adjuvant: 2.5 g spinal cord, 2.2 ml saline, 0.9 ml Arlacel A, 5.4 ml Nujol and 55 mg killed, dried Mycobacterium phlei. Rats received 0.1 ml of this emulsion intradermally in each hind footpad.

Drug administration. Ovalicin was dissolved in ethanol (100 mg/ml), this solution was mixed with an equal volume of Tween 80 and diluted to use with 0.85% NaCl. In several experiments the drug was administered as a suspension in 0.5% carboxymethyl-cellulose in saline. Ovalicin was given intraperitoneally or orally. The treatment schedules for each experiment are given with the results.

Hemagglutination. Hemagglutinin titres in sera were determined for each individual animal by serial 2-fold dilutions with Takatsy's micro-technic.

Jerne's plaque technic. The analysis of the number of anti-sheep red cell antibody-producing cells in mouse spleen was carried out using the original technic of Jerne [JERNE and NORDIN, 1963].

Observation of symptoms of EAE. Signs of EAE appear in control rats 9–15 days after the injection of the encephalitogenic agent; the symptoms are: weakness, paralysis, loss of sphincter control. The animals were inspected twice daily and were considered to have EAE if signs of paralysis were observed in the front or/and hind legs.

Results

Daily ovalicin treatment for five days, starting on the day of immunisation, inhibited hemagglutinin production in mice, measured on day 9 after immunisation. As shown in figure 1, at the lowest dose-level, 30 mg/kg/day, the animals showed an average inhibition of hemagglutinin titer of more than two dilution steps. The inhibition of hemagglutinin production was dose dependent, and oral drug administration had the same effect as intraperitoneal injection. At a dose of 120 mg/kg/day, drug toxicity was minimal with no deaths and

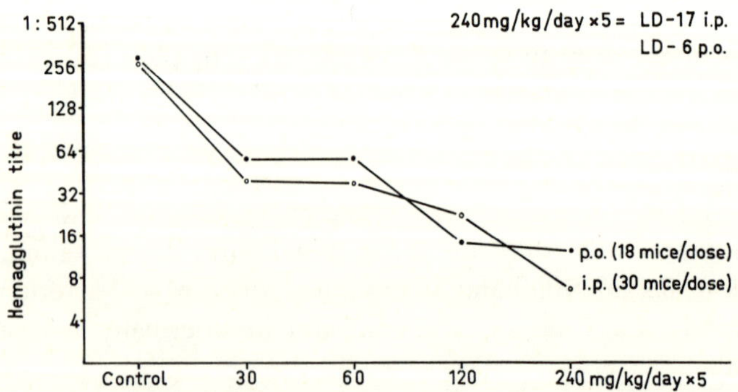

Fig. 1. Effect of ovalicin on hemagglutinin titer in albino mice nine days after i.v. administration of 0.5 ml 10% sheep red cell suspension. Treatment with ovalicin daily for five days, starting on the day of immunisation.

only temporary inhibition of weight gain. At a dose of 240 mg/kg/day
×5 the mortality was 6/30 on intraperitoneal and 1/18 on oral administration. Similar immunosuppressive results were obtained in
analogous experiments with rats.

By using the plaque method of Jerne we determined the optimal
time for injection of a single dose of ovalicin (600 mg/kg), varying
the day of drug treatment in relation to the sheep red cell administration. The number of primary hemolysin forming spleen cells was
determined on day four after immunisation (fig. 2). Ovalicin was
found to be most effective, as manifested by the number of plaque
forming cells, when the drug administration was carried out on the
day of immunisation or one day after it. After drug administration
on the day of immunisation the treated animals had about 98.4 % less
plaque forming cells than controls. After treatment one day after
immunisation the number of hemolysin forming cells in spleen was
lower by 99.7 % than those of the controls. Drug administration one
day before immunisation had only a slight and three day after it no
effect on the number of plaque forming spleen cells as determined on
day four.

In a further experiment we determined the number of primary
hemolysin forming cells at various times after immunisation. The
single drug administration was carried out at two dosage levels one
day after immunisation. In preliminary experiments it had been found

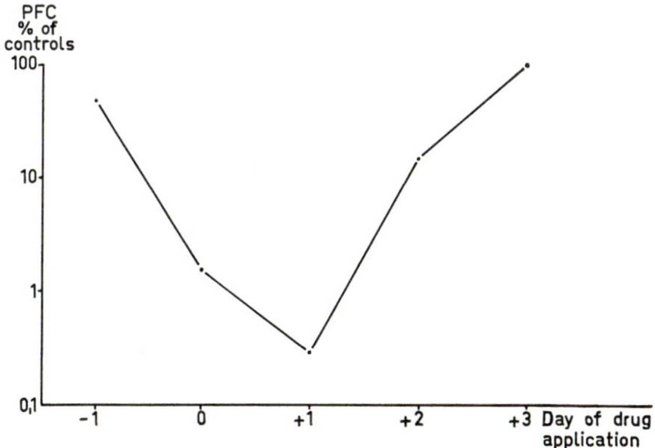

Fig. 2. The effect of ovalicin on the number of plaque forming cells (PFC) on day four
after immunisation. The single drug-treatment, 600 mg/kg i.p., was carried out on
different days in comparison with the sheep red cell administration (day 0). The numbers
of PFC of treated animals are expressed as percentages of the number obtained in the
control animals tested at the same time. The mean values were obtained from 4–20 animals.

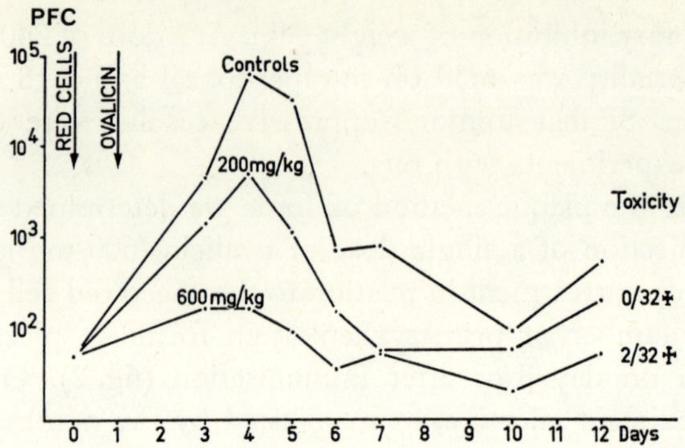

Fig. 3. The effect of ovalicin on the plaque forming cell (PFC) response to sheep red cell immunisation. The single treatment was carried out at two dosage levels one day after the immunisation. The mean values were obtained from four animals in each group.

that non-immunised mice have about 60–80 plaque forming cells producing sheep red cell hemolysin per spleen. As shown in figure 3 the increase of primary hemolysin forming spleen cells after immunisation was very strongly inhibited by the single intraperitoneal treatment of 600 mg/kg ovalicin. We found, on day three and four, 171 and 172 resp. plaque forming cells, in contrast to the controls which had 4420 and 62508 resp.

Relative spleen weight changes after immunisation are influenced by ovalicin treatment in a similar way as the number of plaque forming cells (fig. 4).

In rats, ovalicin reduces considerably the symptoms of EAE. As shown in fig. 5, treatment with 60 mg/kg/day, started on the day of injection of spinal cord-adjuvant emulsion and continued in the manner show in fig. 5, completely inhibited the symptoms of EAE

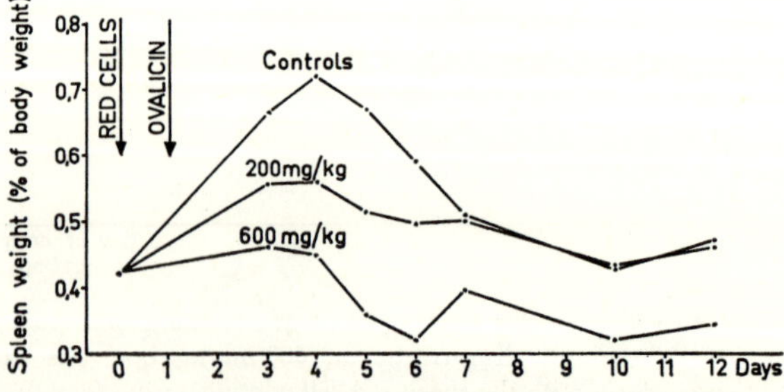

Fig. 4. Effect of ovalicin on the relative spleen weight (average of four mice) after immunisation with sheep red cells (same animals as in fig. 3).

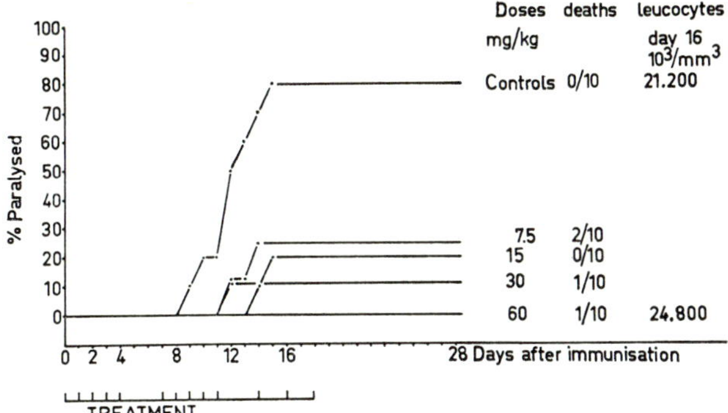

Fig. 5. The effect of ovalicin on the experimental allergic encephalomyelitis in Wistar rats. Treatment started on the day of injection of the spinal cord-adjuvant emulsion.

in all rats. Treatment at lower dosage levels caused a strong diminution of the number of animals with manifestations of EAE.

The absence of any symptoms of EAE combined with the healthy appearance of the animals treated with 60 mg/kg/day of ovalicin in connection with the lack of leucopenia in these and other animals treated with that substance is especially noteworthy.

Summary

Ovalicin was isolated in our chemical laboratories from culture filtrates of *Pseudeurotium ovalis*. This substance was found to inhibit several immunological reactions in animals. A daily dose of 30 mg/kg reduces the hemagglutinin tier of mice immunised with sheep erythrocytes by two to three 2-fold dilution steps, while 120 mg/kg is still completely nontoxic. Similar results were obtained in rats. The influence of ovalicin on antibody production was also investigated with the plaque method of Jerne, using different treatment schedules. Reduction of the number of plaque forming cells with one dose of ovalicin was more than 99% under appropiate conditions. 60 mg/kg/day of ovalicin completely prevents the symptoms of experimental allergic encephalomyelitis in rats; the highest tested doses of ovalicin (120 mg/kg/day) did not produce leucopenia in rats.

References

JERNE, N.K. and NORDIN, A.A.: Plaque formation in agar by single antibody-producing cells. Science *140:* 405 (1963).

NATHAN, H.C.; BIEBER, S.; ELION, G.B. and HITCHINGS, G.H.: Detection of agents which interfere with the immune response. Proc. Soc. exp. Biol., N.Y. *107:* 796–799 (1961).

Authors' address: Dr. S. LAZARY and Dr. H. STÄHELIN, Biological and Medical Research Division, Sandoz Ltd., *4000 Basel* (Switzerland).

Antibiotica et Chemotherapia, vol. 15, pp. 182–198 (Karger, Basel/New York 1969)

Reduction of Immune Responses in Radiation Chimeras
Attempts on Their Restoration[1]

G. Mathé[2], K. Nouza[3], I. Hrsak[4] and V. Kolar[5]

[2] Institut de Cancérologie et d'Immunogénétique, Hôpital Paul-Brousse, 94 Villejuif
[3] Institute of Exp. Biology and Genetics, Czechoslovak Academy of Sciences, Prague
[4] Institute R. Boskovic, Zagreb   [5] Oncological Institute, Brno

Introduction

During attempts to employ allogeneic bone marrow transplantation therapeutically, a serious stumbling block, the secondary syndrome, was encountered [Mathé, 1964; Mathé, Schwarzenberg *et al.*, 1965]. Although its course was variable, the syndrome proved to be fatal in the majority of the patients. The main pathological changes occurring in the syndrome are composed of two main components: (1) infiltration of recipient tissues and organs by the grafted lymphoid cells, which have a direct harmful effect on the host's tissues; (2) atrophy of lymphoid tissues with subsequent immunological insufficiency.

This paper is divided into two parts: firstly a summary of a clinical experience of transplantation of allogeneic bone marrow cells, the analysis of incidence and character of various forms of secondary syndrome, as well as attempts to control this syndrome; secondly report of experimental studies on murine radiation chimeras used as a model system to investigate the immunological deficiencies and methods of treating this condition.

The Clinical Experience

Since 1956, allogeneic bone marrow transplantations have been attempted 24 times in man, mostly in patients suffering from acute

---

[1] Supported by a grant from "E.O.A.R.", contract n° AF. 61 (052) 816.

This work reported in this paper was undertaken during the tenure of a travel fellowship awarded by the international agency for research on cancer.

lymphoblastic leukaemia. Some of these cases were in remission, others in a visible phase of disease.

The patients were given total body irradiation, using a ^{60}Co source. The dose was divided in two sessions separated by 24 h. The total dose varied between 800 and 950 rads. Each patient was given several bone marrow transfusions, from one or several donors.

Immediately after irradiation, the patients were nursed in special pathogen-free wards; the only prophylactic treatment comprised injections of gammaglobulins [Schwarzenberg et al., 1966]. Antibiotics were only used when infectious complications were detected.

In seven cases, the graft failed and six of the patients died; one escaped from aplasia owing to subsequent marrow graft from monozygotic twin.

In 17 cases, the graft took and this was proved by: typing of erythrocytic antigens [Mathé, Jammet et al., 1959], sex-linked granulocyte appendices [Mathé, Bernard, de Vries et al., 1960], sex chromatin of mononuclears [Seman, 1961], sex chromosomes, groups of immunoglobulins, and specificity of immune tolerance [Mathé, Amiel, Schwarzenberg et al., 1963].

In our series, 13 patients died though they had been intensively treated for the secondary syndrome. This syndrome presented itself in various forms, acute, subacute or chronic, the manifestations of which are given in table I.

It is now generally believed, that features of secondary syndrome in man are attributable to the g-v-h reaction, because there exist many

Table I. The various aspects of the secondary syndrome

Acute Syndrome	Subacute Syndrome	Chronic syndrome
Diarrhoea		
Moist oedematous macrodesquamative erythrodermia	Dry microdesquamative erythrodermia	
Hepatic necrosis	Hepatitis	Hepatitis
Bacterial and viral infection	Bacterial and viral infection	Viral infection
30 d	60 d	

analogies with the secondary syndrome occurring in animal radiation chimeras [van Bekkum *et al.*, 1959].

During the first phase of the secondary syndrome, the grafted lymphoid cells react directly against the tissues and organs of the host, giving rise to lymphoid hyperplasia, involvement of liver ("hepatitis"), skin (erythrodermia), intestinal system [Mathé *et al.*, 1965; van Bekkum and de Vries, 1967].

Sometimes, even at this early stage, immunological insufficiency may be demonstrated, attributable to the destruction of host lymphoid cells and "occupation" of grafted cells in the anti-host reaction [Howard and Woodruff, 1961; Blaese *et al.*, 1964; Lawrence and Simonsen, 1967].

In the second phase, lymphoid atrophy with severe immuno-logical insufficiency develops as a result of a mutual lethal hyper-sensitive reaction between donor and recipient lymphoid cells. This insufficiency, which exists even when the lymphoid system appears quantitatively normal, is very dangerous, because it leads probably also in man, to the loss of immunological memory, such as has been demonstrated in mice [Mathé *et al.*, 1961].

Several treatments of the secondary syndrome have been proposed in animals: preventive, such as the pre-incubation of the bone marrow cells for 2 h at 37°C [Mathé, Amiel, Schwarzenberg *et al.*, 1964], or curative, such as the use of immuno-suppressive drugs [Uphoff, 1958; Mathé *et al.*, 1962; Müller-Bérat *et al.*, 1966; Balner *et al.*, 1968], and/or antilymphocyte serum [Ledney and van Bekkum, 1968].

The treatment of the syndrome in man has given disappointing results (table II). This can be seen if a comparison is made of the

Table II. Attempts to control secondary syndrome after bone marrow graft

	Acute secondary syndrome	Subacute secondary syndrome	Absence
I. Treated patients			
Amethopterine	2	3	2
Cyclophosphamide	1	0	0
Amethopterine + Cyclophosphamide	1	1	0
Antilymphocyte serum	1	0	0
Total	5	4	2
II. Non-treated patients	5	3	5

results obtained when such therapy was used and those of earlier grafts before this approach had been tried.

And if one analyses the cause of death, it can be related in all patients to infection (as seen in table III) which suggests that immunological insufficiency is the most important stumbling block to the control of the secondary syndrome.

For this reason, we have started a series of experiments to study the mechanism of a immunological deficiency and to examine the possibility of immunological restoration.

Table III. Infections observed during the secondary syndrome in man

Infections	1	2	3	4	5	6	7	8	9	10	11	12	13	14	15	16	17
Fever	+	+	+	+	+	+	+	+	+	+	+	+	+	+	+	+	+
Staphylococcal	+															+	
Streptococcal		+															
Tuberculosis							+										
Candida albicans			+	+			+								+		
Cytomegalic inclusion disease			+														
Herpes zoster							+										
Virus hepatitis				+													
Chicken pox									+								
Klebsiella										+							
Pseudomonas aeruginosa											+						
B. Coli												+					
Enterococcus													+				

Material and Methods

1. Experimental Animals

Allogeneic radiation chimeras were produced by lethal irradiation (950 rads), of young adult (CBA × C57Br) F1 mice (H-2^k × H-2^k), followed four hours later by the injection of 20 × 10^6 nucleated bone marrow cells from (DBA/2 × C57B/6) F1 donors (H-2^d × H-2^b).

Fifteen to twenty days after irradiation, some chimeras chosen at random received a second injection of 30 × 10^6 living nucleated donor bone marrow cells; other mice received thymic grafts of donor origin, and the others thymic grafts from mice genetically dissimilar to the recipient as well as the donor (Ba*l*b/c) (H-2^d). Thymus donors were 4 to 10 days old and each recipient received i.p. 4–5 thymuses, cut into three to four pieces.

The control group was represented by untreated radiation chimeras.

2. Immunological Tests

The immunological reactivity of untreated and treated chimeras was tested on the 35th day after irradiation (at this time the peak of mortality was observed) and on the 60th day (when the state of chimeras seemed to be stable).

a) Humoral antibody production. The mice tested received i.p. 0.5 ml of 20% suspension of sheep erythrocytes. Four days later they were killed and the blood and spleens harvested. The serum titre of haemagglutinins was determined. In the spleens of animals the number of antibody producing cells (PFC) was determined by the use of Jerne's method.

b) Skin graft survival. Each recipient tested received two tail skin grafts [Bailey and Usama, 1960]. One graft was of bone marrow donor genotype, the other from Balb/c strain mouse. The skin grafts were examined daily; grafts surviving more than 50 days were considered to be tolerated.

c) Foot pad tests. The reactivity to mycobacterium TBC vaccine and fungal antigen was tested. Animals received 7.5 mg of Mycobacterium TBC[1] or 0.1 ml of 1:100 dilution of Candidin+ homogenized with 0.1 ml of complete Freund's adjuvant in one foot pad, and two weeks thereafter, they were reinjected in the other foot pad with the same quantity of antigen without adjuvant. The reactions were examined after 48 h by measuring two diameters, circumference and volume of injected and of control feet. Later because of the great variability of numerical values, the intensity of reaction was expressed by one to four pluses.

d) Graft-versus-host essay. This test was performed in C3H × Balb/c radiation chimeras to ascertain the part of host and donor reactivity. The chimeric and normal (host or donor) spleen cells were injected i.p. into 3-day-old recipients of suitable genetic constitution. After 10 days, Simonsen's assay was used and spleen, liver and thymus indices calculated.

----

[1] Institut Pasteur, Paris.

The groups of untreated and treated chimeras were examined clinically during the 60 days' observation period and the mortality recorded. All dead and killed animals were autopsied and the presence or absence of thymic grafts in the peritoneal cavity noted.

Results

The 60-day survival of animals, treated with the second transplantation of bone marrow cells, and donor as well as "third party" thymus grafts was superior to the survival of untreated chimeras (fig. 1). The difference observed is statistically significant: $\chi^2 = 4.26$; P <0.05.

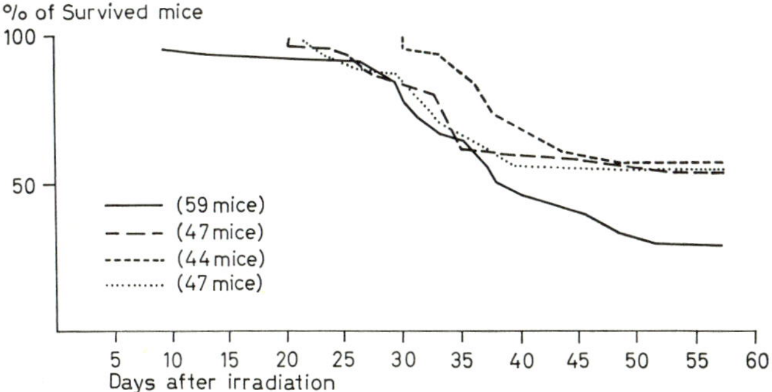

Fig. 1. Survival curves of untreated and treated chimeras.
Group 1: Untreated chimeras
Group 2: Second bone marrow transfusion
Group 3: "Third party" (Balb/c) thymus graft
Group 4: (DBA/2 × C57Bl/6) thymus grafts

The untreated chimeras had very low numbers of plaque forming colonies (PFC) in their spleens and produced low haemagglutinin titres both at the 35th and 60th days after irradiation. In chimeras treated by second marrow injection, no significant changes were observed. The results in animals treated with thymic transplants were similar, where no thymic grafts were found in their peritoneal cavity at 35th day. On the other hand, significant increase of immune reactivity both in the Jerne test and haemagglutinin titre, were found in 35th day in animals with visible thymic grafts. On the 60th day the reactivity of untreated chimeras was only very slightly improved; however, the differences between them and on 35th day successfully influenced chimeras completely disappeared (table IV).

Table IV. Number of plaque forming cells and haemagglutinin titres
in control normal animals, untreated and treated chimeras

Group 1: Normal mice
Group 2: Untreated chimeras
Group 3: Second bone marrow transfusion
Group 4: "Third party" (Balb/c) thymuses
Group 5: Thymuses of donor (DBA/2 × C57B*l*/6)

		Number of PFC per 1.10^6 splenocytes		Haemagglutinin titre	
		35th day	60th day	35th day	60th day
Group 1		991±154 (6)+		8.2±0.8 (6)	
Group 2		30.3± 9.8 (6)	83±17 (3)	2.0±1.0 (6)	1.7±0.5 (4)
Group 3		72 ±19 (4)	40±15 (3)	1.0 (4)	2.2±0.8 (3)
Group 4	Visible thymus grafts	123 ± 7.3 (3)	70±25 (4)	4.0±1.0 (3)	3.3±1.1 (4)
	Not visible thymus grafts	47.2±36 (6)		1.6±1.0 (6)	
Group 5	Visible thymus grafts	186 ±48 (4)	60±18 (4)	5.0 (4)	2.5±1.1 (4)
	Not visible thymus grafts	57.9±37.5 (7)		1.5±1.2 (7)	

+ Number of animals tested

Skin grafts survival of donor and third party strain tail skin is given
in table V. Non-irradiated control recipients rejected Balb/c skin
grafts in 10 ± 0.5 days and (DBA/2 × C57B*l*/6) F1 grafts in 9.1 ±
1.0 days. Untreated chimeras tolerated two from four Balb/c grafts
and three from four donor grafts at 35 days. At 60 days only one out
of four, eventually two out of four were tolerated. In bone marrow
treated chimeras only a few more third party grafts were tolerated.

A higher percentage of chimeras treated with donor thymus
graft tolerated the skin grafts of donor than of third party origin.
Treatment with third party thymus grafts had a similar influence on
donor skin graft retention. However, all third party grafts were rejected, if tested at 35 days, and three out of four, if tested at 60 days.

Reactivity to BCG and Candidin. The results summarized in table VI
indicate that no significant changes could be detected at 35 and 60 days
between control normal mice, and non-treated and treated radiation
chimeras.

Table V. The fate of bone marrow donor and "third party" skin grafts in control normal animals and untreated and treated chimeras (figures indicate the day of complete skin rejection. T = skin grafts tolerated more than 50 days)

Group 1: Normal mice
Group 2: Untreated chimeras
Group 3: Second bone marrow transfusion
Group 4: "Third party" (Balb/c) thymuses
Group 5: Donor (DBA/2 × C57Bl/6) thymuses

		Group 1	Group 2	Group 3	Group 4	Group 5
Balb/c Skin graft	35th day	10.4±0.5 (6)+	18, 28 T, T	14, 18 T, T, T	7, 7, 22, 22	22, 25, 25 T
	60th day		25, 32, 40 T	14 T, T, T	25, 30, 32 T	15, 17 T
(DBA/2 × C57Bl/6) Skin graft	35th day	9.1±1.0 (6)+	20 T, T, T	12, 41, 42 T, T	22, 22 T, T	23 T, T, T
	60th day		12, 31 T, T	25 T, T, T	38, 40 T, T	15, 25 T

+ Number of animals tested

Table VI. Foot pad reactions to BCG vaccine and candidin antigen in normal mice and untreated and treated chimeras

Group 1: Normal mice
Group 2: Untreated chimeras
Group 3: Second bone marrow transfusion
Group 4: "Third party" (Balb/c) thymuses
Group 5: Donor (DBA/2 × C57Bl/6) thymuses

		Group 1	Group 2	Group 3	Group 4	Group 5
BCG	35th day	++++ (3)[1]	++++ (4)	++++ (3)	++++ (3)	++++ (3)
	60th day		++++ (3)	++++ (3)	++++ (3)	++++ (3)
Candinin	35th day	+++ (3)	++ (3)	++ (3)	++ (3)	+++ (3)
	60th day		+ (3)	++ (3)	++ (3)	++ (3)

[1] Number of animals tested

G-V-H assay results are shown schematically in table VII; generally a very low activity or even absence of reactivity of both the host and donor parts of the chimeras were observed. If some degree of reactivity was seen at all after giving chimeric spleen cells, it was exclusively of donor type.

Table VII. The activity of splenocytes from Balb/c → C3H radiation chimeras 30 days after irradiation tested by GVH assay[1]

	3-day-old recipients	No.	Origin of splenocytes injected 10.10⁶ cells per gram of body weight	S I	H I	T I
Activity of recipient's part of chimeras	(C3H × C57B*l*/6) F1	5	C3H normal mice	2.85±0.5	1.56±0.6	0.71±0.05
		5	C3H/Balb chimeras	1.19±0.2	1.07±0.3	0.87±0.06
Activity of donor's part of chimeras	(Balb/c × DBA/2) F1	8	Balb/c normal mice	1.95±0.7	1.58±0.5	0.47±0.05
		7	C3H/Balb chimeras	1.37±0.5	1.13±0.2	0.91±0.1

[1] High mortality during first 30 days caused the low numbers of animals tested.

Discussion

The depression of immune function is a general feature of radiation chimeras. This has been demonstrated by measuring the responses to allogeneic and heterogeneic tumours and skin grafts, G-V-H reactivity and many responses of humoral type. In syngeneic chimeras, treated with a sufficient number of bone marrow cells, the immune reactivity gradually improves whilst in allogeneic chimeras it remains low throughout life [Makinodan *et al.*, 1956; Ilbery *et al.*, 1958; Barnes and Loutit, 1959; Bridges *et al.*, 1960; Cole and Davis, 1961; Doak and Koller, 1961; Lengerovà, 1961; Mathé *et al.*, 1961; van Bekkum, 1962; Doria *et al.*, 1962; Prehn and Thursh, 1962; Thompson *et al.*, 1962 and others].

In our radiation chimeras, pronounced depression of responses to heterologous erythrocytes, allogeneic skin grafts and in G-V-H assay was detected both at 35 and 60 days. On the other hand, the reactivity to mycobacterium TBC vaccine and candidin antigens was not different from response of normal animals, which indicates a surprisingly high resistance of these type responses in chimeras. There is some discrepancy between our findings and demonstration of lowered reactivity to Salmonella and T2 bacteriophage antigens [Blaese *et al.*, 1964; Shevelev, 1965]; perhaps it may be due to the different antigenicity of the bacteria in question; but this difference is more probably due to the different test systems used.

The studies of G-V-H activity, allowing the differenciation between host and donor type of response, had to be performed in other types of chimeras. In the chimeras (C3H × Balb/c), however, the course of secondary syndrome was rapid and they could not be utilized for further studies. The limited data available is in accordance with the general concept that the bulk of immune reactivity in allogeneic radiation chimeras is of donor origin, and a similar development of events could be supposed to occur also in the chimeras we have used routinely.

Many attempts have been made to improve the survival of allogeneic radiation chimeras by supplementary addition of donor cells. Some success was achieved by SIMMONS [1962] with donor lymphocytes and spleen cells and by THOMPSON *et al.* [1967] with spleen cells. In both the cases, the cells were given at 21 days after irradiation and transplantation. However, these attempts seem to be potentially hazardous, because an aggravation of G-V-H reaction cannot be absolutely precluded.

The existence of some malfunction or lability of donor hemopoietic and lymphoid component in radiation chimeras may be presumed. We tried therefore to modify the fate of our chimeras by the supplementary transplantation of donor bone marrow cells. We have obtained some improvement of the 60-day survival, but the animals' immune reactivity was only slightly influenced. It is possible that in some animals the take of primary graft was not perfect or its function was not sufficiently stable. In this case, the second marrow graft could reinforce the donor cells hemopoietic function. The positive influence by lymphoid cells from the bone marrow graft seems to be highly improbable.

The attempts to use thymic grafts in the treatment of allogeneic radiation chimeras were inspired by recent observation of a positive lymphostimulating influence of large amounts of thymic tissue in various experimental situations: (1) some authors succeeded in curing the wasting syndrome after neonatal thymectomy by the transplantation of a high number of thymus grafts [SCHALLER *et al.*, 1967; STUTMAN, 1967]; (2) thymus grafts were able to aid in the restoration of immune reactivity in thymectomized irradiated animals [GLOBERSON and FELDMAN, 1964; MILLER *et al.*, 1964]; (3) thymus tissue *in vitro* enhances the restoration of immune reactivity of irradiated spleen cells [GLOBERSON and AUERBACH, 1967], and potentiates lymph node antibody synthesis [WOLF, 1968]; (4) some recent observations of VAN BEKKUM [1968] on syngeneic supralethally irradiated chimeras seem to indicate a decisive role of thymus in the late phase of secondary syndrome; (5) moreover, the liberation of thymic cells from the grafts to invade the lymphoid tissues of chimera is not to be feared, because of the relative low anti-host reactivity of thymus cells [Mathé, Amiel, Bresin and Choquet, 1964]. It is evident from our results, that in both groups of chimeras, treated by the transplantation of multiple donor or third party thymus grafts, some improvement of the 60-day survival was obtained and increase of immune reactivity in at least a proportion of the animals at 35 days (this time was 15–20 days after thymus transplantation). The increase was evident in the humoral response to heterologous erythrocytes as well as against 3rd party skin grafts. On the other hand, if measured at 60-days (45–50 days after thymic transplantation), no differences were seen between treated and untreated chimeras. Thus, the function of thymic transplants seemed to be only temporary; this is also supported by autopsy findings at 60 days where in none of the mice thymus graft was found in the peritoneal cavity. Because of the donor and third party grafts had the same fate, their immune rejection is improbable; the transient survival was probably due to the physiological conditions prevailing and ultimate resorption of all grafts.

At autopsy on day 35, thymus grafts were found in a certain percentage of animals. If these animals were evaluated separately the number of plaque forming cells in their spleens and haemagglutinins titres were significantly higher than in untreated chimeras, whereas in animals in whom no remaining thymus grafts were found, hardly any effect could be detected. From these results we can postulate that probably in more than half of the animals the thymus grafts did not take or failed early.

The results are derived from animals with successful and unsuccessful graft experiments because it was not possible to control whether a thymus grafts had taken. In other words, it may be supposed that survival as well as the improvement of immune functions might have been better in animals with successful thymus transplants than is apparent from general results from all the grafted animals. This opinion is also supported by the observations of van Bekkum [1968, personal communication], in which subcutaneous grafts failed to give a clear positive effect, whereas grafts put under the capsule of kidney seemed to be beneficial.

In our experiments, the acceptance or at least the temporary acceptance of thymus grafts seemed to be necessary in order to obtain a lymphostimulatory effect, but there is no evidence that the cellular production and migration from the thymic grafts caused this effect. On the contrary, there is a body of evidence in favour of the participation of a humoral factor. If cells had recolonized the lymphoid tissue of chimeras, the improved immunological reactivity should have been more permanent and partially evident at the 60th day. Furthermore, the results of skin grafting tests speak more in favour of a non-specific activity of thymic grafts. Not only did thymus grafts of donor origin, but also third party grafts, support the survival of some donor grafts and limited the survival of third party grafts (the third party thymic grafts were surprisingly even more active in the latter situation). There is evidence that in both situations the immune reactivity of chimeric lymphoid tissue was enhanced, and this probably of donor origin. If third party thymic cells had even temporarily recolonized the lymphoid tissue of chimera, the prolonged survival of skin grafts of their genotype ought to have been expected.

The possible participation of a thymus factor is supported by data from other models: the prevention and even cure of wasting and amelioration of immune functions of neonatally thymectomized animals, the restoration of immune reactivity of thymectomized irradiated animals and even *in vitro* stimulating effects have been achieved not only by thymus grafts, but also by thymus grafts enclosed in millipore chambers and even extracts from thymus tissue [LEVEY *et al.*, 1963; OSOBA and MILLER, 1963; DE SOMER *et al.*, 1963; MILLER *et al.*, 1964, 1965; KLEIN *et al.*, 1965; TRAININ *et al.*, 1966; GLOBERSON and AUERBACH, 1967; SCHALLER and STEVENSON, 1967; SCHALLER *et al.*, 1967; SMALL and TRAININ, 1967; TRAININ and LINKER-ISRAELI, 1967].

Our experiments seem to support the concept that these are two components of the secondary syndrome: a) *the first phase appears* to be thymus independent [FIELD and GIBBS, 1966]. The best therapeutic effect is obtained by immunosuppressive drugs and perhaps also by antilymphocyte serum. However, giving of donor lymphoid cells at this time is very dangerous and leads to increased mortality [VOS *et al.*, 1959; VOS and WEYZEN, 1962]. In our experiments on the G-V-H reaction in young F1 hybrids injected with parental spleen cells, we obtained evidence that thymus grafts and cells are also harmful in this period [NOUZA and DOLEJSKOVÀ]; b) *the late, aplastic phase* of the secondary syndrome is resistant to immunosuppressive drugs and antilymphocyte serum. It may be non-specifically improved by antibiotic therapy [VAN BEKKUM and VOS, 1961], and specifically by donor lymphoid and bone marrow cells. This latter possibility is, however, bound to limited animal experimental conditions. VAN BEKKUM's [1968] and our own observations indicate that this period of the syndrome is partially dependent on the thymus. We think therefore that transplantation of a great amount of thymus tissue may be recommended as a form of therapy. The similar effectiveness of donor and third party grafts enables the effect of thymus grafts also in outbred animal populations to be assessed.

Because the effect of thymus grafts is probably mediated by a humoral factor, purified forms of thymus extracts could be used [TRAININ *et al.*, 1967] and if given in sufficiently high and repeated doses, the development of an immune response against it might be prevented.

It is necessary for us to prolong our studies and to try to find ways to obtain better or even permanent survival of thymus grafts. The importance of lymphoid insufficiency in many clinical situations leads us to think about the possibility of the practical use of such a method for the augmentation of immune reactivity.

Abstract

The secondary syndrome in animal as well as human radiation chimeras comprises two main components: the early, proliferative phase, which seems to be thymus independent and may be best controlled by immunosuppressive drugs or heterologous anti-lymphocyte serum, and the late phase, probably thymus dependant, characterized by profound aplasia of lymphoid tissues, which we are not able to control as yet. We have tried to treat allogeneic murine radiation chimeras with additional i. v. transfusions of donor bone marrow cells or by the i. p. transplantation of multiple thymus grafts from donor or genetically unrelated (third party) mice. The survival at 60 days and immunological reactivity against sheep red cells (SRBC), allogeneic skin grafts, Mycobacterium tuberculosis and Candidin antigen (at the 35th and 60th days) were compared in nontreated and treated animals. Untreated chimeras reacted only feebly to SRBC and skin grafts, whereas the reactions against mycobacterial and fungal antigens were essentially the same as in normal non-irradiated mice.

The second transfusion of donor bone marrow improved the 60 days survival, but had no effect on the immunological activity of chimeras. On the other hand, donor and third party thymus grafts improved at least temporarily the immune responses of some grafted animals. We obtained evidence that at least a temporary take of thymus grafts was necessary for the lympho-stimulating effect to be realized. A humoral factor seems to be involved more probably than the cellular migration of thymus cells to the lymphoid tissues.

The implication of the results to the possible control of the aplastic component of the secondary syndrome in animal experiments as well as in clinical practice is discussed.

References

BAILEY, D. and USAMA, B.: A rapid method of grafting skin on tails of mice. Transplant. Bull. *7:* 424 (1960).

BALNER, H.; VAN BEKKUM, D. W.; DE VRIES, M. J.; DERSJANT, H. and VAN PUTTEN, L. M.: Effect of antilymphocyte sera on homograft reactivity and graft-versus-host reactions in rhesus monkeys. In: Advances in transplantation, p. 449. (Eds.) J. DAUSSET, J. HAMBURGER and G. MATHÉ (Munsgaard, Copenhagen 1968).

BARNES, D. W. H. and LOUTIT, J. F.: Immunological status and longevity of radiation chimaeras. Proc. roy. Soc. *150:* 131–146 (1959).

VAN BEKKUM, D. W.; VOS, O. and WEYZEN, W. W. H.: The pathogenesis of the secondary disease after foreign bone marrow transplantation in X-irradiated mice. J. nat. Cancer Inst. *23:* 75 (1959).

VAN BEKKUM, D. W. and VOS, O.: Treatment of secondary disease in radiation chimaeras. Inter. J. Rad. Biol. *3:* 173 (1961).

VAN BEKKUM, D. W.: Tolerance of donor cells towards the host in radiation chimeras. In: Mechanisms of immunological tolerance, p. 385. (Eds.) HASEK, LENGEROVA, VOJTISKOVA, Prague (1962).

VAN BEKKUM, D. W. and DE VRIES, M. J.: Radiation chimaeras (Logos Press Ltd., London 1967).

VAN BEKKUM, D. W.: Immunological and hematological aspects of recovery: Implications for therapeutic use of bone marrow grafts. Proc. Brookhaven Symp. on Recovery and repair mechanisms in Radiobiology – 5./7. June 1967. (to be published, 1968).

BLEASE, R. M.; MARTINEZ, C. and GOOD, R. A.: Immunologic incompetence of immunologically runted animals. J. exp. Med. *119:* 211 (1964).

BRIDGES, J. B.; LOUTIT, J. F. and MICKLEM, S.: Transplantation immunity in the isologous mouse radiation chimaera. Immunology *3:* 195 (1960).

BUCKLEY, R. H.; LUCAS, Z. J.; HATTLER, B. G.; ZMIJEXSKI, C. M. and AMOS, D. B.: Defective cellular immunity associated with chronic mucocutaneous moniliasis and recurrent staphylococcal botryomycosis: Immunological reconstitution by allogeneic bone marrow. Clin. exper. Immunol. *3:* 153 (1968).

COLE, L. Y. and DAVIS, W. E.: Specific homograft tolerance in lymphoid cells of long-lived radiation chimeras. Proc. nat. Acad. Sci. U. S. *47:* 594 (1961).

COLOMBANI, J.; DAUSSET, J. et PREAUX, J.: Homogreffe de peau chez l'homme en relation avec les isoantigènes leucocytaires. Nouv. franç. Hémat. *4:* 499–505 (1963).

DOAK, S. M. A. and KOLLER, P. C.: Homografts on isologous and homologous radiation mouse chimaeras. Transplant. Bull. *27:* 444 (1961).

DORIA, G.; GOODMAN, J. W.; GENGOZIAN, N. and CONGDON, C. C.: Immunologic study of antibody forming cells in mouse radiation chimeras. J. Immunol. *88:* 20–30 (1962).

FIELD, E. O. and GIBBS, J. E.: Effect of thymectomy and irradiation on graft-versus-host disease. Transplantation *3:* 634 (1966).

GLOBERSON, A. and FELDMAN, M.: Role of the thymus in restauration of immune reactivity and lymphoid regeneration in irradiated mice. Transplantation *2:* 212 (1964).

GLOBERSON, A. and AUERBACH, R.: Reactivation *in vitro* of immunocompetence in irradiated mouse spleen. J. exp. Med. *126:* 223–234 (1967).

HOWARD, J.G. and WOODRUFF, M.F.A.: Effect of the graft-versus-host reaction on the immunological responsiveness of the mouse. Proc. roy. Soc. B. *154:* 532 (1961).

ILBERY, P.L.T.; KOLLER, P.C. and LOUTIT, J.F.: Immunological characteristics of radiation chimaeras. J. nat. Cancer Inst. *20:* 1051 (1958).

KLEIN, J.J.; GOLDSTEIN, A.L. and WHITE, A.: Enhancement of *in vivo* incorporation of labelled precursors into DNA and total protein of mouse lymph nodes after administration of thymic extracts. Proc. nat. Acad. Sci. Wash. *53:* 812 (1965).

LAWRENCE, W. Jr. and SIMONSEN, M.: The property of "strength" of histocompatibility antigens and their ability to produce antigeneic competition. Transplantation *5:* 1304 (1967).

LEDNEY, G.D. and VAN BEKKUM, D.W.: Suppression of acute secondary disease in the mouse with antilymphocyte serum. In: Advance in Transplantation, p. 441. (Eds.) J. DAUSSET, J. HAMBURGER, G. MATHÉ (Munsgaard, Copenhagen 1968).

LENGEROVA, A.; MICKLEM, H.S. and DENT, T.: Graft-versus-graft immunologic tolerance in radiation chimaeras. Folia biol. (Prague) *7:* 309 (1961).

LEVEY, R.H.; TRAININ, N. and LAW, L.W.: Evidence for function of thymic tissue in diffusion chambers implanted in neonatally thymectomized mice. J. nat. Cancer Inst. *31:* 199 (1963).

MAKINODAN, T.; GENGOZIAN, N. and CONGDON, C.C.: Agglutinin production in normal sublethally irradiated mice treated with mouse bone marrow. J. Immunol. *77:* 250 (1956).

MATHÉ, G.; AMIEL, J.L.; BREZIN, C. et CHOQUET, C.: Comparaison de la réactivité contre l'hôte de thymocytes et de cellules ganglionnaires semi-allogéniques. Rev. franç. Et. clin. biol. *9:* 988 (1964).

MATHÉ, G.; JAMMET, H.; PENDIC, B.; SCHWARZENBERG, L.; DUPLAN, J.F.; MAUPIN, B.; LATARJET, R.; LARRIEU, M.J.; KALIC, D. et DJUKIC, Z.: Transfusion et greffes de moelle osseuse homologue chez des humains irradiés à haute dose accidentellement. Rev. franç. Et. clin. biol. *4:* 226–38 (1959).

MATHÉ, G.; BERNARD, J.; VRIES, M.J. DE; SCHWARZENBERG, L.; LARRIEU, M.J.; LALANNE, C.; DUTREIX, A.; AMIEL, J.L. et SURMONT, J.: Nouveaux essais de greffe de moelle osseuse homologue après irradiation totale chez des enfants atteints de leucémie aiguë en rémission. Le problème du syndrome secondaire chez l'homme. Rev. Hémat. *15:* 115–61 (1960).

MATHÉ, G.; AMIEL, J.L. et DAGUET, G.: Etude des agglutinines sériques contre un antigène bactérien chez des radiochimères hématologiques immunisées contre l'antigène avant l'irradiation. Nouv. Rev. franç. Hémat. *1:* 65–71 (1961).

MATHÉ, G.; AMIEL, J.L. et NIEMETZ, J.: Recherche d'un test d'histocompatibilité pour des essais de greffes allogéniques. I. Etude chez la souris. Rev. franç. Et. clin. biol. *6:* 684–687 (1961).

MATHÉ, G. et AMIEL, J.L.: La greffe. Aspects cliniques et biologiques. Vol. 1 (Masson et Cie, Paris 1962).

MATHÉ, G.; AMIEL, J.L.; MATSUKURA, M. et MERY, A.M.: Restauration hématopoïétique de souris irradiées par greffe de moelle osseuse allogénique de plusieurs donneurs de diverses lignées. C.R. Acad. Sci. *255:* 3480–3482 (1962).

MATHÉ, G.; AMIEL, J.L. et NIEMETZ, J.: Greffe de moelle osseuse après irradiation totale chez des souris leucémiques suivie de l'administration d'un produit antimitotique. C.R. Acad. Sci. *54:* 3603–3605 (1962).

MATHÉ, G.; AMIEL, J.L.; SCHWARZENBERG, L.; CATTAN, A. and SCHNEIDER, M.: Hematopoietic chimera in man after allogeneic (homologous) bone marrow transplantation: Control of the secondary syndrome, specific tolerance due to chimerism. Brit. med. J. *2:* 1633–1635 (1963).

MATHÉ, G.: Le syndrome secondaire, pierre d'achoppement du traitement des leucémies par l'irradiation totale suivie de transfusion de cellules hématopoïétiques allogéniques. In: Diagnostic et traitement des radiolésions aigues. pp. 197–230 (Ed.) O.M.S., Genève (1964).

MATHÉ, G.; AMIEL, J.L.; MATSUKURA, M. and MERY, A.M.: Restoration of haemopoietic function in irradiated mouse by means of allogeneic bone marrow grafts from several donors of different strains'. Brit. J. Haemat. *10:* 257–263 (1964).

MATHÉ, G.; AMIEL, J. L.; SCHWARZENBERG, L. et DA COSTA, H.: Effets (selon la durée) de la conservation à 37°C dans du tyrode sur les cellules immunologiquement compétentes et les cellules souches myéloïdes. Rev. franç. Et. clin. biol. *9:* 625 (1964).

MATHÉ, G.; AMIEL, J. L. et SCHWARZENBERG, L.: L'aplasie myélo-lymphoïde de l'irradiation totale. (Gauthier-Villars, Paris 1965).

MATHÉ, G.; AMIEL, J.L.; SCHWARZENBERG, L.; CATTAN, A.; SCHNEIDER, M.; VRIES, M.J. DE; TUBIANA, M.; LALANNE, C.; BINET, J.L.; PAPIERNIK, M.; SEMAN, G.; MATSUKURA, M.; MERY, A.M.; SCHWARZMANN, V. and FLAISLER, A.: Successful allogeneic bone marrow transplantation in man: Chimerism induced specific tolerance and possible antileukaemic effects. Blood. *25:* 179–195 (1965).

MATHÉ, G.; SCHWARZENBERG, L.; VRIES, M.J. DE; AMIEL, J. L.; CATTAN, A.; SCHNEIDER, M.; BINET, J. L.; TUBIANA, M.; LALANNE, C.; SCHWARZMANN, V. et NORDMANN, R.: Les divers aspects du syndrome secondaire compliquant les transfusions allogéniques de moelle osseuse ou de leucocytes chez des sujets atteints d'hémopathies malignes. Europ. J. Cancer. *1:* 75–113 (1965).

MATSUKURA, M.; MERY, A.M.; AMIEL, J.L. and MATHÉ, G.: Investigation on a test of histocompatibility for allogeneic grafts. II. Study on rabbits. Transplantation *1:* 61–64 (1963).

MERY, A.M.; BREZIN, C.; SEKIGUCHI, M.; VAUBEL, W.E.; AMIEL, J.L. and MATHÉ, G.: Investigation on a test of histocompatibility for allogeneic grafts. III. A study in men. Transplantation *4:* 206–207 (1966).

MICKLEM, H.S. and LOUTIT, J.F.: Tissue grafting and radiation (Academic Press, London 1966).

MILLER, J.F.A.P.; LEUCHARS, E.; CROSS, A.M. and DUKOV, P.: Immunologic role of the thymus in radiation chimeras. Ann. N.Y. Acad. Sci *120:* 205 (1964).

MILLER, J.F.A.P.; OSOBA, D.; DUKOR, P.: A humoral thymus mechanism responsible for immunological maturation. Ann. N.Y. Acad. Sci. *124:* 95 (1965).

MULLER-BERAT, C.N. and VAN PUTTEN, L.M.: Cytostatic drugs in the treatment of secondary disease following homologous bone marrow transplantation: Extrapolation form the mouse to the primate. Ann. N.Y. Acad. Sci. *129:* 340 (1966).

OSOBA, D. and MILLER, J.F.A.P.: Evidence for a humoral thymus factor responsible for maturation of immunological faculty. Nature *199:* 653 (1963).

PREHN, R.T. and THORSH, D.R.: The immunologic status of long-term radiation chimeras. p. 397. In: Mechanisms of immunological tolerance. (Eds.) M. HASEK and A. LENGEROVÁ, Prague (1962).

RAMSEIER, H. and STREILEIN, J.W.: Homograft sensitivity reaction in irradiated hamster. Lancet *i:* 622 (1965).

SCHALLER, R.T. and STEVENSON, J.K.: Reversal of post-thymectomy wasting syndrome with multiple thymus grafts in diffusion chambers. Proc. Soc. exp. Biol. Med. *124:* 199 (1967).

SCHALLER, R.T.; SCHALLER, J. and STEVENSON, J.K.: Reversal of wasting syndrome in thymectomized mice by multiple syngeneic or allogeneic thymus grafts. J. nat. Cancer Inst. *38:* 287 (1967).

SCHWARZENBERG, L.; CATTAN, A.; SCHNEIDER, M.; SCHLUMBERGER, J.R.; AMIEL, J.L. et MATHÉ, G.: La réanimation hématologique. II. Correction des désordres graves des leucocytes et des immunoglobulines. Presse méd. *74:* 1061 (1966).

SEMAN, G.: Technique personnelle de coloration des lobules hétérochromatiques des leucocytes (spécialement des mononuclées). Valeur de cette technique dans la détermination du sexe. Rev. franç. Et. clin. biol. *6:* 161–165 (1961).

SHEVELEV, A.S.: Study of the mechanism of immunological unresponsiveness induced by the transplantation of homologous spleen cells to sublethally irradiated animals. Folia biol. (Prague) *11:* 177 (1965).

SIMMONS, E.L.; THOMPSON, J.H. and RANDI, J.M.: Reduction in secondary disease by injection of homologous lymphoid cells. Radiat. Res. *16:* 569 (1962).

SMALL, M. and TRAININ, N.: Increase of antibody forming cells of neonatally thymectomized mice receiving calf thymus extract. Nature *216:* 377 (1967).

DE SOMER, D.; DENYS, P. and LEYTEN, R.: Activity of noncellular calf thymus extract in normal and thymectomized mice. Life Sci. *1:* 810 (1963).

STUTMAN, O.; YUNIS, E.J.; MARTINEZ, C. and GOOD, R.A.: Reversal of post-thymectomy wasting disease in mice by multiple thymus grafts. J. Immunol.

THOMAS, E.D.; COLLINS, J.A.; HERMAN, E.C. Jr. and FERREBEE, J.W.: Marrow transplants in lethally irradiated dogs given Methotrexate. Blood *19:* 217–228 (1962).

THOMPSON, J.S.; SIMMONS, E.L. and HOFSTRA, D.: Studies of the immunologic unresponsiveness during the secondary disease period of lethally irradiated mice protected by homologous bone marrow. J. Immunol. *89:* 62 (1962).

THOMPSON, J.S.; SIMMONS, E.L.; MOY, R.H. and CRAWFORD, M.K.: Studies of immunologic unresponsiveness during secondary disease. II. The effect of added donor and host immunologically competent cells. J. Immunol.

TRAININ, N.; BEJERANO, A.; STRAHILEVITCH, M.; GOLDRING, D. and SMALL, M.: A thymic factor preventing wasting and influencing lymphopoiesis in mice. Israel. J. med. Sci. *2:* 549 (1966).

TRAININ, N.; BURGER, M. and KAYE, A.M.: Some characteristics of a thymic humoral factor determined by assay *in vivo* of DNA synthesis in lymph nodes of thymectomised mice. Biochem. Pharmacol. *16:* 711 (1967).

TRAININ, N.; LINKER-ISRAELI, M.: Restoration of immunologic reactivity of thymectomized mice by calf thymus extracts. Cancer Res. *27:* 309 (1967).

UPHOFF, D.E.: Atteration of homograft reaction by amethopterin in lethally irradiated mice treated with homologous marrow. Proc. Soc. exp. biol. Med. *99:* 651–653 (1958).

VOS, O.; DE VRIES, M.J.; COLLENTEUR, J.C. and VAN BEKKUM, D.W.: Transplantation of homologous and heterologous lymphoid cells in X-irradiated and nonirradiated mice. J. nat. Cancer Inst. *23:* 53 (1959).

VOS, O. and WEYZEN, W.W.H.: Killing effect of injected lymph node cells in homologous radiation chimeras. Transplantation Bull. *30:* 111 (1962).

WOLF, B.: Postulation of lymph node antibody synthesis by normal thymus *in vitro*. Immunology *14:* 235 (1968).

Authors' addresses: Prof. Dr. G. MATHÉ, Institut de Cancérologie et d'Immunogénétique, Hôpital Paul-Brousse, 14 Av. Paul-Vaillant Couturier, *94-Villejuif* (France); Dr. K. NOUZA, Institute of Exp. Biology and Genetics, Czechoslovak Academy of Sciences, *Prague* (Czechoslovakia); Dr. I. HRSAK, Institute R. Boskovic, *Zagreb* and Dr. V. KOLAR, Oncological Institute, *Brno* (Jugoslavia).

Antibiotica et Chemotherapia, vol. 15, pp. 199–212 (Karger, Basel/New York 1969)

The Effect of Plant Mitogens on Humoral and Cellular Immune Responses

M. Landy and L. N. Chessin

National Institute of Allergy and Infectious Diseases,
National Institutes of Health, Bethesda, Md.

There has been a rapid evolution of our understanding of the effects of plant mitogens on peripheral lymphocytes in tissue culture. This has included, e.g., knowledge of the cyto-architectural changes [8] and the series of biochemical events initiated by these agents [6, 7, 24], as well as some of the very early and essential features of the inter-action between mitogen and lymphocyte. Until very recently it had not been established that the mitogens would affect lymphocytes *in vivo* in a manner analogous to the well known effects in tissue culture. However such data, now becoming available, indicate that the effects evoked in experimental animals do indeed relate to the tissue culture work.

From earlier work it could not be predicted with certainty whether the alterations in lymphocytes would subsequently be expressed as augmentation or depression of their immunocompetence. However, as information on this interaction accumulated, this effect seemed to be more in the direction of interference; a growing body of literature now attests to this. It is not unreasonable to assume that such sup-pression of the immune response by mitogens involves at least some of the phenomena so well defined *in vitro*. The purpose of this com-munication is to assess the reports to date on mitogen immunosup-pression, to present data on the nature of the cell receptor for mitogen and, to develop a concept of the means by which mitogen could suppress immunocompetence.

Systemic effects on lymphoid tissues. The fortuitous observation by Nowell in 1960 [29] that crude extracts of the red kidney bean (*Phaseolus vulgaris*—PHA) caused normal mononuclear cells to undergo *in vitro* a series of morphologic changes into a distinctive kind of blast-like cell served as the impetus for a continually expanding series of investigations in lymphocyte biology. This effect, and the type of transformed cell developed, have been of compelling interest to the immunologist inasmuch as the altered cell bears a striking morphologic resemblance to the cell type associated with the histologic response to antigenic stimuli [12]. Later on, the ultrastructural and biochemical events in this process were progressively identified [8]. In retrospect, it is understandable that these remarkable findings on lymphocytes were viewed as having major relevance to an understanding of immunologic phenomena. It was therefore inevitable that the effects of mitogens would also be explored *in vivo,* as detailed elsewhere in this report. In these studies in experimental animals and man, it was tacitly assumed that the host effects evoked by these plant extracts would in some measure correspond to the well documented *in vitro* manifestations.

In studies on experimental animals most of the evidence has been obtained with crude PHA and is consistent with the view that the effects produced *in vivo* are, in a general way, similar to those developed in tissue culture. The most impressive evidence *in vivo* has however been obtained with pokeweed, (PWM) in an experiment of nature. Inadvertant oral ingestion of poke berries by children [2] resulted in a peripheral blood picture of plasmacytosis, absolute eosinophilia, platelet phagocytosis, and thrombocytopenia. In higher dosage, crude PHA, and PWM as well, produce immediate toxicity with predominantly neuromuscular effects including, muscular hyperactivity, followed by paralysis, convulsions and death [28]. Administration of PHA intravenously produces intravascular hemagglutinates which, if they are of sufficient magnitude, lead to emboli in the major organs. A number of investigators [9, 11, 13] have shown convincingly that PHA evokes a stimulatory effect on lymphoid organs. This includes, for example, effects on spleen, lymph nodes, and bone marrow where there is discerned several days after a single dose of mitogen an increase in (a) number of cells synthesizing DNA, (b) the proportion of medium and large lymphocytes and (c) numbers of cells in peripheral blood resembling the blast-like cells obtained in tissue culture.

Highly purified PWM [30] has been administered to BALB/c mice [1]. Amounts of 50 μg i.p. produced CNS effects and proved lethal; 1 μg was sufficient to evoke hematopoietic changes manifested three to seven days later. Some leucopenia was evident and moderate

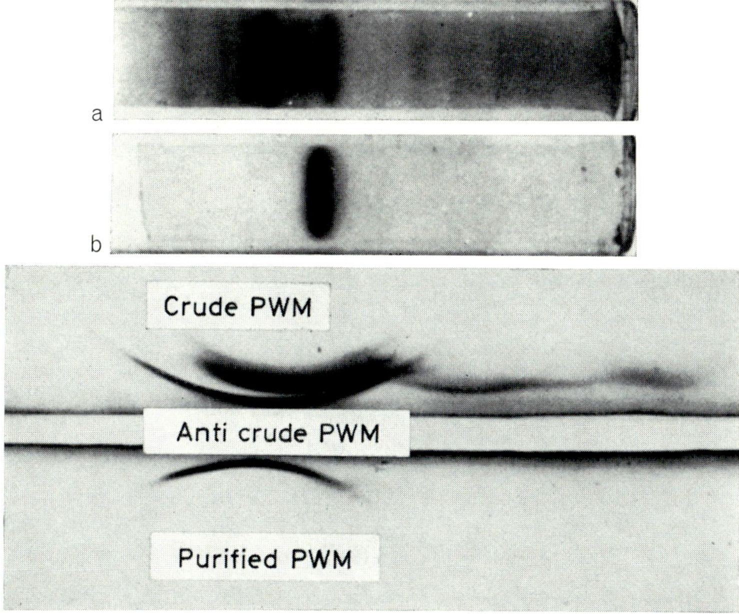

Fig. 1. Analytical multiphase zone electrophoresis on polyacrylamide gel and immuno-electrophoretic patterns of crude (TCA precipitate) and purified homogeneous PWM.

numbers of atypical lymphocytes and blast forms were present in peripheral blood. Thus evidence has been obtained that the same component (fig. 1) causing transformation of lymphocytes in tissue culture does indeed evoke generally similar effects on peripheral lymphocytes *in vivo*.

Assessment of the literature on immunosuppression by plant mitogens. At present the literature on the effects of plant mitogens on humoral and on cellular immunity consists, to the best of our knowledge, of eight and ten reports respectively. Summaries of these studies have been organized in tables I and II to present what we consider the most relevant information concerning the experimental situation explored, the conditions of host treatment with mitogen, and a concise assessment of the results obtained in these two separate forms of the immune response. These effects on humoral and cellular immunity, involving as they do a spectrum of models, are variable. They range all the way from negative to suggestive, to apparently clear-cut demonstrations of suppression or enhancement. Analysis of these diverse findings is rendered difficult by virtue of an exceedingly large number

Table I. Summary of investigations on the effect of plant mitogens on humoral immunity

| Reference | Immunological system | | Mitogen | | | Experimental conditions | | Findings and conclusions |
	Antigen	Mouse strain	Product	Route	Dose	Interval between mitogen and antigen (days)[1]	Immune assay	
Gamble [14]	Rat rbc	A/J	Difco PHA M	i.v.	1.2 mg	–5 to +1	Passive hemagglutination HGG immune elimination	Enhancement of hemagglutinin response; suppression of HGG primary
Spreafico and Lerner [32]	Sheep rbc	BALB/c	PHA P	i.p.	0.5 mg	–5 to +1	PFC	Almost total suppression of primary and secondary response
Hege and Cole [18]	Sheep rbc	CBA	PHA M	i.v.	0.3 ml	–4 to +1	PFC	10-fold reduction in primary immune response
Gengozian and Hubner [15]	S. typhosa flagella	C3BF	PHA M	i.p. s.c.	0.75 ml 0.25 ml	–1 to +1	Bacterial H agglutination	Almost total suppression of primary; reduction in secondary

Golub and Weigle [17]	HGG	C57 Bl	PHA M	i.v.	0.5 ml	−3 to +3	Immune elimination of antigen	No effect on development of immunological tolerance
Singhal *et al.* [31]	Sheep rbc BGG HSA	New Zealand Rabbits	PHA M	i.v.	5 ml	−3 to +3	Hemagglutinins Passive hemagglutination	Enhancement of immune response to HSA and BGG; no effect on response to sheep rbc
Markley *et al.* [25]	Sheep rbc	NIH mice	PHA M PHA P	i.p.	0.1 ml daily	−4 to 0	Hemagglutinins	Almost total suppression of primary response; secondary diminished by multiple doses of PHA
Lerner and Sanders [22]	Sheep rbc	BALB/c	PWM (TCA ppt)	i.p.	0–1.05 mg	−5 to +1	PFC	Virtually complete suppression of primary immune response

[1] Interval: − refers to days before antigen injection; + refers to days post antigen administration.

Table II. Summary of investigations on the effect of PHA on cellular immunity

| Reference | Immunological system | | Mitogen | | | Experimental conditions | | Findings and conclusions |
	Antigen	Experimental animals (strain)	Product	Route	Dose	Interval between mitogen and antigen (days)[1]	Immune assay	
CALNE *et al.* [4]	renal allografts	dog	Crude PHA and azothio-prine	i.v.	2×30 mg 3×15 mg	–1 to +5	graft rejection	Homograft reaction absent in 15/15; 4 survived indefinitely
CASCIANI and CORTESINI [5]	renal allografts	dog	Difco PHA P and azothio-prine	i.v.	3 mg/kg daily	–10 reject	graft rejection	Retention—controls 5 days; experimental 12–44 days
MARKLEY *et al.* [26]	skin allografts	rabbits	Difco PHA P	i.p.	1–5 ml daily	–2 reject	graft rejection	Retention—controls 7 days; experimental 15 days
KEHN and RIGBY [21]	skin allografts	mice Swiss C57 bl	PHA M	i.v.	½–1 ½ ml	–3 to +3	graft rejection	No significant effect on rejection time
ST. PIERRE *et al.* [33]	skin allografts	mice DBA C57 bl	PHA P	i.p.	3×0.1 ml	–3 to +4	graft rejection	Retention—controls 8 days; experimental 12 days

Lozzio [23]	carbon clearance	mice C3H/H2	PHA P	i.p.	0.2–6 mg ×3 or daily	–0 to + ½	blood clearance	Depression of RES phagocytic activity
Gillette *et al.* [16]	skin allografts	mice Sta C57 bl	PHA M Freund's Adjuvant	i.p.		–6 to 0	graft rejection	PHA and Freund's Adjuvant produced prolonged graft retention
Elves [10]	skin allografts GVH	rats mice	Burroughs Wellcome PHS	i.p.	3×4 mg	–3	mortality splenomegaly	No significant changes from controls in either system
Hunter and Millman [19]	GVH	Mice BALB/c CAF	Difco PHA P	i.p.	1 mg	–5 to +1	carbon clearance splenomegaly	PHA 1 day prior to challenge led to diminution in GVH manifestations
Moore and Stefani [27]	skin allografts	Mice C/57 bl C3H	Difco PHA P	i.p.	0.1–3 mg	–4 to 0	graft rejection	Maximum retention 24 days; PHA-dose dependent

[1] Interval: – refers to days before challenge; + refers to days post challenge.

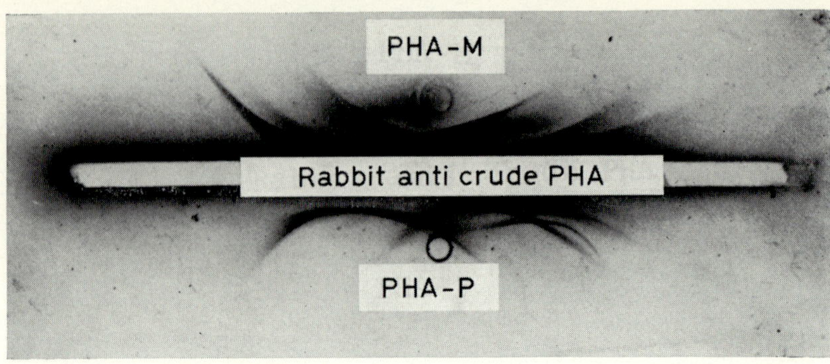

Fig. 2. Comparative immunoelectrophoretic patterns for Difco PHA M vs PHA P. Developed with antiserum prepared by immunization of rabbits with saline extract of *Phaseolus vulgaris.*

of variables. For example, the PHA mitogen itself, has been in virtually every instance, a crude and complex commercial product; in this laboratory it has been shown to contain at least eight to ten components (fig. 2). As is attested in many of these reports it is certainly toxic in at least some of the dose levels used. It is a potent hemagglutinin which, unless it has been absorbed with erythrocytes, is capable of producing intravascular hemagglutinates with consequent emboli. In none of these publications has evidence been adduced that the effects seen are necessarily attributable to the mitogenic component. There is the additional complication of the immunogenic action of the product [28] and the possibility that it could conceivably be exerting suppressive effects on the basis of competition of antigens. Finally, there has been a lack of awareness that non-lymphoid tissue probably binds a large proportion, or perhaps even most of the administered dose—in which case either the product has remarkable biologic potency, or at appropriate sites very little is required.

In some of these reports suitable controls are conspicuously absent, in others administration of mitogen has been combined with antimetabolite or with adjuvant. In a number of instances the findings obtained involved an insufficient number of animals to yield data of acceptable quantitative significance. Moreover any interpretation is affected by the exceedingly large number of variables that are likely to be operative in the 20 or so individual investigations which constitute the body of literature under review. As example may be cited the particular mitogen used, the dose, whether individual or multiple, route, time elapsed between mitogen and antigen administration, species of animal, immunologic model used and the test parameter for ascertaining results, to mention only the major factors. Any of these could affect profoundly the outcome, and indeed it is likely that one or another was operative in each of the series of studies thus far performed. Despite the complexity of these experimental situations, it appears that suppression of immunity can be effected by mitogens; however the findings more clearly attest to effects exerted on humoral than on cellular immunity. This interference is normally seen only when mitogen was administered before the test antigen.

Characterization of the erythrocyte receptor. Studies on the hemagglutination produced by PHA and PWM disclose that both are pan-hemagglutinins [3], the former expressing this effect in saline, while the latter requires high molecular weight substances such as dextran or albumin for this effect to be manifested. PWM binding to erythrocytes can also be detected by Coombs reaction with an anti PWM serum. Working with an array of human iso-antigenic red cell types it became clear that PWM hemagglutination is primarily directed against the 0(H) and/or I antigenic determinants. Erythrocytes were treated with a variety of enzymes to determine which, if any, altered, modified, or destroyed the receptor for mitogen. As seen in table III only the glycosidases were effective in this regard.

A considerable literature attests to the polysaccharide character of many erythrocyte antigens [20]. Moreover the 0(H) and the I receptors appear to be implicated in the binding of mitogen to erythrocytes.

Table III. Characterization of erythrocyte receptor for mitogen

	PHA	PWM
Specificity	Panagglutinin (complete, saline)	Panagglutinin (incomplete, dextran-dependent)-reacts in the presence of the 0 (H) and I determinants
Inhibition reactions		
Vi antigen	Complete	Complete
H substance	None	Partial
Le^a substance	None	Partial
Type XIV Pneumococcal polysacch.	Partial	Complete
N-acetyl-D-galactosamine	Complete	Complete
N-acetyl-D-glucosamine	None	Complete
Effect of enzymes on rbc receptor		
Neuraminadase	None	None
Trypsin (Ficin, Bromelin)	None	Enhancement of agglutination
Glycosidases	—	Destruction of receptor

Accordingly, inhibition experiments were performed with relevant polysaccharide antigens and their recognized constituents. Table III shows that inhibition of PHA is effected by type XIV SSS and N-acetyl-d-galactosamine. In the case of PWM, partial inhibition was produced by H and by Lewis (Le^a) substances; complete inhibition was effected by type XIV SSS, as well as N-acetyl-d-galactosamine and N-acetyl-d-glucosamine. These studies suggest that the erythrocyte receptors for mitogen are generally similar to the recognized blood groups.

Relevance to lymphocytes of erythrocyte receptor findings. The information presently available on the attributes of the lymphocyte receptor to PWM is summarized in table IV. Glycosidases, which remove completely the mitogen receptor on erythrocytes, also destroy the receptor for PWM on lymphocytes as judged by loss of leucoagglutination and transformation by mitogen. Sialic acid is not involved inasmuch as neuraminidase produces no destruction of receptor. Binding is viewed as essential for biologic effects, but binding *per se* does not necessarily lead to agglutination, *viz* the effect of PWM on erythrocytes. With respect to lymphocytes, this distinction may be even more marked. It is a reasonable assumption that the percentage of erythrocytes carrying the receptor is much greater than in lymphocytes. Moreover it is possible that, per cell, the number of receptors on erythrocytes is much greater than on lymphocytes. While admittedly fragmentary the foregoing suggests that lymphocytes possess a common receptor (s), analogous to the identifiable blood groups, which could account for attachment of PWM. To simultaneously ascertain the magnitude of binding, and its kinetics for both mitogens, H^3 thymidine incorporation into newly synthisized DNA was utilized in connection with purified PHA and PWM. The results of these

Table IV. The properties of the lymphocyte receptor for PWM

---

1. Binding of mitogen is unaffected by Neuraminidase-(30′)

2. Binding of mitogen is unaffected by Trypsin-(30′)

3. Binding of mitogen is destroyed by Glycosidases-(15′)

4. Binding site is blocked by (a) Ulex (Lectin Anti-H)
         (b) Human Bombay Anti-H

5. Absorption of purified PWM with human rbc has no discernible effect on mitogenicity

6. Absorption of purified PWM with lymphocytes removes hemagglutinating, leucagglutinating and mitogenic activities

---

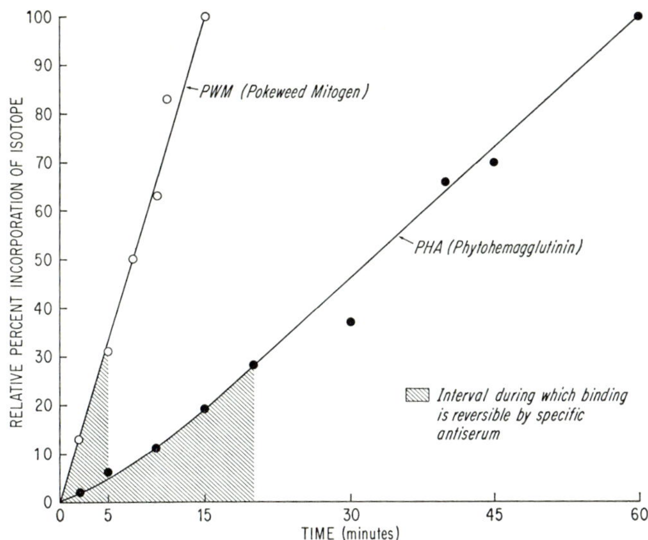

Fig. 3. Kinetics of binding of mitogen to peripheral blood lymphocytes.

labeling studies are shown in fig. 3. At 5 μg PWM and 20 μg PHA, amounts previously established as providing maximal transformation [6], binding of PWM to human peripheral blood lymphocytes was complete within 15 min. During the first 5 min it was still possible to prevent or reverse this process with antiserum specific for the mitogen. In contrast, PHA required 60 min for complete binding; in this case binding could be annulled by specific anti-PHA during the first 20 min. These data attest to the significantly greater affinity of purified PWM for lymphocytes.

Although the plant mitogens are immunogenic, it does not at present seem reasonable that this property *per se* accounts for their effect on immunocompetent cells. Simply stated, the reason is as follows: The reaction of antigen with competent cells, to the extent that binding or fixation occurs, is conceded to required preformed immunoglobulin, or its subunits, in or on the cell. In contrast, at least a considerable proportion of immunocompetent cells naturally possess quite different but nonetheless effective, surface receptors which may be unrelated to immunoglobulin, but capable of leading to cell fixation of mitogen.

Concept of mode of action. In seeking to account for the manner in which mitogen, administered parenterally, could lead to a state of general unresponsiveness to antigen by host lymphoid cells, all significant clues derive from the investigations based on *in vitro* lymphocyte culture methodology. The first requirement almost certainly is that of binding of mitogen to the immunocompetent cells that carry the natural receptor for these plant components. Unlike an array of protein antigens which appear to involve a modest proportion of cells, mitogens have a much broader affinity for lymphoid cells, presumably because many—perhaps even a majority—of these cells carry natural receptors for these structures. Occupying or pre-empting these sites on lymphocytes could have far-reaching consequences as regards the capacity of such cells subsequently to react to otherwise effective antigenic stimuli. Such sites could be crucial by virtue either of location, number or configuration. An appropriate kind of analogy may be that of antigenic competition where, under the right circumstances of time and dose, a single antigen is capable selectively of producing immunosuppression to another antigen.

In a similar vein, heterologous antilymphocyte serum (ALS) can be viewed as a polyvalent agent capable of reacting with an array of natural receptors, components, determinants, etc. on lymphocytes. In this context—except for quantitative considerations—these two otherwise quite dissimilar agents may modify the competence of lymphocytes in a parallel fashion. The very means by which ALS is prepared assures its consisting of a collection of specific antibodies individually directed against host tissue antigens shared by lymphocytes. Because of the multiple nature of the involvement of these cells, i.e. more than one antibody specificity and more than a single kind of receptor site, ALS would be expected to be by far the more effective suppressant of immunologic competence, as indeed it is.

We have obtained evidence (table IV) that the mitogens have a more limited spectrum of reactivity with lymphoid cells; that is, they are viewed as capable of reacting with a significant proportion of lymphocyte populations, but in all probability with only a single kind of receptor on these cells. This is not to imply that binding of mitogen is of itself equated with suppression of competence. Rather it is emphasized that binding or occupation of appropriate sites is a first and essential requirement for all subsequent events, concerning which regretably little is known.

Provided certain requirements are met, such as for example structural features of antigen or mitogen, or the antibody composition of a given ALS, and perhaps even more importantly the matter of complementariness of the cell receptor, there then occurs promptly the activation of new RNA and protein synthesis, followed by DNA synthesis; mitosis and cell division then occur sequentially. Whatever the actual nature of the fit, between these varied effector agents and the key cells, the process activated is broadly similar. Perhaps the major point now to be made is that as regards the capacity of the affected cells then to respond to another *antigen,* each of these otherwise unrelated agents has, in a similar fashion, temporarily nullified the capacity of these cells to respond.

Concluding Statement. The literature on immunosuppression by plant mitogens is uncommonly heterogeneous as regards the kinds of experimental situations studied. The results obtained have been widely variable and indeed conflicting. Nonetheless, in a significant number of instances, immunosuppression or unresponsiveness to antigenic challenge was of such magnitude as to indicate that these plant glycoproteins are effective in this regard and are worthy of further, better controlled, investigation.

References

1. ASOFSKY, R.; FINERTY, J. and CHESSIN, L.N.: (unpublished data).
2. BARKER, B.E.; FARNES, P. and MARCHE, P.J.: Hemagglutinin effects of pokeweed. Lancet *i:* 437 (1967).
3. BORJESON, J.; REISFELD, R.A.; CHESSIN, L.N.; WELSH, P.D. and DOUGLAS, S.D.: Studies on human peripheral blood lymphocytes *in vitro:* I. Biological and physiochemical properties of the pokeweed mitogen. J. exp. Med. *124:* 859–872 (1966).
4. CALNE, R.Y.; WHEELER, J.R. and HURN, B.A.A.: Combined immunosuppressive action of phytohemagglutinin and azathioprine (imuron) on dogs with renal homotransplants. Brit. med. J. *2:* 154–155 (1965).
5. CASCIANI, C.T. and CORTESINI, R.: Phytohaemagglutinin action on renal homograft survival. In: Histocompatability Testing, pp. 83–89 (Munksgaard, Copenhagen 1967).
6. CHESSIN, L.N.; BORJESON, J.B.; WELSH, P.D.; DOUGLAS, S.D. and COOPER, H.C.: Studies on human peripheral blood lymphocytes in vitro: II. Morphological and biochemical studies on the transformation of lymphocytes by pokeweek mitogen. J. exp. Med. *124:* 873–884 (1966).
7. COOPER, H.L. and RUBIN, A.D.: RNA metabolism in lymphocytes stimulated by phytohemagglutinin: Initial responses to phytohemagglutinin. Blood *25:* 1014–1027 (1965).
8. DOUGLAS, S.D.; HOFFMAN, P.F.; BORJESON, J.B. and CHESSIN, L.N.: Studies on human peripheral blood lymphocytes *in vitro:* III. Fine structural features of lymphocyte transformation by pokeweed mitogen. J. Immunol. *98:* 17–30 (1967).
9. ELVES, M.W.; ROATH, S. and ISRAELS, M.C.G.: Effects of phytohemagglutinin on homograft rejection. Nature *198:* 494 (1963).
10. ELVES, M.W.: The *in vivo* effect of phytohemagglutinin on homograft reactions. Transplantation *5:* 1532–1534 (1967).
11. EPSTEIN, L.B. and SMITH, C.W.: The *in vivo* induction of mouse lymphocyte transformation by phytohemagglutinin. J. Immunol. *100:* 421–435 (1968).

12. FAGRAEUS, A.: In Cellular aspects of Immunity. (Eds.) WOLSTENHOLME, G.E. and M. O'CONNOR (Little, Brown and Co., Boston 1959).
13. GAMBLE, C.N.: The effects of phytohemagglutinin in mouse spleen *in vivo*. Blood *28:* 175–187 (1966).
14. GAMBLE, C.N.: The effect of phytohemagglutinin on the primary antibody response of mice to rat erythrocytes and human gamma globulin. Int. Arch. Allergy *29:* 470–477 (1966).
15. GENGOZIAN, N. and HUBNER, K.F.: Effect of phytohemagglutinin (PHA) on an antibody forming system. J. Immunol. *99:* 184–190 (1967).
16. GILLETTE, R.; GOULIAN, D. and CONWAY, H.: Abstr. 1st Int. Congr. Transpl. Soc., Paris 1967 (personal communication).
17. GOLUB, E.S. and WEIGLE, W.O.: Studies on the induction of immunologic unresponsiveness. I. Effects of endotoxin and phytohemagglutinin. J. Immunol. *98:* 1241–1247 (1967).
18. HEGE, J.S. and COLE, L.J.: Antibody plaque-forming cells in unsensitized mice. Specificity and response to neonatal thymectomy, X-irridiation and PHA. J. lmmunol. *99:* 61–70 (1967).
19. HUNTER, R.L., JR. and MILLMAN, R.B.: (unpublished data).
20. KABAT, E.A.: Blood group substances; their chemistry and immunochemistry (Academic Press Inc., New York 1956).
21. KEHN, B. and RIGBY, P.: Effects of phytohaemagglutinin on homograft rejection. Nature *216:* 182–184 (1967).
22. LERNER, E.M. and SANDERS, E.: (unpublished data).
23. LOZZIO, B.B.: Depression of reticuloendothelial phagocytic activity by phytohemagglutinins (32469). Soc. exp. Biol., N.Y. *126:* 435–438 (1967).
24. MACKINNEY, A.A.; STOHLMAN, F., JR. and BRECHER, G.: The kinetics of cell proliferation in cultures of human peripheral blood. Blood *19:* 349–358 (1962).
25. MARKLEY, K.; SMALLMAN, E. and EVANS, G.: Decrease of mouse circulating antibodies to sheep erythrocytes by phytohemagglutinins. Int. Arch. Allergy *32:* 482–489 (1967).
26. MARKLEY, K.; EVANS, G. and SMALLMAN, E.: Prolongation of skin allograft survival time by phytohemagglutinin. Transplantation *5:* 1535–1537 (1967).
27. MOORE, C.D. and STEFANI, S.S.: The effect of phytohemagglutinin on skin allograft survival in mice. Fed. Proc. *27:* 432 (1968). (Personal communication.)
28. NORINS, L.C. and MARSHALL, W.H.: Phytohemagglutinin. Lancet *ii:* 647–648 (1964).
29. NOWELL, P.C.: Phytohemagglutinin: An initiator of mitosis in cultures of normal human leukocytes. Cancer Res. *20:* 462–466 (1960).
30. REISFELD, R.A.; BORJESON, J.B.; CHESSIN, L.N. and SMALL, P.A., JR.: Isolation and characterization of a mitogen from pokeweed (Phytolacca Americana). Proc. nat. Acad. Sci. *58:* 2020–2027 (1967).
31. SINGHAL, S.K.; NASPRITZ, C.K. and RICHTER, M.: The action of phytohemagglutinin in rabbits. I. The enhancement of the primary immune response to human serum albumin, bovine gamma globulin and sheep erythrocytes. Int. Arch. Allergy *31:* 390–398 (1967).
32. SPREAFICO, F. and LERNER, E.M.: Suppression of the primary and secondary immune response of the mouse by phytohemagglutinin. J. Immunol. *98:* 407–416 (1967).
33. ST. PIERRE, R.L.; YOUNGER, J.B. and ZMIJEWSKI, C.M.: Effects of phytohemagglutinin on skin allograft survival in mice. Proc. Soc. exp. Biol., N.Y. *126:* 687–690 (1967).

Authors' address: Dr. M. LANDY and Dr. L.N. CHESSIN, National Institute of Allergy and Infectious Diseases, National Institutes of Health, *Bethesda, Md.* (USA).

Antibiotica et Chemotherapia, vol. 15, pp. 213–233 (Karger, Basel/New York 1969)

Immunosuppression by Carcinogens

J. STJERNSWÄRD

Department of Tumorbiology, Karolinska Institutet, Stockholm

Tumor Specific Antigens and Chemical Carcinogenesis

Oncogenesis may be influenced by two decisive events the *induction* of neoplastic cells, either by a virus, chemical carcinogen or spontaneous cellular variations leading to malignancy, and by a *selection* stage e. g. by the subsequent interaction between the proliferative tendency of the changed cells and the restricting mechanisms of the host, including conventional immunological and hormonal regulation mechanisms. The final outcome will be the resultant of this balance and the added probability of the tumor cell escape by variation and selection.

The well documented difference between the antigenic cross-reactivity of tumors induced by the same virus in contrast to the antigenic individuality of the chemically induced tumors [41, 43, 57, 69] suggests that the induction stage may proceed along different pathways in the two systems, already at the very first stage, the induction.

Specific transplantation antigens capable of inducing rejection reactions in genetically compatible hosts are present and relatively stable in all virus induced tumors so far investigated [41, 43, 57, 69]. They are characteristic and differ in specificity for different oncogenic viruses. There is direct evidence, at least as far as the Rous and polyoma viruses are concerned [16, 70, 78] that the neoplastic transformation is the direct result of an interaction between the oncogenic virus and the target cells. Neoplastically transformed tumor cells that no longer produce infectious virus have been shown to contain virus specific messenger RNA in the polyoma and adeno-12 systems [8] and in addition to the specific transplantation antigen, they also contain antigenic complement fixing "neoantigens". This indicates that at least some viruses induce the neoplastic change directly by introducing new genetic information. The immunodepressive effect found for four experimentally selected viruses, the Friend, Moloney, Rauscher and Gross passage A viruses [66, 55, 17, 67, 68, 23 and 58] may also suggest an inherent ability of the viruses to affect the selection phase, the host surveillance mechanisms. Moloney and Gross may also induce specific tolerance if transmitted to the newborn [42].

Chemical carcinogens possibly also may be capable of inducing a neoplastic change by direct action on the target cell, involving the alterations at the hereditary information level. The theory that an early event in carcinogenesis may be an alteration in the expression of genetic information which would reflect itself in an altered metabolism of messenger RNA as suggested by Jacob and Monod [35], is supported by recent findings [21, 22, 47]. Not only with proteins [31] but also with DNA, do the hydrocarbons interact [12, 24].

Chromosomal changes were found in MCA-induced tumors although there was no correlation to malignancy [32]. Recently it has been claimed by Berwald and Sachs [10] that *in vitro* cell transformation with BaP and MCA may occur. Thus both empirical and theoretical data exist to lend support to the possibility that the carcinogenic hydrocarbons may act directly on the induction level.

The antigenicity of the induced tumors represents somewhat of a paradox. A possible explanation is interference with the hosts ability to cope with the arising tumor. Another possibility is that the neoplastic cells have changed in some way that renders them capable of escaping the defense mechanisms of the host. Regarding this selection stage, the carcinogens may not only interfer with it at the host level, as demonstrated and discussed below, by interfering with the hosts defense mechanisms, but also act through the changes at target cell level. Neoplastic cells arising after hydrocarbon carcinogenesis are possibly less sensitive to the toxic effect of the carcinogens than normal non-neoplastic cells as reviewed by Vasiliev and Guelstein [84].

Theoretically the most potent carcinogen among the ones that induce antigenic tumor cells would be a substance capable of changing not only normal cells into neoplastic by direct action but also of interfering with the surveillance mechanisms of the host. The carcinogen's oncogenic power, or rather ability to induce antigenic neoplastic cells would thus be dependent on their ability to influence both levels, induction and selection.

The individual antigenic specificity of the tumors arising after exposure to aromatic hydrocarbons permits us only to speculate about the induction stage. The possibility cannot be excluded that the effect of some carcinogens is purely selective [13, 39, 61], rather than inductive.

Spontaneous cellular changes may be responsible for the malignant transformation proceeding along slightly different pathways in the different cases, and the function of the carcinogen would be merely to interfere with host surveillance mechanisms and thus allow their selective outgrowth. It is relevant in this context that certain tumors induced by aromatic hydrocarbons show a relatively strong tumor specific antigenicity and can induce rejection reactions in syngeneic and autochthonous hosts as well, whereas spontaneously arising tumors of similar type are more weakly antigenic or entirely non-antigenic [3, 4, 41, 59]. This further emphasizes the question whether there exists a correlation between the antigenicity of the induced tumor and the ability of the inducing agents to interfere with the immunological defense mechanisms of the host.

A related question concerns the mechanisms whereby strongly antigenic tumors are allowed to develop, and the ways in which they escape rejection and the nature of the primary tumor bearing host's immune status against its own tumor.

On a random basis both antigenic gain and loss mutations can be expected to occur. This would be compatible with the findings that it is sometimes possible to show gain of antigens, specific for the neoplastic cells, but often only in a certain percent of the tested tumors within the same carcinogenic system. Loss of already existing tissue specific antigens or differentiation products related to the variation in cell function may possibly occur. It cannot be ruled out definitely at present that the concept of tumor specific antigens may be a laboratory artifact of this century, selected for by the experimentalists. Fortunately—indications exist that spontaneous tumors, both in human and experimental host may contain tumor-specific antigens or at least some factor that differentiate them from the normal cells of its host [3, 14, 42].

The question of antigenicity is thus of importance as well as the factors causing variations in it. Analyses of the latter factors, that will say, those factors that influence the degree of antigenicity, qualitatively as well as quantitatively, may reveal what causes the variations and give a clue to how the antigenic neoplastic cells escape the host's defence mechanisms thereby killing him.

Inducing Agents

A review of substances, chemical carcinogens, physical agents as well as viruses demonstrated to induce antigenic tumors in experimental host is given in table I, as well as a summary of the substances ability to effect the host's immune status when tested.

Table I. Tumor specific antigens in experimental tumors. Inducing agents and their effect on the immune reactivity of the host

Tumor induction by:	Relative degree of antigenicity	Immune status of the host found depressed after carcinogen exposure as measured by:
Chemical carcinogens		
3-Methylcholanthrene	++	PFC[1], AB:S[2], autochthonous and syngeneic tumor grafts, skin grafts
1, 2, 5, 6-Dibenzanthracene		
9, 10-Dimethylbenzanthracene		PFC
3, 4, 9, 10-Dibenzpyrene		
3–4 Benzpyrene	+	PFC
P-Dimethylaminoazobenzene		
Diethylnitrosamine		
Physical carcinogens		
Ultraviolett Light		
Strontium -90	+	PFC, AB:S
Cellophane film	±	
Millipore filter	±	
Viruses		
Polyoma		
SV 40		
Adenovirus 12, 18		
Shope papilloma		
Mammary tumor agent [BITTNER]		
Gross	+	PFC
Moloney	++	PFC, γ-Globulin levels
Rauscher		PFC, AB:S
Friend		PFC, AB:S
Graffi		
Rous [SCHMIDT-RUPPIN]		PFC
Spontaneous (?)		Age

[1] PFC = hemolytice plaque-forming spleen cells.
[2] AB:S = humoral antibody response to injected antigens, e.g. sheep erythrocytes T-2 phage.

Factors Determining Variations in Antigenicity

Both depending on the type of inducing agent, its way of administration and dose and on the host, particularly its species, strain, sex and age—the frequency of tumors, their appearance and possibly also their antigenic strength may vary. Antigenicity is measured by the degree of resistance that can be built up in an immunized host in relation to appropriate controls and by the number of viable cells required to break through this. Within groups of tumors induced by the same carcinogen the antigenic "strength" of the individual tumors, measured by the level of resistance that could be built up against them by specific immunization, was variable and inversely related to the *duration of the latency period* after carcinogen administration [56]. The data of Klein *et al.* [44, 45] show a clear difference in antigenicity between tumors induced by MCA and tumors induced by cellophane films. The latter tumors are only slightly antigenic and their latency period is much longer than that for the MCA-induced sarcomas [44, 45]. With longer latency periods Prehn found an inverse correlation between antigenicity of MCA, DBA, millipore and spontaneous occuring tumors and their antigenicity [63, 64]. Probably due to an insufficient spread in the latency time of the tested MCA and dibenz (a, h) anthrazene-induced tumors, no clear correlation between latency period and antigenicity was found for tumors induced by these two substances by Prehn. Furthermore well documented correlations between dose of inducing carcinogen and latency period before appearance of the antigenic cells exist [11, 27, 28, 81].

Another factor, which seems to be of importance for the degree of tumor antigenicity is the *immune status of the host*. This is best demonstrated by the findings of Balner and Dersjant [7] who found that tumors induced by MCA in mice thymectomized as newborn had an increased antigenicity although tumor frequency or latency period or type of tumor did not change with thymectomy. In agreement with the concept that the more antigenic tumors are rejected by the intact primary host, Miller *et al.* [51] found that thymectomy of newborned increased the frequency of primary BaP induced sarcomas. Grant and Miller [29] furthermore found that neonatal thymectomy in C57BL mice shortened the latency period of the arising sarcomata after MCA-exposure. Data by Defendi and Roosa [20] indicate that thymectomized mice, particularly females, get an increased and earlier incidence of subcutaneous fibrosarcomas after MCA-exposure. Yasu-

Hira [86] described "chemical thymectomy" after intraperitoneal injection of MCA in newborn mice. Both homograft and delayed hypersensitivity reaction [2, 49] as well as the number of PFC and humoral antibody response were shown to decrease after thymectomy [52, 26]. Nishizuka et al. [54] could show that thymectomy increases the frequency of hepatic tumors after MCA-exposure.

More indirect findings of Davidsohn and Stern [18] also suggest a correlation between immunological reactivity and tumor incidence. They studied eleven strains of inbred mice. Of these, five showed a low tumor incidence and a vigorous immune response to SRBC. Of the remaining six strains which showed a very low capacity to form antibodies, five showed a low capacity to form antibodies. The low immunological capacity of the DBA/2 and C3H strains, which have a high incidence of spontaneous tumors, was confirmed by others too when testing for immune reactivity by different antigens [33, 34], as well as the genetic background for the high reactivity of the C57BL mouse [40], a strain with low tumor incidence.

A clear difference exists between spontaneous tumors and chemically induced tumors with regard to antigenic strength. The most rapidly acting carcinogens used in experimental work may well be the ones that induce the most strongly antigenic tumors by producing the most drastic cellular changes in the induction phase and/or excerting the strongest immunodepressive effect to permit their outgrowth.

The increased incidence of many forms of spontaneous cancer with *age* is an unquestionable fact. It was found that immunological reactivity decreased with age [73, 85] both when measured by humoral antibody production and rejection of small, graded doses of tumor cells carrying tumor specific antigens. It is possible that the age-dependent decrease of immune responsiveness and increase of tumor incidence are more than superficially related. No clear evidence exists, indicating if the tumors induced or arising spontaneously in different age groups vary in their degree of antigenic strength. Expressed as tumor incidence we know that newborns are more sensitive to the oncogenic power of both carcinogenic hydrocarbons [38, 82, 83] and viruses [30].

Host—Carcinogen Relationship

a) Immunosuppressive effect of MCA. The observed antigenicity of MCA, BaP and DMBA-induced tumors may be related either to a direct action of the carcinogenic hydrocarbon on the target cells as discussed above, and/or an indirect effect on some host resistance mechanism, leading to a failure to eliminate antigenic neoplastic cell variants. The latter explanation is favoured by the demonstrated existence of host resistance mechanisms in immunologically undisturbed hosts, capable of preventing the outgrowth of small antigenic tumor grafts. The immunological nature of this host resistance is indicated by its radiosensitivity, its strengthening after preimmunization and the regular and specific tumor inhibiting ability of sensitized host lymphoid cells. In what way can antigenic tumors develop at all? The increased tumor incidence and the increased antigenicity of the developing tumors in recipients exposed to carcinogenic hydrocarbons and which had been thymectomized when newborn [7, 20, 51] indicates that at least certain tumors are naturally rejected and that the host immune status may be of critical significance. Based on this reasoning, the effect of the carcinogens on host immune status was the main subject of the present investigation.

Earlier investigations on carcinogens and immune responses [19, 48, 66], differed in their results and are on the basis of the data given not absolutely conclusive. Malmgren et al. [48] found that two carcinogenic hydrocarbons depressed the antisheep haemolysin antibody titers as compared to non-carcinogenic analogues. The test substances were given in relatively high doses between two to three mg and haemolysin titers against SRBC were measured only at a single point on the 5th day after the administration of the test antigen. This study did not clarify the question whether the carcinogens caused a real depression or merely a delay in antibody response or whether the carcinogens depressed the immune response when given in the lower doses used in tumor induction experiments. Although no data was given, Davidsohn et al. [19] claimed that skin painting of MCA depressed the antibody response in one strain, but was without effect in another, but no details of their experiments were given. Rubin [65] claimed that subcutaneous administration of the carcinogenic hydrocarbons did not depress the humoral antibody response towards SRBC. However, the experimental design in the administration of the testantigen, SRBC, given seven times intraperitoneally as 0.5 ml of a 5% SRBC solution as well as 0.4 ml intravenously seven times and bleeding ten days after the last injection certainly may mask any differences in haemagglutinating and haemolysing antibody response between MCA-exposed and unexposed hosts [65].

In view of these rather inconclusive previous results, the present study was undertaken to investigate in more detail whether MCA, the first carcinogen shown to induce strongly antigenic sarcomas after subcutaneous administration, was capable of affecting the immune status of the exposed animal to a serious extent. The dose given (0.5 mg) was within the range routinely used for induction experiments. To study the effect of MCA on the cell population engaged in antibody formation, the number of individual antibody forming spleen cells, PFC, was determined during the oncogenesis by a haemolytic agar plaque technique *in vitro* [36, 37] at different time intervals after carcinogen exposure.

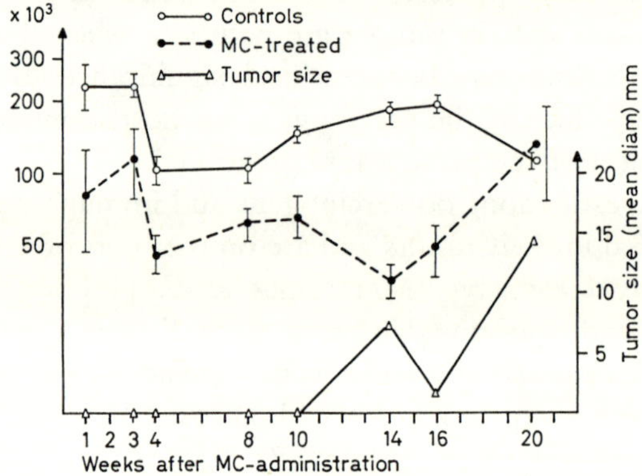

Fig. 1. Depressive effect of 3-methylcholanthrene on the number of plaque-forming spleen cells (PFC) per spleen. Arithmetic means and standard error of the mean are given at the different test intervals for mice inoculated with antigen four days previously. Mean tumor diameters in mm are given on the righthand abscissa.

After a single MCA exposure prior to antigen administration the number of PFC reached lower levels than in the untreated controls and remained depressed for a period of several months, *corresponding in length to the latency period* prior to the appearance of the antigenic primary MCA-induced sarcomas (figs. 1 and 2). A depression was also evident both when comparing to the total number of PFC/spleen and their relative number, expressed as proportion of PFC per 10^6 nucleated spleen cells. There was also a reduction in the humoral haemolysing and haemagglutinating antibody titers towards the same test antigen, sheep erythrocytes. The primary and the secondary anamnestic immune response were both affected [71]. The survival of skin grafted across a monospecific weak histocompatibility barrier (H-1), was not affected during the earlier part of the tumor latency period. The transplants did show a prolonged survival in tumor bearing hosts or at the time of appearance of primary tumors.

Although different mechanisms are probably responsible, it should be mentioned that an immuno depressive effect also has been found after exposure to five experimentally oncogenic selected viruses, that induce antigenic tumors, as discussed in detail in this symposium by Salaman [pages 393–406].

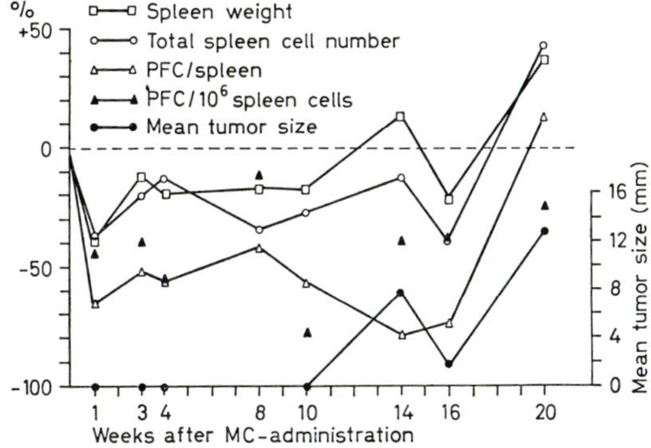

Fig. 2. Effect of exposure to 0.5 mg MCA on the host's spleen weight, total spleen number, PFC/spleen and PFC/10⁶ nucleated spleen cells measured at different time intervals after MCA-exposure, expressed as difference in percent between MCA-treated and trioctanoin treated controls (0 %).

b) Immunosuppressive specificity as correlated to carcinogenicity. In further studies [72] an attempt was made to investigate whether the carcinogenic and immunodepressive effect were correlated when comparing different hydrocarbons (table II). Three carcinogenic and three

Table II. Compounds tested and their degree of carcinogenicity

Test compound	Abbreviations used in text	Degree of carcinogenicity
Trioctanoin	Tri	—
Anthracene	Ae	—
Benzo[*e*]pyrene	BeP	—
7-Methyldibenzanthracene	MDBA	±
Benzo[*a*]pyrene	BaP	+
7,12-Dimethylbenz[*a*]anthracene	DMBA	+
3-Methylcholanthrene	MCA	+

non-carcinogenic hydrocarbons were tested. BaP, DMBA and MCA, all potent carcinogens capable of inducing antigenic neoplastic cells, showed a clear immunodepressive effect on the number of PFC in the haemolytic agar plaque assay. DMBA had a slight but not significant effect, and the non-carcinogenic hydrocarbons Ae and BeP showed no immunodepressive effect. This lends support to the assumption of a possible correlation between the carcinogenic power inducing antigenic tumor cells and the immuno depressive effect (fig. 3).

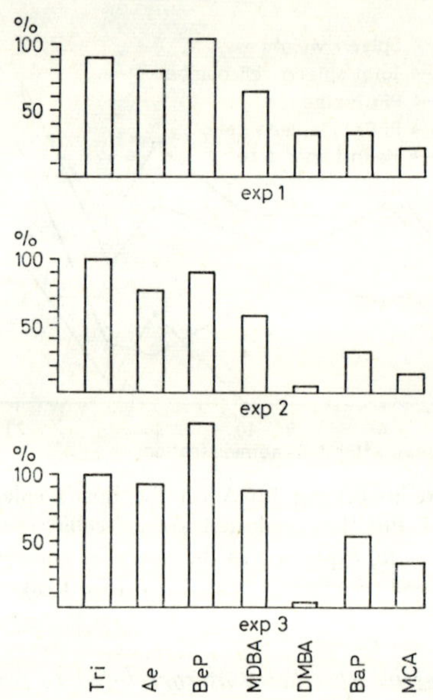

Fig. 3. Effect of Ae, BeP, MDBA, DMBA, BaP and MCA compared to that of Tri on the number of plaque forming cells per spleen.

More important than a substance's ability to work at the induction stage in a host with intact selection mechanism may be the observed long lasting immunodepression, for the fact that strongly antigenic tumor cells were found [71]. Lots of substances causing immune depression are not carcinogenic [9]. Our findings of the long lasting immuno depressive effect of a single MCA exposure have been confirmed later for another carcinogen DMBA [5] and also after the exposure of newborn mice to as little as 150 μg MCA [6]. Also in another oncogenic system, where weakly antigenic tumor cells arise after experimental induction a similar long lasting depression of the

Table III. Prolonged depression of PFC number after a single Sr^{90}-exposure [77]

No. of mice	Treatment	Total number of nucleated cells $\times$ 10^6	Number of PFC/spleen $\times$ 10^3	Number of PFC/10^6 nucleated spleen cells
5	Untreated	137.0 ± 10.2	43.3 ± 7.0	313.7 ± 35.7
5	Sr^{90}-7 months-SRBC	84.0 ± 13.1	11.7 ± 3.2	59.5 ± 15.6

Table III. Statistically, the differences were significant at the following percent levels, between untreated and strontium-90, Sr^{90}, exposed: for PFC/spleen 0.01 (t = 4.1) and for PFC/10^6 nsc 0.001 (t = 6.5).

host's immune response was found after a single exposure to 0.9 μC of strontium^{90}, Sr^{90} [77]. The number of PFC was significantly depressed up to seven months after the Sr^{90} administration (table III). At this time about 20 % of the injected Sr^{90} dose still may be demonstrated in the skeleton [53].

Tumors induced by urethane were rarely or not at all found to possess detectable tumor-specific antigens [62]. It is uncertain whether tumor inducing doses of urethane have any immunodepressive effect of long duration. MALMGREN *et al.* [48] used excessively high doses and found an immunodepression on the 5th day after antigen administration, and DAVIDSOHN *et al.* [19] did not find any immunodepressive effect of urethane. The latter result is further supported by the finding that urethane administration failed to facilitate the take of an antigenic tumor transplant as compared to some carcinogenic polycyclic hydrocarbons that were highly efficient in this respect. Nor did urethane administered before, concurrently or at various times after DMBA administration have any effect on the incidence of sarcomas induced by DMBA [80].

c) Dose response studies. Dose-response studies of the immunodepressive effect of the carcinogen appeared to be of interest in view of available information concerning the relationship between carcinogen dose and tumor frequency and latency period as well as between the length of the latency period and antigenic strength of the tumors that arise. The effect of MCA was studied therefore in the dose range between 0.1 mg and 5 mg, including fractionated exposure to multiple small doses [75] (fig. 4).

The dose-effect relationship studies of MCA dose versus PFC depression showed that PFC dropped sharply when the dose was increased from 0.1 to 1.0 mg MCA. Further increase up to 5.0 mg

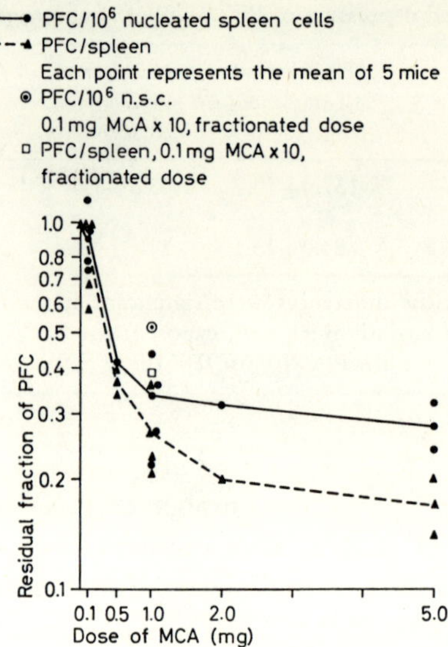

Fig. 4. The mean number of plaque-forming spleen cells, PFC, for 13 different groups, each consisting of five or six mice exposed to MCA in doses between 0.1 and 5.0 mg. The immunodepressive effect is always related to a control group, always beeing 1.0 tested at the same time.

had little effect. Repeated exposure to small doses of the carcinogen led to a cumulative immunodepressive effect. This may agree with the long lasting immunodepressive effect found earlier for a single dose. In addition to the subcutaneous route of administration skin painting of MCA was found to decrease immune reactivity as well [75].

As with earlier studies [19, 48, 65] doubts can be raised whether the results reflect any real immune depression, or the documented differences were only due to a delay in time of the appearance of the maximal immune response, which would mean that no real change in the total reactivity occurred. To investigate whether the effects observed merely represented a delay in the time of appearance of maximal response, the number of PFC was determined 2, 3, 4, 5, 6 and 12 days after exposure to MCA. A decrease of the total immune response was found both when expressed as PFC/spleen and PFC per relative unit nucleated spleen cells [75] (fig. 5).

d) Influence of the carcinogen-exposure on host resistance. It was considered of importance to explore if the demonstrated immuno depression by the carcinogen also affected the host's immune responts towards the carcinogen-induced tumors. Specially as the earlier resulse

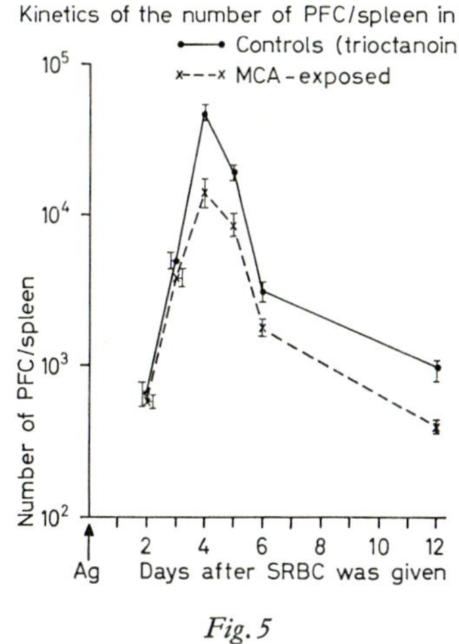

Fig. 5

only reflects the effect of the carcinogens on the humoral antibody response. To test if the cellular immune response also was affected, the outgrowth of small graded doses of antigenic tumor transplants was investigated in MCA-exposed and unexposed hosts [73]. In view of the antigenic variations characteristic for MCA-induced tumors as many different tumors as feasible was tested. Seventy-five different primary MCA-induced sarcomas were tested as first generation transplants by grafting cell doses varying between 10^3 and 10^6 cells to untreated and MCA-exposed hosts. Fifty-five of the 75 tested tumors grew significantly better in the latter category of recipients (tables IV and V).

These findings are in good agreement with the previous results of PREHN [60] and they support the conclusion that MCA-exposure of the host facilitates the outgrowth of MCA-induced tumors. PREHN found furthermore a certain relationship between the growth facilitation of a transplanted tumor in the MCA treated host and the immuno-

Table IV. Takes of first-generation transplants of sarcomas induced by MCA in MCA-exposed and unexposed syngeneic recipients

	Number of mice with tumor/no. inoculated			
Number of tumor cells inoculated	10^3	10^4	10^5	10^6
MCA-exposed hosts	32/39	90/102	56/56	9/9
Untreated hosts	17/40	56/104	55/56	9/9

Table V. Difference in growth of MCA-induced sarcomas in MCA-exposed hosts and in controls

Growth in MCA-exposed host compared to unexposed	Number of viable tumor cells transplanted subcutaneously			
	10^3	10^4	10^5	10^6
Better	13/18	31/42	11/25	2/7
Same	5/18	8/42	7/25	5/7
Worse	—	3/42	1/25	—
Number of different tumors tested	18	42	25	7

genicity of the same tumor in syngeneic hosts. No growth facilitation was observed if MCA was given simultaneously with the tumor graft. This corresponds well with the present findings and could be explained by our findings below of the dramatic difference in MCA's immuno depressive effect depending on whether it is given before or after the antigen [75].

A decreased reactivity towards normal and tumor tissue homografts was observed after MCA-exposure [46, 60, 65, 71]. Skin graft survival was only facilitated in MCA-exposed hosts, at the time when primary tumors appeared [46, 71]. A decreased reactivity also has been documented in the human cancer patient both in regard to delayed hypersensitivity skin reactions and ability to respond to heteroantigens. The rejection of skin and cancer homografts was delayed and in lymphocyte transfer tests lymphocytes from normal donors produced a stronger reaction than did those obtained from cancer patients. It is still uncertain whether this is a secondary result of the tumor burden or may be a primary event in the oncogenic process. A prolonged survival of tumor homografts was observed in mice bearing a MCA-induced tumor transplant [50].

e) Relationships between carcinogen dose, immunodepression, tumor latency and antigenicity. Data exist [27, 28, 81] showing a clear correlation between dose of hydrocarbon injected and latency period prior to tumor development. An inverted relationship also was found between the length of the latency period and antigenicity of the arising tumor, both when comparing tumors induced by the same agent [56] and for groups of tumors induced by different agents [44, 45, 63]. A dose-effect study was undertaken to investigate the effect of various doses of MCA as well as small fractionated doses of PFC number [75].

The dose-effect relationship studies of MCA dose versus PFC depression showed that PFC dropped sharply when the dose was increased from 0.1 to 1.0 mg MCA. Further increase up to 5.0 mg had little effect (fig. 4).

In contrast to the experimental induction of tumors by large doses of strong carcinogens in the laboratory, chemical carcinogenesis under natural conditions is more likely to result from fractionated exposure to small doses of chemicals over long periods of time. Fractionated exposure to the carcinogen MCA, led to a cumulative immunodepressive effect in our tests, perhaps comparable to the total dose [75]. The same is known to be true with regard to the carcinogenic effect of this compound.

The data thus suggests that an inverse relationship between a tumor's immunizing capacity in syngeneic host, and length of its latency period exists. Comprehensive data demonstrate correlation between dose of inducing hydrocarbons and tumor latency period [27, 28, 81]. The observed immunological dose-effect relationship between MCA dose and PFC [75] together with the effect of such an induced immunodepression on the host's ability to reject small antigenic tumor transplants, suggests that the induced depression may be of importance for the ability of antigenic tumor cells to arise. In a slightly depressed host only tumors of weak antigenicity can develop while more strongly antigenic clones may fail. The relatively low or missing ability of spontaneous tumors to specifically immunize may thus reflect that they arosen through an intact selection pressure.

This conclusion is supported by the increased carcinogenic power of hydrocarbon in newborn as compared to adult [38, 82, 83] seen in the light of the variation of the immune status with age [73, 85] as well as the increased incidence of spontaneous tumors with senescence [15, 25].

f) Possible immunosuppressive specificity and first target. The question arises whether the immuno depressive effect of the carcinogen was an expression of a general toxicity or had a more specific component. The effect of MCA on PFC was very different, depending on the time of MCA administration in relation to the introduction of antigen. The immune depressive effect was much less pronounced if MCA was given 1 ½ h after than 1 ½ h before the antigen as seen in figures 6 and 7, showing the summary of the results from four different experiments. The results indicates that a very early step, possibly related to the uptake of the antigen, is most sensitive to MCA. Once the process leading to a PFC has begun, MCA seems to have a much smaller effect. If indeed the first cells processing the antigen

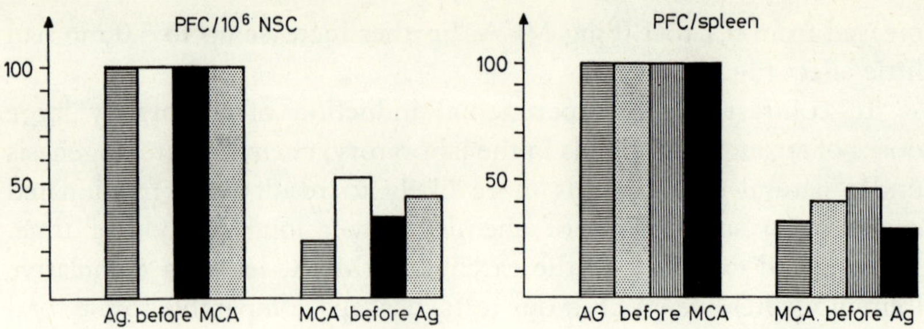

Figs. 6 and 7. Effect of MCA on PFC/spleen and PFC/10⁶ nucleated spleen cells when given 1 ½ h before the antigen, SRBC, compared to the effect of MCA given 1 ½ h after the antigen (100 %).

are affected and if these cells are also the first actively engulfing MCA, in parallel with the findings of, e. g. Dr. White in this symposium, demonstrating that similar cells in the chicken spleen collect and preserve injected antigen as well as non-antigenic carbon particles, a remarkable effect would be achieved even by low doses of carcinogen when given before the antigen.

As described above, MCA seems to affect the immune cells within the spleen cell population specifically, as the relative number of PFC/10⁶ nucleated spleen cells is depressed. This, as well as the unchanged doubling time in PFC number in unexposed as compared to MCA exposed hosts, together with the dramatic decrease in the effect of the carcinogen if given 1 ½ h after the antigen instead of 1 ½ h before, suggests that the immune system and especially a very early step in the process leading to a PFC after antigen exposure is particularly sensitive to the carcinogens.

Summary

A quantitative haemolytic agar plaque technique was adopted to study the effect of a carcinogenic hydrocarbon, 3-methylcholanthrene, MCA, on the immune response of the exposed host. A single exposure to the carcinogen rapidly depressed the number of plaque-forming spleen cells, PFC, during a long period of time, corresponding to the latency period of tumor development.

In addition to a depression of the number of PFC per total spleen there was also a specific decrease of PFC within the nucleated spleen cell population, after host exposure to the carcinogenic hydrocarbons benz(a)pyrene (BaP), 7,12-dimethyl-benz(a)-anthracene (DMBA) or MCA. The non-carcinogenic hydrocarbons anthracene (Ae) and benz(e)pyrene (BeP) had no such immunodepressive effect. 7-methyldibenzanthracene (MDBA) had a slightly depressive effect on PFC. BaP, DMBA and MCA are all potent carcinogens, and the tumors they induce carry tumor specific antigens. It was suggested that a correlation may exist between the ability of a carcinogen to induce antigenic tumor and its inhibitory effect on host immune responses.

MCA administration also affected the host's ability to reject small cell doses from syngeneic MCA-induced sarcomas, known to carry tumor specific antigens. A significantly higher incidence of takes and/or earlier tumor appearance was seen in the MCA-exposed hosts.

Analysis of the MCA-induced immune depressions as a function of time after administration of the carcinogen showed that it was not due merely to a delay in time of the appearance of the maximum immune response. The relatively greater decrease in the proportion of antibody forming spleen cells as related to the total number of nucleated spleen cells indicated furthermore that antibody forming cells were affected in a rather specific manner.

The effect of MCA on PFC was very different, depending on the time of MCA administration in relation to the introduction of the antigen. The immunodepressive effect was much less pronounced if MCA was given 1 ½ h after than 1 ½ h before the antigen. The doubling time of PFC numbers was the same in MCA-exposed and in untreated hosts. This was interpretated to mean that a very early step in the process leading, to the formation of PFC, possibly related to antigen uptake, was a particularly sensitive target for MCA action.

Acknowledgements

The investigation was made possible by generous financial support from the Swedish Cancer Society.

References

1. ABELEV, G.I.: Antigenic structure of chemically-induced hepatomas. Prog. exp. Tum. Res. *7:* 104–157 (1965).
2. ARNASON, B.G.; JANKOVIC, B.D. and WAKSMAN, B.H.: Effect of thymectomy on delayed hypersensitivity reactions. Nature *194:* 99–100 (1962).
3. BALDWIN, R.W.: Tumour-specific immunity against spontaneous rat tumours. Int. J. Cancer *1:* 257–264 (1966).
4. BALDWIN, R.W.: Immunity to methylcholanthrene-induced tumours in inbred rats following atrophy and regression of the implanted tumours. Brit. J. Cancer *9:* 652–657 (1955).
5. BALL, J.K.; SINCLAIR, N.R. and McCARTER, J.A.: Prolonged immuno-suppression and tumor induction by a chemical carcinogen injected at birth. Science *152:* 650–651 (1966).
6. BALL, J.K.: (Personal communication).
7. BALNER, H. and DERSJANT, H.: Neonatal thymectomy and tumor induction with methylcholanthrene in mice. J. nat. Cancer Inst. *36:* 513–521 (1966).
8. BENJAMIN, T.L.: Virus specific RNA in cells productively infected or transformed by polyoma virus. J. mol. Biol. *16:* 359–365 (1966).
9. BERENBAUM, M.C.: Effects of carcinogens on immune processes. Brit. med. Bull. *20:* 159–164 (1964).
10. BERWALD, Y. and SACHS, L.: *In vitro* cell transformation with chemical carcinogens. Nature *200:* 1182–1184 (1963).
11. BRYAN, W.R. and SHIMKIN, M.B.: Quantitative analysis of dose response data obtained with carcinogenic hydrocarbons. J. nat. Cancer Inst. *1:* 807–833 (1941).
12. BROOKES, P. and LAWLEY, P.D.: Evidence of the binding of polynuclear aromatic hydrocarbons to the nucleic acids of mouse skin: Relation between carcinogenic

power of hydrocarbons and their bindings to deoxyribonucleic acid. Nature *202:* 781–789 (1964).

13. Burnet, F.M.: Immunological factors in the process of carcinogenesis. Brit. med. Bull. *20:* 154–158 (1964).

14. Chu, E.H.Y.; Stjernswärd, J.; Clifford, P. and Klein, G.: Reactivity of human lymphocytes against autochthonous and allogeneic normal and tumor cells *in vitro.* J. nat. Cancer Inst. *39:* 595–617 (1967).

15. Clemmesen, J.: Statistical studies in malignant neoplasms. I. Review and results. II. Basic tables, Denmark, 1943–1957 (Munksgaard, Köpenhamn 1965).

16. Crawford, L.; Dulbecco, R.; Fried, M.; Montagnier, L. and Stocker, M.: Cell transformation with different forms of polyoma virus DNA. Proc. nat. Acad. Sci. *52:* 148–152 (1964).

17. Cremer, N.E.; Taylor, D.O.N. and Hagens, S.J.: Antibody formation, latency and leukemia: Infection with Moloney virus. J. Immunol. *96:* 495–508 (1966).

18. Davidsohn, I. and Stern, K.: Heterohemoantibodies in inbred strains of mice. II. Immune agglutinins and hemolysins for sheep and chicken red cells. J. Immunol. *72:* 216–223 (1954).

19. Davidsohn, I.; Stern, K. and Sabet, L.: Immune response in mice and rats exposed to carcinogens. Amer. Ass. Cancer Res. *2:* 102 (1956).

20. Defendi, V. and Roosa, R.A.: The role of the thymus in carcinogenesis. In: The thymus, pp. 121–128 (Eds.) V. Defendi and D. Metcalf, Wistar Inst. Symp. Monogr. No. 2 (1964).

21. DeMayer-Guignard, J. and DeMayer, E.: Effect of carcinogenic and noncarcinogenic hydrocarbons on interferon and virus plaque development, J. nat. Cancer Inst. *34:* 265–276 (1965).

22. DeMayer, E. and DeMayer-Guignard, J.: Effect of polycyclic aromatic carcinogens on virus replication: similarity to actinomycin D. Science *146:* 650–651 (1964).

23. Dent, P.B.; Peterson, R.D.A. and Good, R.A.: A defect in cellular immunity during the incubation period of passage a leukemia in C3H mice. Proc. Soc. Exp. biol. Med. *119:* 869–871 (1965).

24. Diamond, L.; Defendi, V. and Brookes, P.: The interaction of 7-12-dimethylbenz-(a)anthracene with cells sensitive and resistant to toxicity induced by this carcinogen. Cancer Res. *27:* 890–897 (1967).

25. Dorn, H.F. and Cutler, S.J.: Morbidity from cancer in the United States. Public Health Monogr. no. 56, U.S. Dept. of Health, Education and Welfare, Washington, D.C., U.S. Govt. Print. Off. (1959).

26. Fichtelius, K.E.; Laurell, M. and Philipson, L.: The influence of thymectomy on antibody formation. Acta path. microbiol. scand. *51:* 81–86 (1961).

27. Graffi, A.: In: Probleme der Krebsforschung und Krebsbekämpfung. Abh. Dtsch. Akad. Wiss., Berlin *1:* 1–28 (1953).

28. Graffi, A. and Bielka, H.: Probleme der experimentellen Krebsforschung (Akademische Verlagsgesellschaft, K.G. Geest und Portig, Leipzig 1959).

29. Grant, G.A. and Miller, J.F.A.P.: Effect of neonatal thymectomy on the induction of sarcomata in C57BL mice. Nature *205:* 1124–1125 (1965).

30. Gross, L.: Oncogenic viruses (Pergamon Press, 1961).

31. Heidelberger, C.: The relation of protein binding to hydrocarbon carcinogenesis. In: Carcinogenesis, mechanisms of action, pp. 179–192 (Ciba Found. Symp. J.A. Church, Ltd., London 1959).

32. Hellström, K.E.: Chromosomal studies on primary methylcholanthrene-induced sarcomas in the mouse. J. nat. Cancer Inst. *23:* 1019–1033 (1959).

33. Ipsen, J.: Inherent immunizability to tetanustoxoid, based on studies in pure inbred mice. J. Immunol. *72:* 243–247 (1954).

34. IPSEN, J.: Difference in primary and secondary immunizability of inbred mice strains. J. Immunol. *83:* 448–457 (1959).
35. JACOB, F. and MONOD, J.: On the regulation of gene activity. Cold Spring Harbor Symp. Quant. Biology *26:* 193–211 (1961).
36. JERNE, N.K. and NORDIN, A.A.: Plaque formation in agar by single antibody-producing cells. Science *140:* 405 (1963).
37. JERNE, N.K.; NORDIN, A.A. and HENRY, C.: The agar plaque technique for recognizing antibody-producing cells. (Eds.) B. AMOS and H. KOPROWSKI. Cellbound antibodies, pp. 109–111 (Wistar Institute Press, Philadelphia 1963).
38. KELLY, M.G. and O'GARA, R.W.: Induction of tumors in newborn mice with dibenz(a, h)anthracene and 3-methylcholanthrene. J. nat. Cancer Inst. *26:* 651–679 (1961).
39. KLEIN, E.: Transplantation antigens as markers in somatic cell genetics. Symp. Quant. Biol. *29:* 273–283 (1964).
40. KLEIN, E. and LINDER, O.: Factorial analysis of the reactivity of C57BL females against isologous male skingrafts. Transplant. Bull. *27:* 457–460 (1961).
41. KLEIN, G.: Tumor antigens. Ann. Rev. Microbiol. *20:* 223–252 (1966).
42. KLEIN, G.; CLIFFORD, P.; KLEIN, E. and STJERNSWÄRD, J.: Search for tumor specific immune reactions in Burkitt lymphoma patients by the membrane immunofluorescence reaction. Proc. nat. Acad. Sci. *55:* 1628–1636 (1966).
43. KLEIN, G. and KLEIN, E.: Antigenic properties of other experimental tumors. Symp. Quant. Biol. *27:* 463–470 (1962).
44. KLEIN, G.; SJÖGREN, H.O. and KLEIN, E.: Demonstration of host resistance against sarcomas induced by implantation of cellophane films in isologous recipients. Cancer Res. *23:* 84–92 (1963).
45. KLEIN, G.; SJÖGREN, H.O.; KLEIN, E. and HELLSTRÖM, K.E.: Demonstration of resistance against methylcholanthrene-induced sarcomas in the primary autochthonous host. Cancer Res. *20:* 1561–1572 (1960).
46. LINDER, O.E.A.: Survival of skin homografts in methylcholanthrene-treated mice and in mice with spontaneous mammary cancers. Cancer Res. *22:* 380–383 (1962).
47. LOEB, L.A. and GELBOIN, H.V.: Stimulation of amino-acid incorporation by nuclear ribonucleic acid from normal and methylcholanthrene-treated rats. Nature *199:* 809–810 (1963).
48. MALMGREN, R.A.; BENNISON, B.E. and MCKINLEY, T.W.: Reduced antibody titers in mice treated with carcinogenic and cancer chemotherapeutic agent. Proc. Soc. exp. biol. Med. *79:* 484–488 (1952).
49. MARTINEZ, C.; KERSEY, J.; PAPERMASTER, B.W. and GOOD, R.A.: Skin homograft survival in thymectomized mice. Proc. Soc. exp. biol. Med. *109:* 193–196 (1962).
50. MATSUYAMA, H. and NAKAMURA, T.: Homologous tumour growth in methylcholanthrene-induced sarcoma bearing mice. Nature *202:* 200 (1964).
51. MILLER, J.F.A.P.; GRANT, G.A. and ROE, F.J.C.: Effect of thymectomy on the induction of skin tumours by 3,4-benzopyrene. Nature *199:* 920–922 (1963).
52. MILLER, J.F.P.A.; DE BURGH, P.M. and GRANT, G.A.: Thymus and the production of antibody-plaque-forming cells. Nature *208:* 1332–1334 (1965).
53. NILSSON, A. and ULLBERG, S.: Uptake and retention of strontium[90] in mouse tissues studied by whole animal autoradiography and impulse counting. Acta Radiol. *58:* 81–98 (1962).
54. NISHIZUKA, K.; NAKAKUKI, K. and USUSI, M.: Enhancing effect of thymectomy on hepatotumorigenesis in Swiss mice following neonatal injection of 20-methylcholanthrene. Nature *205:* 1236–1238 (1965).
55. ODAKA, T.; ISHII, H.; YAMAURA, K. and YAMAMOTO, T.: Inhibitory effect of Friend leukemia virus infection on the antibody formation to sheep erythrocytes in mice. Jap. J. exp. Med. *36:* 277–290 (1966).

56. Old, L. J.; Boyse, E. A.; Clarke, D. A. and Carswell, E. A.: Antigenic properties of chemically induced tumors. Ann. N. Y. Acad. Sci. *101:* 80–106 (1962).
57. Old, L. J. and Boyse, E. A.: Immunology of experimental tumors. Ann. Rev. Med. *15:* 167–186 (1964).
58. Peterson, R. D. A.; Hendrickson, R. and Good, R.: Reduced antibody forming capacity during the incubation period of passage A leukemia in C3H mice. Proc. Soc. exp. biol. Med. (N. Y.) *114:* 516–521 (1963).
59. Prehn, R. T. and Main, J. M.: Immunity to methylcholanthrene-induced sarcomas. J. nat. Cancer Inst. *18:* 769–778 (1957).
60. Prehn, R. T.: Function of depressed immunologic reactivity during carcinogenesis. J. nat. Cancer Inst. *31:* 791–805 (1963).
61. Prehn, R. T.: A clonal selection theory of chemical carcinogenesis. J. nat. Cancer Inst. *32:* 1–17 (1964).
62. Prehn, R. T.: Specific isoantigenicities among chemically induced tumors. Ann. N. Y. Acad. Sci. *101:* 107–113 (1962).
63. Prehn, R. T.: The role of immune mechanisms in the biology of chemically and physically induced tumors. In conceptual advances in immunology and oncology. 16th Ann. Symp. Fund. Cancer Res., pp. 475–485 (Hoeber, New York 1963).
64. Prehn, R. T.: Tumor immunity to nonviral tumors. Canad. Cancer Conf. *5:* 387–395 (1963).
65. Rubin, B. A.: Carcinogen-induced tolerance to homotransplantation. Progr. exp. Tumor Res. *5:* 217–292 (1964).
66. Salaman, M. H. and Wedderburn, N.: The immunodepressive effect of Friend virus. Immunology *10:* 445–458 (1966).
67. Siegel, B. V. and Morton, J. I.: Serum agglutinin levels to sheep red blood cells in mice infected with Rauscher virus. Proc. Soc. exp. biol. Med. *123:* 467–470 (1966).
68. Siegel, B. V. and Morton, J. I.: Depressed antibody response in the mouse infected with Rauscher leukemia virus. Immunology *10:* 559–562 (1966).
69. Sjögren, H. O.: Transplantation methods as a tool for detection of tumor specific antigens. Progr. exp. Tum. Res. *6:* 289–322 (1965).
70. Stoker, M. G. P.: Neoplastic transformation by polyomavirus and its wider implications. Brit. med. J. *i:* 1305–1311 (1963).
71. Stjernswärd, J.: Immunodepressive effect of 3-methylcholanthrene. Antibody formation at cellular level and reaction against weak antigenic homografts. J. nat. Cancer Inst. *35:* 885–892 (1965).
72. Stjernswärd, J.: Effect of non-carcinogenic and carcinogenic hydrocarbons on antibody-forming cells measured at cellular level *in vitro*. J. nat. Cancer Inst. *36:* 1189–1195 (1966).
73. Stjernswärd, J.: Age-dependent tumor host barrier and the effect of carcinogen-induced immunodepression on rejection of isografted methylcholanthrene-induced sarcoma cells. J. nat. Cancer Inst. *37:* 505–512 (1966).
74. Stjernswärd, J.: Immune status of the primary autochthonous host towards its own methylcholanthrene-induced sarcoma. J. nat. Cancer Inst. *40:* 13–22 (1968).
75. Stjernswärd, J.: Further immunological studies of chemical carcinogenesis. J. nat. Cancer Inst. *38:* 515–526 (1967).
76. Stjernswärd, J.: Effect of Bacillus-Calmette-Guérin and/or methylcholanthrene on the antibody forming cells measured at cellular level by a hemolytic plaque test. Cancer Res. *261:* 1591–1595 (1966).
77. Stjernswärd, J.; Révész, L. and Nilsson, A.: Antigenicity of strontium[90]-induced tumors and immunological tumor-host relationships in Sr[90] carcinogenesis (to be published).
78. Temin, H. M. and Rubin, H.: Characteristics of an assay for Rous sarcoma virus and Rous sarcoma cells in tissue culture. Virology *6:* 669–688 (1958).

79. TELLER, M.N.; STOHR, G.; CURLETT, W.; KUBISEK, M.L. and CURTIS, D.: Aging and carcinogenesis. I. Immunity to tumor and skin grafts. J. nat. Cancer Inst. *33:* 649–656 (1964).

80. TOMATIS, L.: Suncutaneous carcinogenesis by implants and by 7,12-dimethyl(a) anthracene. Tumori *52:* 1–16 (1966).

81. TOTH, B. and SHUBIK, P.: Carcinogenesis in Lewis rats injected at birth with 7,12-dimethylbenz(a)anthracene. Brit. J. Cancer *17:* 540–545 (1963).

82. TOTH, B.; RAPAPORT, H. and SHUBIK, P.: Influence of dose and age on the induction of malignant lymphomas and other tumors by 7,12-dimethylbenz(a)anthracene in Swiss mice. J. nat. Cancer Inst. *30:* 723–741 (1963).

83. WALTERS, M.A.: The induction of lung tumours by the injection of 9,10-dimethyl-1,2-benzanthracene (DMBA) into newborn suckling and young adult mice. A dose response study. Brit. J. Cancer *20:* 148–160 (1966).

84. VASILIEV, J.M. and GUELSTEIN, V.I.: Sensitivity of normal and neoplastic cells to the damaging action of carcinogenic substances. A review. J. nat. Cancer Inst. *31:* 1123–1143 (1963).

85. WIGZELL, H. and STJERNSWÄRD, J.: Age-dependent rise and fall of immunological reactivity in the CBA-mouse. J. nat. Cancer Inst. *37:* 513–517 (1966).

86. YASUHIRA, K.: Damage to the thymus and other lymphoid tissues from 3-methylcholanthrene, and subsequent thymoma production in mice. Cancer Res. *24:* 558–569 (1964).

Author's address: Dr. J. STJERNSWÄRD, Department of Tumorbiology, Karolinska-Institutet, *Stockholm* (Sweden).

Antibiotica et Chemotherapia, vol. 15, pp. 234–249 (Karger, Basel/New York 1969)

Antilymphocytic Serum

M. F. A. WOODRUFF

Department of Surgical Science, University of Edinburgh, Edinburgh

Historical Introduction

My interest in the lymphocyte, and its possible role in immunological reactions, goes back more than twenty years to the time when I first read MURPHY's remarkable monograph [36], "The Lymphocyte in Resistance to Tissue Grafting, Malignant Disease and Tuberculous Infection". This was already a classic, having been published in 1926, but it was not widely known and indeed is not widely known today though it is still well worth reading.

MURPHY showed, *inter alia,* that the resistance to tumour homografts and heterografts was diminished in animals whose lymphoid tissue had been depleted by whole body irradiation or by the intraperitoneal injection of a large amount of olive oil. In order to avoid the widespread damage caused by a single large dose of irradiation he used repeated small doses and by this means succeeded in producing a much more selective effect on lymphoid tissue.

It seemed possible that an even greater degree of selectivity might be achieved by substituting for irradiation injection of an antiserum which was specifically active against lymphoid tissue.

The notion that it might be possible to prepare a serum specifically active against one type of cell was first put forward by METCHNIKOFF [30]. METCHNIKOFF had postulated that various atrophic conditions were caused by an undue preponderance of macrophages, and had in consequence suggested that in such cases the integrity of the body might be preserved by administering an antimacrophage serum. In a series of experiments designed to test this hypothesis he prepared antisera by immunizing guinea-pigs with either rat spleen or rabbit lymph node. The sera he obtained were not in fact specifically anti-macrophage, although they did appear to possess a high degree of species specificity.

Metchnikoff's investigations were extended by many other investigators. In the light of more recent developments the work of Pappenheimer, and of Chew and Lawrence, is of particular interest. Pappenheimer [39] immunized rabbits with rat thymus or human tonsil, and showed that the sera thus produced, after absorption with erythrocytes, caused both agglutination and, in the presence of complement, cytolysis of lymphocytes. Chew and Lawrence [8] immunized rabbits with guinea-pig lymph node cells and showed that the resulting antiserum caused a marked fall in the blood lymphocyte count when injected intraperitoneally to guinea-pigs.

In the light of the growing realization of the importance of lymphocytes in the homograft reaction, we decided *inter alia* to study the effect of ALS administration on the behaviour of homografts of skin and other tissues. These experiments [46] which were performed in rats using rabbit antirat ALS, yielded only negative results, and we were discouraged from pursuing the matter by our failure to maintain a prolonged lymphopenia in the treated animals, since at that time we assumed (erroneously, as is now apparent) that the only way in which ALS might conceivably exert an immunosuppressive effect would be by causing severe and prolonged lymphocyte depletion. Some years later however Woodruff and Anderson [48, 49] obtained decisive prolongation of skin homograft survival in rats treated with much more potent serum prepared by immunizing rabbits with rat thoracic duct lymphocytes.

Immunosuppressive Properties of ALS and Fractions in Vivo

The homograft reaction. Administration of ALS or globulin derived therefrom has been shown to prevent or delay the rejection of homografts of various kinds including skin homografts in rats [48, 49, 37], mice [15, 32, 28, 29], monkeys [4] and man [34] and kidney homografts in dogs [1, 31, 34, 10] and rats [18]. There is moreover evidence, as we shall see later, which suggests that it may be advantageous in human kidney homograft recipients to give antilymphocytic globulin in addition to azathioprine and prednisone instead of relying on the latter two agents alone. It has also been shown by Levey and Medawar [28] and by Russell's group [32] that ALS causes prolonged

survival of second-set skin homografts in mice, a finding which, as
Levey and Medawar [28] have remarked, distinguishes ALS from
all other immunosuppressive agents yet studied, at any rate when
used in innocuous dosage.

The effect of ALS on the homograft reaction may be increased by
a variety of procedures including lymphocyte depletion by means of
a thoracic duct fistula [48, 49], whole body irradiation prior to administration of serum [28] and administration of corticosteroids [29].
Conversely, whole body irradiation after administration of ALS, and
adrenalectomy, have both been found to shorten homograft survival
[29]. Thymectomy has been found by some investigators to potentiate
the effect of ALS [33, 25] and by others to make no difference or
actually weaken it [29]. It would seem, as Jeejeebhoy [26] has suggested, that the apparent discrepancy between these findings is due
simply to differences in the experimental protocols.

Prolonged survival of rat skin heterografts in mice treated with
ALS was reported by Monaco *et al.* [32]. Heterografts of human and
guinea-pig skin have also been reported to survive for two weeks in
ALS-treated mice [28].

Humoral antibody formation. Heterospecific ALS has been shown to
inhibit humoral antibody formation in rodents injected for the first
time with a wide variety of antigens including sheep erythrocytes
[15, 32, 12, 11, 51, 22] and alum-precipitated bovine serum albumin
[51, 23]. On the other hand ALS appears to have much less effect
on the secondary antibody response in previously immunized animals
[15, 32, 22, 23].

Heterospecific antilymphocytic globulin is itself strongly antigenic.
Thus it has been shown that animals which have received injections
of such material develop antibody to globulins of the species in which
the serum was raised [11, 21] and also show rapid immune elimination
of isotopically labelled normal and antilymphocytic IgG from this
species [9].

Other immunological reactions. It was demonstrated by Inderbitzin
[20] as long ago as 1956 that ALS inhibits delayed-type hypersensitivity reactions and this has been confirmed by many investigators
[45, 44, 42, 34].

ALS inhibits all components of the normal lymphocyte transfer
reaction in guinea-pigs [28]. Moreover, lymphocytes from mice previously injected with ALS fail to cause graft-versus-host (GVH) reaction under conditions in which this does occur when lymphocytes

from untreated mice are used [5, 6, 38]. The capacity of lymphocytes from normal mice to cause GVH reaction may also be reduced by incubation with ALS *in vitro,* but this procedure appears to be less effective than pre-treatment of the lymphocyte donor [5].

ALS has also been shown to suppress experimental polyarthritis in rats [11] to prevent the development of a positive Coombs test in mice of the NZB strain [13] to protect mice against lymphocytic choriomeningitis [14] and to reduce the inflammatory reaction resulting from staphylococcal infection [35].

Effect of ALS on Lymphocytes and Lymphoid Tissue in Vivo

As already mentioned a single injection of ALS is followed by a sharp but transient fall in the blood lymphocyte count. In our experience in both rats and dogs a dose of serum well within the limits of safety can produce a lymphopenia which is still quite marked after 24 h, though not as profound as it was 4 h after injection [48, 49, 1, 3]. The effects of repeated administration are more variable. There may be sustained lymphopenia associated with depletion of lymphoid tissue [16] but this is not always maintained when treatment is prolonged [49, 40, 37, 1, 2]. Moreover, Levey and Medawar [28] observed blast transformation of peripheral blood lymphocytes associated with hypertrophy of lymphoid tissue. Turk and Willoughby [44] found that administration of anti-thymocyte serum to guinea-pigs for 6 days caused a persisting lymphopenia associated with lymphocyte depletion of the paracortical or thymus-dependent region of the lymph nodes but without depletion of the lymphoid follicles.

Effect of ALS on Lymphocytes in Vitro

Antilymphocyte serum is commonly found to contain erythrocyte agglutinins in quite high titre, but it has been found in various laboratories that these may be absorbed out with erythrocytes of the species concerned without loss of immunosuppressive activity or of the properties *in vitro* discussed below.

Antilymphocyte serum which has been inactivated by heating to 56°C for 30 min, irrespective of whether or not it has been subsequently absorbed with erythrocytes, agglutinates lymphocytes [2, 16, 21] and also destroys lymphocytes in the presence of complement [2, 16].

These reactions show a considerable degree of specificity. Thus rabbit-anti-rat ALS had no demonstrable effect on dog lymphocytes, and sheep-anti-dog ALS had no effect on rat lymphocytes; moreover, rat peritoneal macrophages proved to be much more resistant than rat lymphocytes to rabbit-anti-rat ALS [50]. Some degree of cross-reaction with lymphocytes of species other than the one whose lymphocytes were used for the immunization has however been reported by Gray *et al.* [16] and others.

It has been shown by immunofluorescent procedure that lymphocytes exposed to ALS *in vitro* become coated with antibody [29, 50].

It was reported by Grasbeck, Nordman and de la Chapelle [17] that rabbit-anti-human ALS caused blast transformation and mitosis of human lymphocytes in tissue culture. This work was based on morphological observations, but more recently various workers [19, 51] have shown that lymphocytes exposed to ALS raised in various species show increased uptake of isotopically-labelled (^{3}H or ^{14}C) uridine and thymidine, and there is good evidence that this is associated with accelerated synthesis of RNA and DNA respectively.

In most of the experiments referred to in the last paragraph, complement was excluded so far as possible from the culture medium; in particular all serum in the medium (including added ALS) was previously inactivated by being heated to 56°C for half an hour. It was reported by Holt *et al.* [19] that in the presence of complement increased thymidine incorporation occurred at low concentrations of antiserum, but that at high concentrations there was extensive cell destruction and thymidine uptake was small. We [52] have confirmed and extended these observations. We found that when lymphocytes were suspended in medium 199, and ALS and complement (in the form of raw autologous plasma) were added later, there was extensive cytolysis, and stimulation of uridine uptake was completely inhibited. When, on the other hand, the cells were suspended in a mixture of medium 199 and autologous plasma, and ALS was added 30 min or so after the suspension had been prepared, the degree of inhibition was very much less.

Characterisation and Purification of Antilymphocytic Antibody

Both the *in vivo* immunosuppressive activity, and the *in vitro* agglutinin, cytotoxic and stimulating activity, have been found to be largely concentrated in the IgG fraction of the sera we have raised in rabbits and horses [51]. This finding, which is consistent with data from other laboratories [24, 34, 18] is scarcely surprising in view of the prolonged course of immunization employed, but it is of interest that even under these conditions much of the erythrocyte agglutinin activity was in the IgM fraction. In consequence, the quantity of erythrocytes needed to absorb out these unwanted agglutinins could be greatly reduced by preliminary fractionation of the serum.

The $F(ab')_2$ portion of the antibody molecule, obtained by digestion with pepsin, contains both antibody combining sites but does not bind complement. We have found that $F(ab')_2$ prepared from horse-anti-human ALS IgG agglutinates human lymphocytes, and stimulates the uptake of uridine and thymidine by lymphocytes in culture, but, as would be expected, it has no cytotoxic activity [52]. $F(ab')_2$ from horse-anti-rat IgG failed to prolong the survival of skin homografts in rats and produced only a transient lymphopenia under conditions in which an equivalent dose of IgG increased the survival by a factor of 2.5 [3]. The same material also failed to inhibit the primary antibody response of rats to sheep erythrocytes [22] and alum precipitated bovine serum albumin while $F(ab')_2$ prepared from rabbit-anti-mouse IgG did not influence the graft-versus-host reaction (as judged by relative spleen weight) in (C57B1 $\times$ CBA)F_1 hybrid mice injected with parent line (C57B1) spleen cells [38]. There is some evidence from the work of GUTTMAN *et al.* [18] that $F(ab')_2$ (prepared from antithymocyte IgG) may have an immunosuppressive effect when given in very large dosage, but it seems possible that there may have been sufficient whole antibody remaining in the preparation to have accounted for this. Univalent fragment Fab', prepared by reduction of $F(ab')_2$ with cysteine, has proved to be inactive in all *in vitro* tests.

The amount of IgG taken up by lymphocytes exposed to various concentrations of ALS IgG has been determined by using isotopically-labelled (^{131}I) material, and found to range from one million to just over five million molecules per lymphocyte.

It would be expected *a priori* that only a proportion of the IgG molecules obtained by chemical fractionation of ALS would be anti-lymphocytic, since the animal in which the serum was raised cannot be expected to have lacked all previous immunological experience. We [53] have attempted to estimate the ratio (R) of antilymphocytic to total IgG molecules in preparations of horse-anti-human ALS IgG by combining measurements of the uptake of ^{131}I-labelled material with experiments in which the stimulating effect of the preparation was determined before and after it had been absorbed with a known number of human lymphocytes. In these experiments, a dose-response curve was first established in which the uptake of tritiated uridine by a fixed number of lymphocytes from a particular donor was plotted against the total amount of IgG added to the culture medium. The stimulating activity remaining after standard amounts of the same preparation had been absorbed for one hour with a known number of lymphocytes from the same donor was then determined by using the absorbed material as a culture medium for fresh lymphocytes. Tritiated uridine was added to these cultures and the degree of stimulation was determined as usual. The amount (E) of unabsorbed IgG per culture which would produce the same degree of stimulation was read from the dose-response curve.

To calculate R it is necessary to make some assumptions about the types of IgG molecule present in the preparation and their properties. The simplest set of assumptions is as follows: (a) The preparation contains only two classes of IgG molecule: antilymphocytic molecules which bind to lymphocytes and stimulate them to an equal extent (as measured by increase in uptake of tritiated uridine) and non-antilymphocytic molecules which neither bind nor stimulate; (b) The degree of stimulation produced in tests with a standard number of lymphocytes is a function of the number of antilymphocytic molecules in the preparation but independent of the number of non-antilymphocytic molecules. On this basis, if G denotes the amount of IgG per culture (expressed in the same units as E), n = the number of lymphocytes used for the absorption, m = molecular weight of IgG and N = Avogadro's number, it is clear that the unabsorbed preparation contained $\frac{Gn}{m}$ molecules of IgG, of which $\frac{GNR}{m}$ were antilymphocytic and $\frac{GN(1-R)}{m}$ were non-antilymphocytic. After absorption the medium must have contained $\frac{ENR}{m}$ antilymphocytic molecules to cause the observed uptake of tritiated uridine, so that M, the mean number of molecules taken up per cell, is given by $\frac{(G-E)NR}{nm}$ (because, *ex hypothesi*, only antilymphocytic molecules are taken up). Hence $R = \frac{Mnm}{(G-E)N}$.

If the assumptions underlying this calculation were correct the value obtained for R should be the same for different values of G and n; it was found, however, that this was not so but that R was inversely proportional to $\frac{G}{n}$. It seemed that the most likely explanation was that the ALS IgG used in the experiments, far from containing just two types of molecule as postulated, was much more heterogeneous. Such heterogeneity might take various forms, but the simplest hypothesis is that the antilymphocytic molecules are heterogeneous only in respect of their avidity, and that all IgG molecules which become attached to a lymphocyte exert an equal stimulating effect. Heterogeneity of this type may be defined in an operational way as implying simply that when ALS IgG is absorbed with lymphocytes the stimulating capacity of the absorbed solution is less than the stimulating capacity of a dilution of the unabsorbed solution containing the same total number of antilymphocytic IgG molecules, because the more avid molecules are preferentially absorbed whereas during dilution the population distribution remains the same.

The next step seemed to be to try to prepare antilymphocytic antibody of greater purity by elution from lymphocytes previously incubated with either ALS IgG or crude ALS. Several methods of elution were tried, including exposure for various times to buffered solutions of differing pH at 37°C and 56°C, and also to high concentrations of urea. The method [47] which was finally adopted was to elute at 37°C for 20 min in a buffered solution of pH 3.3.

The lymphocyte agglutinating and cytotoxic activity of eluted antibody preparations were determined in the usual way. Lymphocyte stimulating activity was assessed by measuring the uptake of ^{3}H uridine by lymphocyte cultures containing various amounts of the preparation. Capacity to bind to lymphocytes was measured with eluates prepared from isotopically (^{131}I) labelled antilymphocytic IgG. The protein content was estimated from the N content (determined by a micro-Kjeldahl estimation) or, in the case of isotopically-labelled preparations, by radioactive counting.

From 12 to 50% of the agglutinating activity of the original material was recovered and the activity per g protein was increased by a factor of 30 to 60. The preparations were also extremely potent in respect of lymphocyte binding and stimulating activity, but showed little or no cytotoxic activity. Further investigations have shown that the same sort of change occurs, i.e. cytotoxic activity is lost but agglutinating and stimulating activity are preserved, when ALS IgG is exposed to pH 3.0 at 37°C for 20 min. Whatever the explanation of the loss of cytotoxicity it is clear that acid-treated antibody resembles divalent antibody fragment F(ab')$_2$ in respect of its observed effects on lymphocytes *in vitro*. Since, as we have shown [3] the immunosuppressive capacity of antilymphocytic F(ab')$_2$ is small in comparison with that of the ALS IgG from which it is prepared, it would clearly be of interest to measure the immunosuppressive capacity of acid-treated or eluted antibody. This is being undertaken in rats with material prepared from horse-anti-rat ALS.

The dose response curves relating uridine uptake by lymphocytes in culture to the amount of antibody in the medium given by antibody eluted at optimal pH are markedly different in form from those obtained with either crude ALS or ALS IgG [47]. Thus at a level of uridine uptake which is maximal or near-maximal for cells exposed to ALS or ALS IgG the slope of the curve for eluted antibody is both steep and increasing. A possible reason for this difference is suggested by experiments with ^{131}I-labelled antibody [47] in which it was found that the uridine uptake per molecule of antibody absorbed was greater in lymphocyte cultures containing eluted antibody than in those con taining the IgG solution from which the eluted antibody was prepared. It would seem therefore that our hypothesis concerning the heterogeneity of antilymphocytic antibody requires further revision. We began by postulating that ALS IgG contains only two classes of molecule, namely, antilymphocytic molecules which bind to and stimulate lymphocytes and non-antilymphocytic molecules which neither bind nor stimulate. It became apparent that this was an over simplification and that antilymphocytic IgG molecules formed a heterogeneous population; the previous experimental findings could however be accounted for by postulating heterogeneity in respect of avidity only and retaining the assumption that all IgG molecules which become attached to a lymphocyte exert an equal stimulating effect. It would now seem that individual antilymphocytic IgG molecules may differ also in respect of their stimulating activity.

Mechanism of Immunosuppression by Antilymphocytic Antibody

It has been pointed out by several groups of investigators [28, 45, 1, 49] that, contrary to what was at first expected [46], the level of immunosuppression is not entirely dependent on the degree of lymphoid depletion which is produced. It would seem, therefore, that ALS does not produce its effects simply by destroying lymphocytes or their precursors, although this is almost certainly one important factor since preparations which are completely lacking in cytotoxic activity, whether of whole antibody or of antibody fragments, do not appear to be immunosuppressive.

It was suggested by Monaco *et al.* [33] that ALS in association with an antigen produces a form of central inhibition of immunological responsiveness akin to specific immunological tolerance, on the ground that normal reactivity could be restored by adoptive immunization with isogeneic normal or pre-immunized lymphoid cells. The ALS-treated animal, however, differs from the typical tolerant animal in that, as a rule, it does not remain non-reactive indefinitely (even though antigen remains present) after administration of ALS is stopped, although later work by Monaco *et al.* [32] suggests that animals which have also been subjected to thymectomy may do so.

Another hypothesis is that lymphocytes become coated with ALS and in consequence are rendered immunologically ineffective. Coating certainly does occur when lymphocytes are exposed to ALS *in vitro* [50] and there seems no reason to doubt that this also happens *in vivo*. Levey and Medawar [29] have rejected this explanation however on two grounds: (a) experiments in which lethally irradiated mice are repopulated with spleen and marrow cells from isogeneic mice pretreated with ALS suggest that the descendants of lymphocytes which have been exposed to ALS remain unreactive for one or more cellular generations; and (b) chronic treatment of mice with ALS in their experiments did not lead to lymphoid atrophy but to hypertrophy and hyperplasia accompanied by the formation of blast cells. They have, therefore, suggested that ALS acts by causing a generalized sterile activation of lymphoid cells, perhaps analogous to that produced by phytohaemagglutinin.

The demonstration that ALS stimulates lymphocyte transformation and uptake of uridine and thymidine *in vitro* would seem at first sight to provide support for the sterile activation theory, though this cannot be the whole explanation since $F(ab')_2$ preparations show little immunosuppressive activity in relation to their capacity to stimulate lymphocytes *in vitro*. As has been mentioned, however, this stimulation is inhibited when complement is added to the system, and if the concentration of ALS is high lysis occurs. It would scarcely be surprising if similar ambivalence were also manifested *in vivo,* where the balance between stimulation and lysis in lymphoid tissue might depend on such factors as the local concentration of ALS and complement, and the degree of anticomplementary activity. The fact that in some of our own experiments [49, 1] prolonged administration of ALS resulted in lymphoid atrophy, whereas in the experiments of Levey and Medawar [28] lymphoid hyperplasia occurred, suggests that this is indeed the case.

Clinical Applications of ALS

Antilymphocytic globulin has been used in conjunction with azathioprine and prednisone in more than 50 kidney allotransplant recipients by Starzl *et al.* [27], in 18 such patients and 15 others who had not received transplants by Traeger and his colleagues in Lyon [43] and in six kidney transplant recipients by our group in Edinburgh [54]. Nineteen of the first 20 patients treated in this way by Starzl [41] were alive and showed good graft function 10–16 months after receiving transplants from living closely related donors, whereas the expected death rate, in the light of previous experience, without antilymphocytic globulin, would have been about 30%.

Thirteen of Traeger's 18 transplant recipients were alive when the cases were reported, two more than 14 months after operation. No claim was made of prolonged survival as compared with survival of patients treated elsewhere without antilymphocytic antibody, but infection appeared to present a less serious problem, perhaps because of the relatively low dosage of corticosteroids which Traeger and his colleagues found to be sufficient in their more recent cases.

Our own experience is small, and is difficult to evaluate because in four of the six patients antilymphocytic globulin was not used as a primary treatment but was given later when it was proving difficult to arrest a process of chronic rejection with acceptable doses of azathioprine and steroids (3 cases) or to compensate for a reduction in the dose of azathioprine in a patient who had developed a serious infection. In at least one patient however a marked reduction in prednisone dosage, which had not been possible before antilymphocytic globulin was given, was achieved without detriment to the transplant.

While the clinical results are encouraging it is apparent that they do not compare with those obtained in experimental animals. This may well be due at least in part to the fact that the dose of antilymphocytic globulin used in man per kg body weight has been relatively small. Despite the relatively low dosage employed, however, administration of antilymphocytic globulin to man has been found to have some serious disadvantages. Nearly all patients have experienced pain, sometimes severe, at the site of injection (intramuscular or subcutaneous). Fever, and anaphylactoid reactions of various types, are quite common. Severe thrombocytopenia has occurred in two of our patients and has been reported also by STARZL. One of our patients died from a malignant lymphoma, but it appears possible in retrospect that this may have been present before administration of antilymphocytic globulin was begun.

Most of the ALS used in animal experiments has been raised by injecting rabbits, sheep, goats or horses with xenogeneic thoracic duct lymphocytes, lymph node cells or thymocytes without adjuvants; sometimes as few as two injections have been given, sometimes many injections spread over months or even years. ALS for clinical use in Denver and Edinburgh has been raised by chronic immunization of horses with human spleen cells. In Lyon, TRAEGER and his colleagues have used human thoracic duct lymphocytes, but have suspended these in a mixture of equal parts of Eagle's medium and Freund's adjuvant [7].

It seems possible that safer and more potent preparations for clinical use might be obtained by immunizing the serum-producing animals with lymphocytes obtained from blood or other sources apart from spleen without adjuvants, or alternatively by further treatment of material obtained by current methods of immunization and fractionation. Three procedures which we are currently investigating are (a) absorption of ALS IgG with human platelets, (b) further fractionation of ALS IgG by electrophoresis, and (c) modification of antibody molecule by treatment at various temperatures with acid or alkali.

Another modification of current practice which might possibly lead to better results would be to inject the material intravenously instead of intramuscularly. Our experience of this in man is limited to a short course of injections in one patient; we were however impressed by the absence of pain and other untoward symptoms. If preparations of antilymphocytic antibody contain antibody complexed with, or capable of reacting with, human serum protein, intravenous injection is likely to result in the deposition of antigen-antibody complexes in the kidney and elsewhere, but it should be possible to avoid this danger by absorbing the preparation with serum proteins and then subjecting it to ultracentrifugation. Intravenous administration might also increase the risk of renal damage due to some component of the preparation reacting with glomerular basement membrane, but this could conceivably be avoided by prior absorption and by infusing the preparation sufficiently slowly to enable all the antibody to become bound to lymphocytes in the peripheral blood. There are other obvious dangers, such as acute anaphylactic shock, but preliminary skin testing and the simultaneous administration of corticosteroids should go far to prevent this.

The potential value of antilymphocytic antibody as an immunosuppressive agent has been abundantly demonstrated in experimental animals. There are clearly many difficulties to be overcome before this potential can be fully realised in the clinical field, but there seems no reason to suppose that any of these difficulties will prove to be insuperable.

References

1. ABAZA, H.M.; NOLAN, B.; WATT, J.G. and WOODRUFF, M.F.A.: The effect of antilymphocytic serum on the survival of renal homotransplants in dogs. Transplantation *4:* 618–632 (1966).
2. ABAZA, H.M. and WOODRUFF, M.F.A.: *In vitro* assay of antilymphocytic serum. Rev. franc. Et. clin. biol. *11:* 821–827 (1966).
3. ANDERSON, N.F.; JAMES, K. and WOODRUFF, M.F.A.: Effect of antilymphocytic anti: body on skin homograft survival and the blood lymphocyte count in rats. Lancet. *i:* 1126–1128 (1967).
4. BALNER, H. and DERSJANT, H.: Effects of antilymphocyte sera in primates. In: WOLSTENHOLME and O'CONNOR's Ciba Foundation Study Group No. 29 on Antilymphocytic Serum, pp. 85-96 (Churchill, London 1967).
5. BEKKUM, D.D. VAN; LEDNEY, G.D.; BALNER, H.; PUTTEN, L.M. VAN and VRIES, M.D. DE: Suppression of secondary disease following foreign bone marrow grafting with antilymphocyte serum. In: WOLSTENHOLME and O'CONNOR's Ciba Foundation Study Group No. 29 on Antilymphocytic Serum, pp. 97–107 (Churchill, London 1967).
6. BOAK, J.L.; FOX, M. and WILSON, R.E.: Activity of lymphoid tissues from antilymphocyte-serum-treated mice. Lancet. *i:* 750–752 (1967).
7. CARRAZ, M.; TRAEGER, J.; FRIES, D.; PERRIN, J.; SAUBIER, E.; BROCHIER, J.; VEYSSEYRE, C.; PRÉVOT, J.; BRYON, P.; JOUVENCEAUX, A.; ARCHIMBAUD, J.P.; BONNET, P.; MANUEL, Y.; BERNHARDT, J.P. and TRAEGER FOUILLET, Y.: Préparation, propriétés et activité d'immunoglobines de cheval antilymphocytes humains. Rev. Inst. Pasteur de Lyon. *1:* 17–53 (1967).
8. CHEW, W.B. and LAWRENCE, J.S.: Antilymphocytic serum. J. Immunol. *33:* 271–278 (1937).
9. CLARK, J.G.; JAMES, K. and WOODRUFF, M.F.A.: Elimination of normal horse IgG labelled with Iodine-131 in rats receiving horse anti-rat lymphocytic IgG. Nature (Lond.) *215:* 869–870 (1967).
10. CLUNIE, G.J.A.; NOLAN, B.; JAMES, K.; WATT, J.G. and WOODRUFF, M.F.A.: Prolongation of canine renal allografts with antilymphocytic serum. Transplantation *6:* 459–467 (1968).
11. CURREY, H.L.F. and ZIFF, M.P.: Suppression of experimentally induced polyarthritis in the rat by heterologous anti-lymphocyte serum. Lancet. *ii:* 889–891 (1966).
12. DENMAN, A.M.; DENMAN, E.J. and HOLBOROW, E.J.: Effect of anti-lymphocyte globulin on kidney disease in (NZB×NZW)F$_1$ mice. Lancet. *ii:* 841–843 (1966).

13. DENMAN, A.M.; DENMAN, E.J. and HOLBOROW, E.J.: Suppression of Coombs-positive haemolytic anaemia in NZB mice by antilymphocyte globulin. Lancet. *i:* 1084–1086 (1967).

14. GLEDHILL, A.W.: Protective effect of anti-lymphocytic serum on murine lymphocytic choriomeningitis. Nature (Lond.) *214:* 178–179 (1967).

15. GRASBECK, R.; NORDMAN, C.T. and CHAPELLE, A. DE LA: The leucocytemitogenic effect of serum from rabbits immunized with human leucocytes. Acta med. scand. Suppl. *412:* 39–47 (1964).

16. GRAY, J.G.; MONACO, A.P. and RUSSELL, P.S.: Heterologous mouse anti-lymphocyte serum to prolong skin homografts. Surg. Forum *15:* 142–144 (1964).

17. GRAY, J.G.; MONACO, A.P.; WOOD, M.L. and RUSSELL, P.S.: Studies on heterologous anti-lymphocyte serum in mice. J. Immunol. *96:* 217–228 (1966).

18. GUTTMAN, R.D.; CARPENTER, C.B.; LINDQUIST, R.R. and MERRILL, J.P.: An immuno-suppressive site of action of heterologous antilymphocyte serum. Lancet. *i:* 248–249 (1967).

19. HOLT, L.J.; LING, N.R. and STANWORTH, D.R.: The effect of heterologous antisera and rheumatoid factor on the synthesis of DNA and protein by human peripheral lymphocytes. Immunochemistry *3:* 359–372 (1966).

20. INDERBITZIN, T.: The relation of lymphocytes, delayed cutaneous allergic reactions and histamine. Int. Arch. Allergy *8:* 150–159 (1956).

21. IWASAKI, Y.; PORTER, K.A.; AMEND, J.R.; MARCHIORO, T.L.; ZUHLKE, V. and STARZL, T.E.: The preparation and testing of horse antidog and antihuman antilymphoid plasma or serum and its protein fractions. Surg. Gynec. Obstet. *124:* 1–24 (1967).

22. JAMES, K. and ANDERSON, N.F.: Effect of anti-rat lymphocyte antibody on humoral antibody formation. Nature (Lond.) *213:* 1195–1197 (1967).

23. JAMES, K. and JUBB, V.S.: Effect of anti-rat lymphocyte antibody on humoral antibody formation. Nature (Lond.) *215:* 367–371 (1967).

24. JAMES, K. and MEDAWAR, P.B.: Characterization of anti-lymphocytic antibody. Nature (Lond.) *214:* 1052–1053 (1967).

25. JEEJEEBHOY, H.F.: Immunological studies on the rat thymectomized in adult life. Immunology (Lond.) *9:* 417–425 (1965).

26. JEEJEEBHOY, H.F.: The relationship of lymphopenia production and lymphocyte agglutinating and cytotoxic antibody titers to the immunosuppressive potency of heterologous antilymphocyte plasma. Transplantation *5:* 1121–1126 (1967).

27. KASHIWAGI N.; BRANTIGAN, C.; BRETTSCHNEIDER, L.; GROTH, C.G. and STARZL, T.E.: Clinical reactions and serologic changes after the administration of heterologous antilymphocyte globulin to human recipients of renal homografts. Ann. intern. Med. *68:* 275-286 (1968).

28. LEVEY, R.H. and MEDAWAR, P.B.: Some experiments on the action of anti-lymphoid antisera. Ann. N.Y. Acad. Sci. *129:* 164–177 (1966a).

29. LEVEY, R.H. and MEDAWAR, P.B.: Nature and mode of action of antilymphocytic antiserum. Proc. nat. Acad. Sci., Wash. *56:* 1130–1137 (1966b).

30. METCHNIKOFF, E.: Etudes sur la resorption des cellules. Ann. Inst. Pasteur *13:* 737–769 (1899).

31. MONACO, A.P.; ABBOTT, W.M.; OTHERSON, H.B.; SIMMONS, R.L.; WOOD, M.L.; FLAX, M.H. and RUSSELL, P.S.: Antiserum to lymphocytes: prolonged survival of canine renal allografts. Science *153:* 1264–1267 (1966).

32. MONACO, A.P.; WOOD, M.L.; GRAY, J.G. and RUSSELL, P.S.: Studies on heterologous anti-lymphocyte serum in mice. II. Effect on the immune response. J. Immunol. *96:* 229–238 (1966).

33. MONACO, A.P.; WOOD, M.L. and RUSSELL, P.S.: Adult thymectomy: effect on recovery from immunologic depression in mice. Science *149:* 432–435 (1965).

34. MONACO, A.P.; WOOD, M.L.; WERF, B.A. VAN DER and RUSSELL, P.S.: Effects of antilymphocyte serum in mice, dogs and man. In: WOLSTENHOLME and O'CONNOR's Ciba Foundation Study Group No. 29 on Antilymphocytic Serum, pp. 111–134 (Churchill, London 1967).

35. MORRIS, P.J. and BURKE, J.F.: Antilymphocyte serum and staphylococcal infection. Nature (Lond.) *214:* 1138–1139 (1967).

36. MURPHY, J.B.: The lymphocyte in resistance to tissue grafting, malignant disease, and tuberculous infection. Monographs of Rockefeller Institute for medical research, No. 21 (1926).

37. NAGAYA, H. and SIEKER, H.O.: Allograft survival: effect of antiserums to thymus glands and lymphocytes. Science *150:* 1181–1182 (1965).

38. NAYSMITH, J.D. and JAMES, K.: Effect of F(ab')$_2$ from rabbit anti-mouse lymphocyte IgG on the graft versus host reaction in F$_1$ hybrid mice. Nature (Lond.) *217:* 260–261 (1968).

39. PAPPENHEIMER, A.M.: Experimental studies upon lymphocytes. I. The reactions of lymphocytes under various experimental conditions. J. exp. Med. *25:* 633–650 (1917).

40. SACKS, J.H.; FILLIPPONE, D.R. and HUME, D.M.: Studies of immune destruction of lymphoid tissue. I. Lymphocytotoxic effect of rabbit-anti-rat lymphocyte antiserum. Transplantation *2:* 60–74 (1964).

41. STARZL, T.E.; GROTH, C.G.; TERASAKI, P.I.; PUTNAM, C.W.; BRETTSCHNEIDER, L. and MARCHIORO, T.L.: Heterologous antilymphocyte globulin, histoincompatibility matching, and human renal homotransplantation. Surg. Gynec. Obstet. *126:* 1023–1035 (1968).

42. STARZL, T.E.; PORTER, K.A.; IWASAKI, Y.; MARCHIORO, T.L. and KASHIWAGI, N.: The use of heterologous antilymphocyte globulin in human renal homotransplantation: in WOLSTENHOLME and O'CONNOR's Ciba Foundation Study Group No. 29 on Antilymphocytic Serum, pp. 4–34 (Churchill, London 1967).

43. TRAEGER, J.; PERRIN, J.; FRIES, D.; SAUBIER, E.; CARRAZ, M.; BONNET, P.; ARCHIMBAUD, J.P.; BERNHARDT, J.P.; BROCHIER, J.; BETUEL, H.; VEYSSEYRE, C.; BRYON, P.A.; PRÉVOT, J.; JOUVENCEAU, A.; BANSSILLON, V.; ZECH, P. and ROLLET, A.: Utilisation chez l'homme d'une globuline antilymphocytaire: Résultats cliniques en transplantation rénale. Lyon méd. *5:* 307–369 (1968).

44. TURK, J.L. and WILLOUGHBY, D.A.: Central and peripheral effects of antilymphocyte sera. Lancet. *i:* 249–251 (1967).

45. WAKSMAN, H.B.; ARBOUYS, S. and ARNASON, B.C.: Use of specific "lymphocyte" antisera to inhibit hypersensitive reactions of the "delayed" type. J. exp. Med. *114:* 997–1022 (1961).

46. WOODRUFF, M.F.A.: The transplantation of tissues and organs (Thomas, Springfield 1960).

47. WOODRUFF, M.F.A.: Purification of antilymphocytic antibody. Nature (Lond.) *217:* 821–824 (1968).

48. WOODRUFF, M.F.A. and ANDERSON, N.F.: Effect of lymphocyte depletion by thoracic duct fistula and administration of antilymphocytic serum on the survival of skin homografts in rats. Nature (Lond.) *200:* 702 (1963).

49. WOODRUFF, M.F.A. and ANDERSON, N.F.: The effect of lymphocyte depletion by thoracic duct fistula and administration of antilymphocytic serum on the survival of skin homografts in rats. Ann. N.Y. Acad. Sci. *120:* 119–128 (1964).

50. WOODRUFF, M.F.A.; ANDERSON, N.F. and ABAZA, H.M.: Experiments with antilymphocytic serum: in YOFFEY's The lymphocyte in immunology and haemopoiesis, pp. 286–291 (Edward Arnold, London 1966).

51. WOODRUFF, M.F.A.; JAMES, K.; ANDERSON, N.F. and REID, B.L.: *In vivo* and *in vitro* properties of antilymphocytic serum: in WOLSTENHOLME and O'CONNOR's Ciba

Foundation Study Group No. 29 on Antilymphocytic Serum, pp. 57–68 (Churchill, London 1967).
52. Woodruff, M.F.A.; Reid, B.L. and James, K.: Quantitative *in vitro* studies with antilymphocytic antibody. Nature (Lond.) *216:* 758–762 (1967).
53. Woodruff, M.F.A.; Nolan, B.; Robson, J.S.; and Macdonald, M.K.: Experience with renal transplantation in man. (Awaiting publication.)

Author's address: Prof. M.F.A. Woodruff, University of Edinburgh Medical School Department of Surgical Science, *Edinburgh* (Scotland).

Antibiotica et Chemotherapia, vol. 15, pp. 250–266 (Karger, Basel/New York 1969)

Lymphocyte Kinetics and Lymphoid Tissue Morphology Accompanying Immunosuppression by Antilymphocyte Serum (ALS)

R. N. Taub

National Institute for Medical Research, London

Introduction

Antilymphocyte serum, or ALS, is now recognized as a potent immunosuppressive agent with potential clinical value [4, 20, 8, 15]. The precise mode of action of ALS has not yet been fully agreed upon; some of the possibilities entertained in this regard have been summarized by Levey and Medawar [8] and include lymphocytolytic action, "sterile activation" of lymphoid tissue, prevention of antigen recognition by a "blindfolding" action, or inhibiting the usual activities of the thymus.

Any of the hypothesized mechanisms, if operative, might be expected to give rise to characteristic and specific alterations in lymphoid tissues. However, while a number of observers have noted widespread marked changes in lymphoid tissue after ALS treatment, the changes that have been reported have been quite variable, ranging from generalized lymphatic depletion [12] or discrete lymphoid tissue lesions [7, 13, 18] to overt lymphoid hyperplasia [8].

We have carried out a detailed investigation of the histological effects and deleterious consequences of both acute and protracted ALS administration, the results of which have been submitted elsewhere [17]. The present report will be largely concerned with changes occurring after a single dose or relatively brief course of antiserum, with a view toward delineating those invariably linked to immunosuppression by ALS. Other observations are reported which bear on the possible pathogenesis of some of these changes and their relationship to the unique immunosuppressive properties exhibited by ALS.

Methods and Materials

a) Mice. CBA mice of either sex, weighing between 25 and 35 g obtained from the National Institute for Medical Research breeding unit, were used throughout these studies.

b) Preparation and assay of antisera. Rabbit anti-mouse lymphocyte antiserum (RAMLS) was prepared by the method of Levey and Medawar [8] by immunizing New Zealand white rabbits with two intravenous injections of 10^9 mouse thymocytes spaced a fortnight apart. Serum was obtained one week after the last injection, heated to 56° C for 30 min, Seitz filtered, and stored at –20° C. Normal rabbit serum (NRS) obtained from unimmunized rabbits was processed and stored similarly.

Horse anti-mouse lymphocyte gamma globulin (HALGG) was kindly supplied by the Wellcome Foundation.

Duck anti-mouse lymphocyte serum (DAMLS) was raised by a similar method [6].

C57Ks-anti-CBA thymocyte antiserum was raised by immunizing C57Ks mice with two intraperitoneal inoculations of CBA thymocytes using Freund's adjuvant. A detailed description of the preparation and properties of this antiserum will be reported elsewhere.

The immunosuppressive potency of each antiserum was assayed by the ability of two subcutaneous injections of 0.5 ml to prolong the survival of A strain skin grafted to CBA mice, when given on day $+2$ and $+5$ after grafting. Skin grafting was performed according to the method of Billingham and Medawar [1].

In vitro lymphocytotoxic assays were performed by Dr. M. Ruszkiewicz using Cr-51 labelled lymphocytes, according to the method of Wigzell [19].

c) Administration of antisera. Mice were given single or repeated doses of 0.5 ml of antiserum subcutaneously in the region of the right axilla. Control mice were given similar amounts of normal rabbit serum. Mice were usually sacrificed three at a time from each treatment group at various intervals after the last injection for hematologic and histologic study.

d) Hematologic and histologic studies. Microhematocrit, total leukocyte count, and Wright-stained smears for differential leukocyte counts and platelet estimations were obtained from caudal arterial blood or by cardiac puncture.

For histologic study, mice were sacrificed by cervical dislocation and peripheral lymph nodes (brachial, axillary, inguinal), mesenteric lymph nodes, thymus, spleen, and sternal bone marrow were fixed in 10% neutral formalin for further processing. Cut sections were stained routinely with hematoxylin-eosin and methyl green-pyronine.

e) Radioautographic studies. Groups of four to six mice were left untreated or given three doses of either RAMLS or NRS at 2-day intervals. Two to five days after the last dose, a caudal vein of each mouse was cannulated with a finely-drawn, indwelling nylon catheter, and mice were perfused for the ensuing 36 h with 0.1 ml/h of phosphate-buffered saline (pH 7.2) containing tritiated thymidine (Radiochemical Centre, Amersham, Bucks—specific activity 5 mC/mM) in a concentration of 25 microcuries/ml. Two to three hours after perfusion had been stopped, the animals were sacrificed, and smears were made of samples of peripheral blood. Portions of lymphoid tissue were fixed in 10% neutral formalin and sectioned at five microns. Autoradiography of smears was carried out using Kodak AR-10 stripping film for blood smears, and Ilford L-4 nuclear emulsion for the sectioned material. Development time ranged from two to four weeks. Processed tissues were stained with either Giemsa's or neutral red stain.

Observations

1. Lesions Accompanying Immunosuppression by ALS

a) Lymphopenia. Antisera capable of prolonging skin homograft survival were also capable of producing sustained lymphopenia for at least 48 h after a single subcutaneous injection (fig. 1). The duration of lymphopenia produced after a single dose of these antisera seemed related to their immunosuppressive potency. The extent to which the lymphocyte count was depressed within the first 24 h did not correlate with later lymphocyte levels: 0.5 ml of normal rabbit serum caused a fall comparable to that in ALS treated animals during the first 24 h, but the lymphocyte level had been fully restored after 48 h.

There was little correlation between *in vitro* cytotoxic titres and the ability to maintain lymphopenia *in vivo,* except that sera devoid of cytotoxic activity such as DAMLS produced no lymphopenia. On the other hand, RAMLS, HALGG, and C57Ks-anti-CBA antiserum all showed high cytotoxic titres yet differed widely in their ability to maintain lymphopenia *in vivo.*

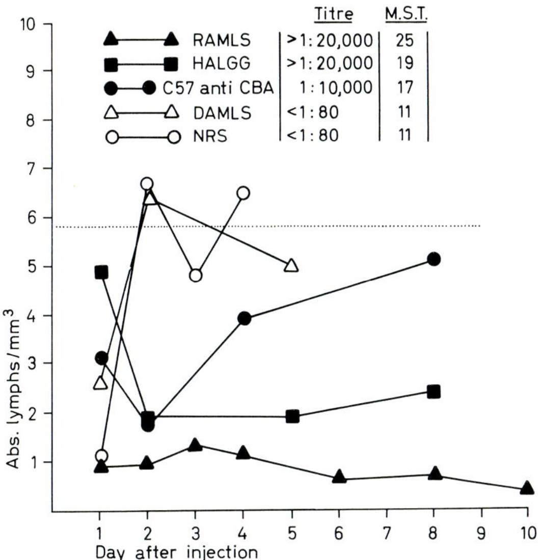

Fig. 1. Lymphopenia produced after a single 0.5 ml dose of various anti-lymphocyte antisera, including rabbit anti-mouse (RAMLS), horse anti-mouse lymphocyte gamma globulin (HALGG), duck anti-mouse lymphocyte antiserum (DAMLS), C57Ks anti-CBA thymocyte isoantiserum and normal rabbit serum (NRS). Each point on the graph represents the mean value obtained from three to four animals.

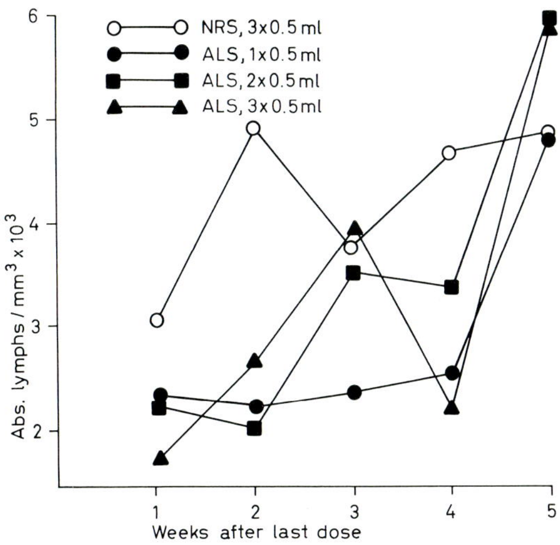

Fig. 2. Persistence of lymphopenia after one, two or three doses (0.5 ml each) of a powerful rabbit antiserum, or of NRS. Lymphocyte counts were determined at weekly intervals after the last dose of serum. Each point represents the mean value obtained from three animals.

One rabbit-anti-mouse serum tested (serum 37, MST 31 days) given subcutaneously in a dose of 0.5 ml produced marked lymphopenia which stabilized at about one-half normal lymphocyte levels for two weeks before returning to normal (fig. 2). The degree and duration of lymphopenia was approximately the same, however, whether one, two or three doses of antiserum were given; so that although the immunosuppressive potency of an antiserum may also be reflected in the lymphopenic activity of a single dose, the actual lymphocyte counts obtaining during a course of treatment are not indicative of the degree of immunosuppression that has been achieved.

An attempt was made to further classify the type of lymphopenia with regard to the proportions of short-lived or long-lived lymphocytes remaining after ALS treatment.

One group of four mice was treated with two doses of 0.5 ml RAMLS given two days apart. Five days after the last injection, these mice were perfused with intravenous tritiated thymidine for 36 h. The proportions of labelled peripheral blood lymphocytes in these mice were compared with those of normal mice similarly perfused (table I). The absolute lymphocyte count of the ALS-treated group averaged less than half of the control group. The labelling index of circulating lymphocytes was two to three times greater, however, in the ALS-treated group. In thus seems that ALS treatment

Table I. Thymidine labelling of peripheral lymphocytes after ALS

	Total WBC	(%) Lymphocytes	Absolute lymphocytes	(%) Labelled lymphocytes	Absolute labelled lymphocytes
Normals	5 950	44	2618	6.0	157
	12 250	48	5880	3.4	200
	5 100	66	3366	4.2	141
	8 450	51	4310	4.3	185
	7939$\pm$3190		4043$\pm$1397	4.5$\pm$1.1	171$\pm$27
ALS-treated	5 850	46	2701	12.8	346
	2 800	40	1120	12.3	138
	4 550	47	2138	18.6	398
	4 600	57	2622	19.6	514
	4450$\pm$1244		1995$\pm$723	15.8$\pm$3.3	349$\pm$156

Absolute lymphocytes per cmm^3 and per cent labelled lymphocytes in normal animals and after two doses of rabbit anti-mouse ALS (*see* text). All animals were perfused with 90 microcuries each of tritiated thymidine over a 36-hour period.

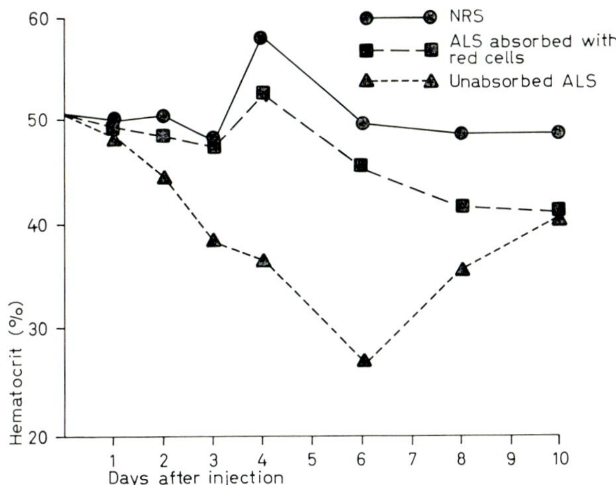

Fig. 3. Hematocrit values after treatment with a single 0.5 ml dose of unabsorbed ALS or ALS previously absorbed against 4:1 mouse red blood cells, or normal rabbit serum. Each point represents the mean of duplicate determinations from three animals

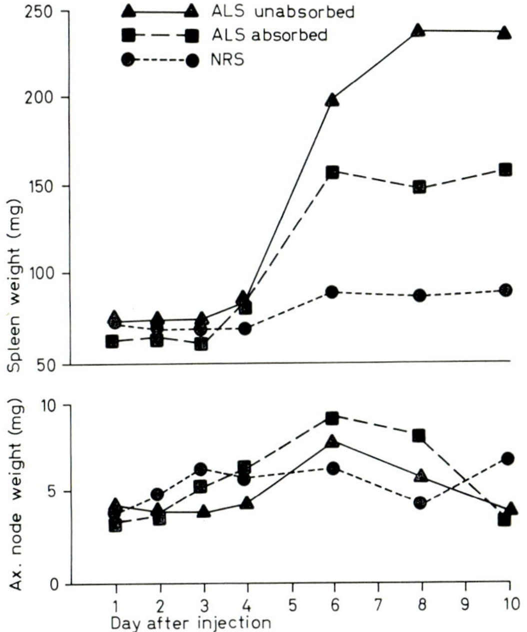

Fig. 4. Wet weights of spleens and both axillary lymph nodes following a single subcutaneous dose of unabsorbed ALS, absorbed ALS, or NRS. – (Same animals as used for experiment depicted in fig. 3). Each point represents the mean value obtained from three animals.

causes a shift in the normal circulating lymphocyte population from predominantly long-lived to predominantly newly-formed cells.

b) Lymphoid depletion. Following the administration of a single subcutaneous dose of an immunosuppressive antiserum, a well-defined sequence of changes occurs within lymphoid tissues.

Lymph nodes. Between 12 and 24 h after injection, damaged lymphocytes with pyknotic nuclei may appear within capillaries and venules in the paracortical areas of lymph nodes and in intestinal Peyer's patches. By 48 h, a striking depletion of small lymphocytes, sharply localized to paracortical areas, is observed in lymph nodes both adjacent to or distant from the site of injection (fig. 5, 7). No depletion is observed after NRS treatment (fig. 6, 8). Within the depleted paracortical areas, a few small lymphocytes remain, closely adjacent to post-capillary venules, but the majority of cells remaining in this area are large lymphocytes, a few immunoblasts, and reticular cells (fig. 9). After a single dose of a potent rabbit antiserum this depletion lasts one week or more. Antisera which are less immunosuppressively active seem to produce lesser degrees of depletion, as judged by the appearance of the paracortical areas (table II).

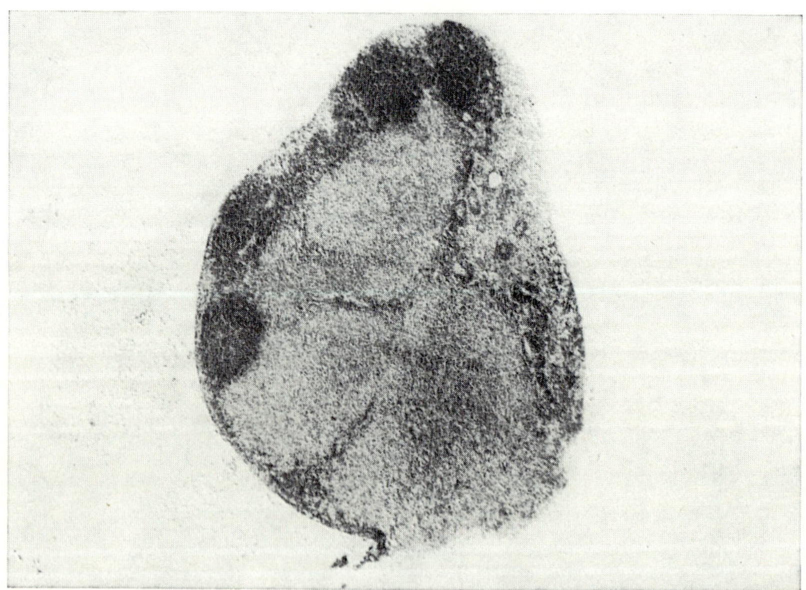

Fig. 5. CBA mouse axillary lymph node 48 h after a single subcutaneous dose of 0.5 ml rabbit anti-mouse ALS. Note extensive depletion of cells from paracortical areas. The cortex and medulla are well preserved. Hematoxylin and eosin. × 52

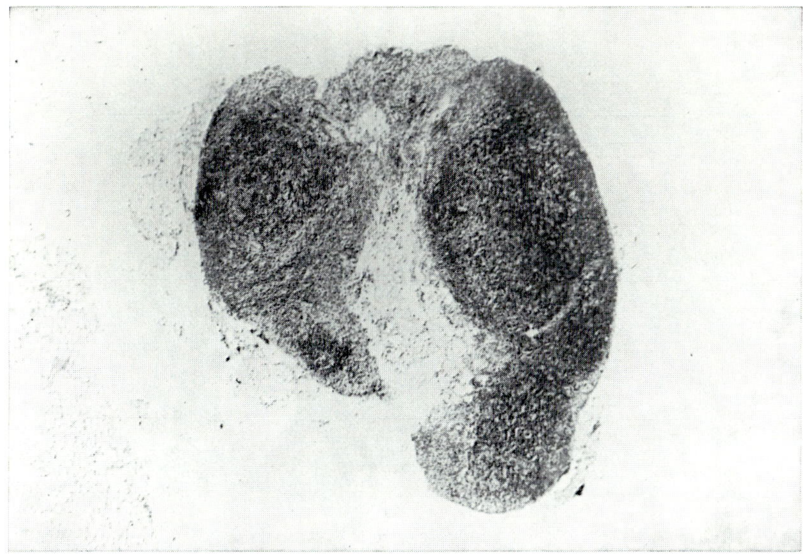

Fig. 6. Axillary lymph node 48 h after a single subcutaneous injection of 0.5 ml normal rabbit serum. The node presents a normal appearance. Hematoxylin and eosin. × 52

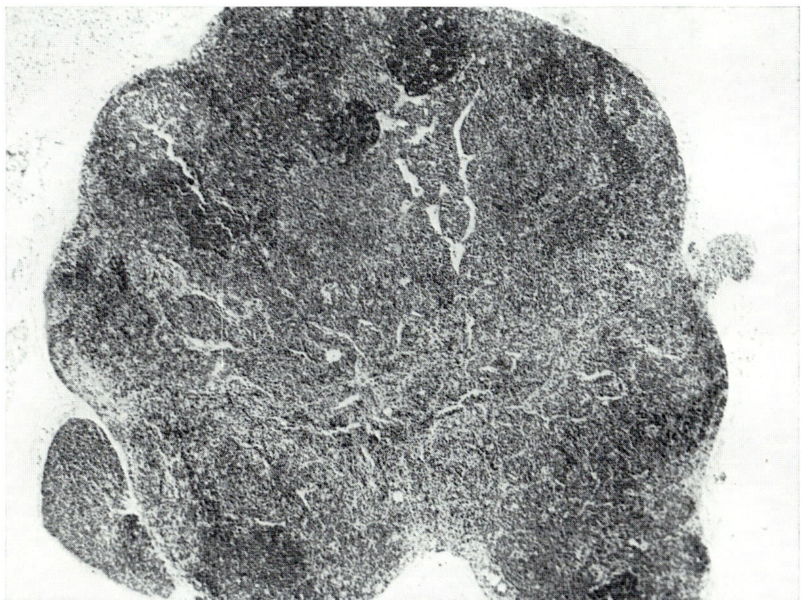

Fig. 7. Axillary lymph node eight days after a single subcutaneous injection of ALS. Note marked increase in size of node (magnifications as in fig. 5). Paracortical depletion still persists. There is extensive medullary hyperplasia and secondary follicle formation. Hematoxylin and eosin. × 52

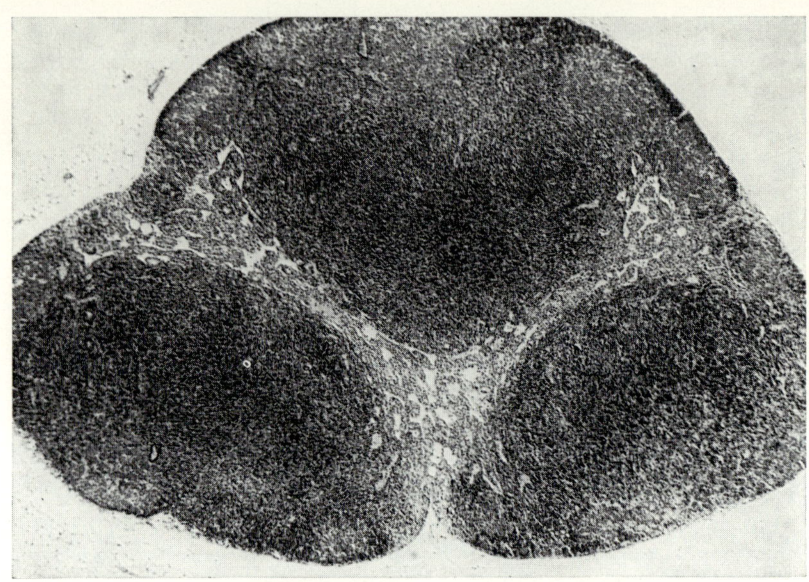

Fig. 8. Axillary lymph node eight days after a single subcutaneous injection of normal rabbit serum. (Magnifications as in fig. 6). There is marked medullary hyperplasia as in figure 7. The paracortical region is densely populated and shows no depletion. Hematoxylin and eosin. × 52

Table II. Lymphoid depletion observed after subcutaneous ALS

Serum	Days after injection		
	2	6	10
RAMLS	++++	++	++
HALGG	++	—	—
C57 anti-CBA	±	—	N.E.
DAMLS	—	—	N.E.
NRS	—	—	—

Summary of histologic observations on the extent of lymph node paracortical area depletion at 2, 6 and 10 days following a single subcutaneous injection of 0.5 ml of various antilymphocyte antisera. RAMLS = rabbit anti-mouse ALS; DAMLS = duck anti-mouse antiserum; HALGG = horse anti-mouse lymphocyte gamma globulin fraction; NRS = normal rabbit serum; C57Ks anti-CBA = mouse anti-mouse thymocyte iso-antiserum. Degrees of lymphoid depletion are recorded as: ++++ severe; +++ marked; ++ moderate; + minimal; ± questionable; — absent; N.E. not examined.

Spleen. A single subcutaneous dose of even a potent antiserum does not usually produce significant lymphoid depletion in the spleen; however, after three repeated doses, a striking depletion of small lymphocytes develops, sharply localized to the periarteriolar areas of the lymphoid follicles (fig. 9). A collection of immunoblasts and plasma cell precursors usually persists as a rim of cells just surrounding the central follicular arteriole (fig. 10, 11).

Thymus. Occasionally the thymus shows a decrease in weight following a short course of antiserum, but this is inconstant. Usually thymic architecture and callularity appear surprisingly well-preserved, even at a time when the lymph nodes and spleen have been severely depleted of lymphocytes.

Bone marrow. No obvious changes seem to result from a single dose of antiserum. Multiple injections usually bring about a hyperplasia of erythroid elements, with a relative decrease in the numbers of small lymphocytes present.

Thus a characteristic pattern of lymphoid depletion is seen to emerge after ALS treatment, involving primarily the paracortical areas of lymph nodes and the periarteriolar regions of splenic follicles, while the thymus is relatively unaffected.

The depletion of lymphocytes from lymph node paracortical areas was further characterized autoradiographically in mice given three

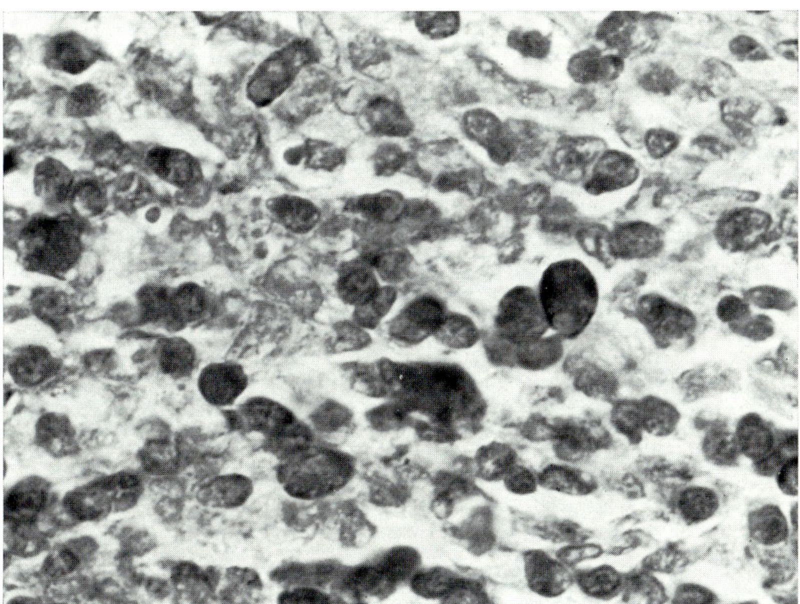

Fig. 9. Paracortical area of axillary lymph node 48 h after a single dose of 0.5 ml ALS. A few small lymphocytes remain, associated with vascular channels, but the content of this region consists largely of reticulum cells with pale nuclei. A few darkly-stained immunoblasts are also present. Methyl green-pyronine. × 1250

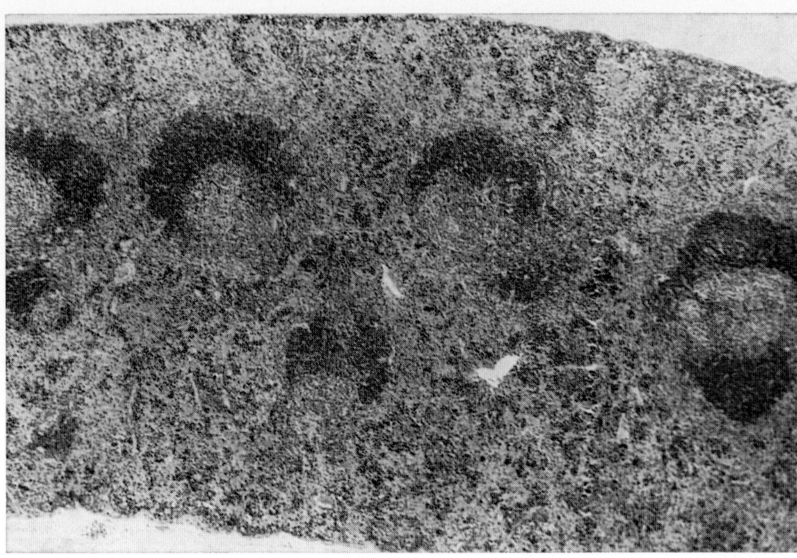

Fig. 10. Longitudinal section of spleen from mouse treated with three subcutaneous doses of ALS, five days after the last dose. Note the sharply defined zones of lymphocyte depletion within splenic follicles, surrounding follicular arterioles. Hematoxylin and eosin. × 138

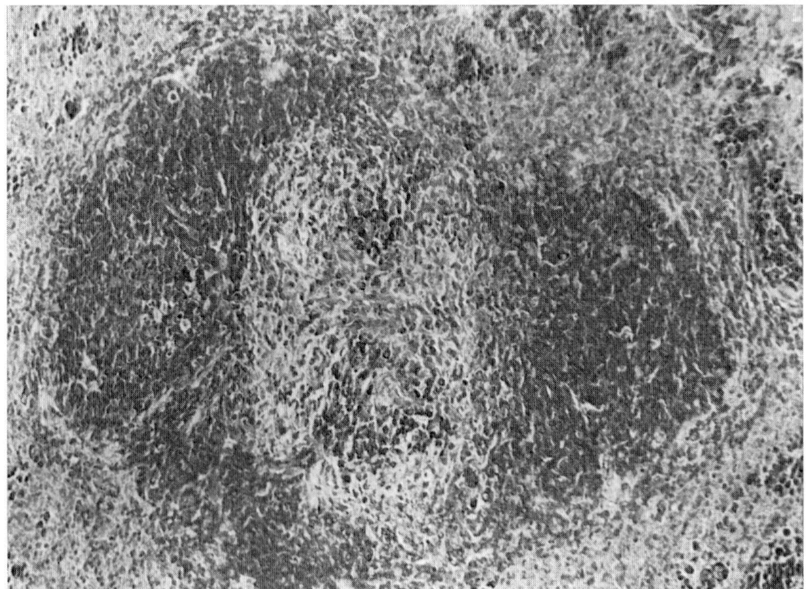

Fig. 11. Higher power of a single splenic follicle shown in figure 10. Note the rim of pyroninophilic cells surrounding central arterioles in an area otherwise markedy depleted of lymphocytes. Methyl green pyronine. × 480

doses (0.5 ml + 0.25 ml + 0.25 ml on alternate days) of either RAMLA or NRS. Two days after the last dose, both groups were infused intravenously with tritiated thymidine for 36 h.

Autoradiographs of lymph node sections showed striking differences in the paracortical regions of the two groups (figs. 12 and 13).

NRS-treated mice showed a preponderance of unlabelled (presumably long-lived) lymphocytes in these areas, and several labelled large lymphocytes and immunoblasts. Little label was deposited within reticular cells.

ALS-treated animals showed depletion of unlabelled, small lymphocytes; virtually every cell remaining within the paracortical area had taken up tritiated thymidine during the period of perfusion. In addition, large amounts of label were seen within reticular cells.

2. Lesions Irrelevant to the Immunosuppressive Activity of ALS

a) Immune response to constituents of rabbit serum. Between four and ten days after the administration of either RAMLS or NRS the features

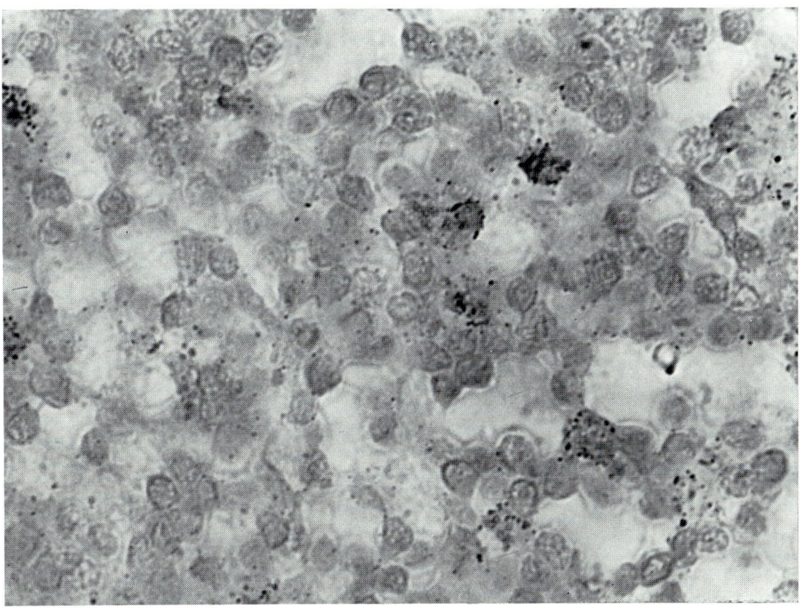

Fig. 12. Autoradiograph of paracortical area of axillary lymph node after three doses of normal rabbit serum, followed by intravenous infusion of tritiated thymidine. (See text.) Note the preponderance of long-lived unlabelled lymphocytes in this area and little or no label within reticulum cells. Ilford L-4 nuclear emulsion; neutral red stain; × 1250

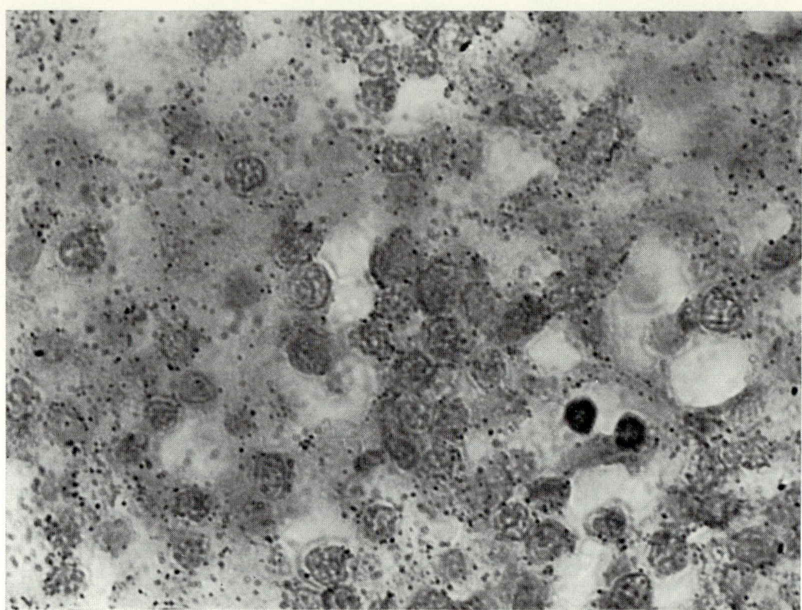

Fig. 13. Autoradiograph of paracortical area of axillary lymph nodes after three doses of rabbit anti-mouse ALS, followed by intravenous infusion of tritiated thymidine (see text). There is a marked increase in the number of labelled lymphocytes present, when compared with figure 12. Note the heavy deposition of radioactivity within reticulum cells. Ilford L-4 nuclear emulsion; neutral red stain; × 1250

of immunization develop within lymph nodes and spleen, both of these tissues showing an increase in weight (fig. 4). In the lymph nodes, which are considerably enlarged (figs. 7, 8), marked medullary hyperplasia develops, with increased numbers of immunoblasts and plasma cell precursors. In the ALS-treated nodes, paracortical depletion persists despite the hyperplasia seen in other areas. In the spleen, follicular hyperplasia develops after either ALS or NRS with numerous periarteriolar immunoblasts and plasma cells at the follicular periphery and within the red pulp. All of these changes recede gradually during the second to fourth week after antiserum injection.

b) Anemia. If RAMLS is not absorbed with mouse erythrocytes prior to use it may contain sufficient anti-red-cell activity to produce anemia (fig. 3). There is usually accompanying splenic enlargement due to erythroid hyperplasia (fig. 4). The anemia can be considerably ameliorated and the splenic hyperplasia lessened by prior red-cell absorption. Absorption with red cells does not impair the ability of the antiserum to prolong skin homografts.

Discussion

Several kinds of antilymphocyte antisera, differing in immunosuppressive potency and *in vitro* activity, were chosen for these studies. Rabbit antimouse serum (RAMLS) was strongly cytotoxic *in vitro* and strongly immunosuppressive *in vivo;* horse anti-mouse gamma globulin (HALGG) was equally cytotoxic *in vitro,* but rather less effective as an immunosuppressive; C57Ks anti-CBA thymocyte antiserum was still less effective. Duck anti-mouse antiserum (DAMLS), although strongly lymphagglutinating [6] possessed minimal *in vitro* cytotoxicity and no immunosuppressive activity. Normal rabbit serum is neither lymphagglutinating, lymphocytotoxic, nor immunosuppressive.

The data presented indicate that the immunosuppressive potency of these antisera seems reflected in the ability of a single dose to cause a lymphopenia which is sustained. That immediate or transient lymphopenia gives no clue to immunosuppressive capabilities is apparent from the observation that normal rabbit serum may also produce lymphopenia which is, however, quickly reversed.

The observation that two or three doses of a powerful antiserum do not produce a much more profound or lasting lymphopenia than a single dose is of interest, as it raises the possibility that the lymphopenia produced by ALS may be largely limited to one sub-population of circulating lymphocytes. This idea is lent some further support by data derived from tritiated thymidine labelling studies (table I). After ALS treatment the proportion of newly-formed cells is increased threefold, even when the total lymphocyte count has been reduced by one-half. It thus seems that ALS treatment may cause a shift in the normal lymphocyte population to one of predominantly newly-formed cells, either by selectively removing long-lived lymphocytes, by increasing the turnover of new cells, or by both mechanisms. If ALS is equally capable of destroying all lymphocytes in a population of lymph node cells, as seems to be the case *in vitro* [Ruszkiewicz, personal communication, 1968,] then the net effect of repeated doses of ALS might be expected to be more pronounced on the cells which would regenerate more slowly, resulting in their selective removal.

In addition to lymphopenia, the histologic changes in lymphoid tissues that correlate best with the immunosuppressive effects of ALS constitute a characteristic pattern of selective depletion of small lymphocytes, restricted to paracortical areas of lymph nodes and peri-arteriolar regions of splenic follicles, leaving the thymus and bone marrow lymphocytes relatively unaffected. Within the limits of precision attainable in any test system dependent on morphologic criteria, the more immunosuppressively potent antisera produced the greater degree of lymphoid tissue depletion, while ineffective antisera produced no such changes.

This pattern of depletion has been commented on previously by several workers [3, 13, 18], and noted consistently by Lance [7] in mice bearing allogeneic skin grafts after chronic treatment with ALS for six months or longer.

The paracortical and periarteriolar areas are known to be colonized by cells of the long-lived, rapidly recirculating lymphocyte pool [5, 13]. Depletion of this pool of cells by manoevres such as thoracic duct drainage [11] or by extracorporeal irradiation of the circulating blood [2] will also produce histologic signs of depletion in these areas, although these signs develop more slowly than with ALS treatment.

The radioautographic observations of these areas after treatment with ALS and NRS (figs. 12, 13) strongly suggest that a selective depletion of long-lived cells, presumably recirculating cells because of their localization within specific lymph node areas, results from antiserum treatment.

It therefore seems reasonable to hypothesize that a primary action of ALS in achieving immunosuppression may involve a rapid and drastic depletion of the long-lived recirculating pool of small lymphocytes from blood and lymphoid tissues. Such a depletion might also be expected to involve thoracic duct lymphocytes as well, and indeed Gowans and Lance [personal communication] have noted a reduced output of cells from the thoracic duct of rats after ALS administration.

While thoracic duct drainage *per se* is a relatively weak immunosuppressive manipulation [11], it is possible that a more rapid and extensive depletion such as that produced by ALS could operate in a qualitatively similar but much more intense fashion to allow prolongation of homografts.

Levey and Medawar [9] suggested initially that ALS acts in the first instance on peripheral lymphocytes. Lance [7] proposed that chronic ALS treatment selectively depletes the pool of long-lived recirculating lymphocytes, because their migratory life-cycle results in their greater exposure to ALS antibody. The present observations would tend to favour these concepts.

Additional support for this hypothesis may be provided by our previous studies on the migration of Cr-51 radioactively labelled lymphocytes, which suggested that the *in vivo* cytotoxic effects of ALS are largely restricted to circulating lymphocytes at a time when they have not yet "homed" to lymph nodes [17].

Although the lymphocytoxicity and observed lymphoid depletion suggest these and similar mechanisms as a mode of action of ALS, other possibilities cannot be ruled out from these studies. Certain ones seem, however, to be rendered more remote than others: e.g., the observation that the thymus suffers little morphologic damage in the face of extensive lymphoid depletion in other organs suggests that ALS probably does not act by duplicating the effects of thymectomy. There is also little evidence from these studies that would support a theory of action based on the mechanisms of either "blind-folding" or "sterile activation". The predominant change observed which appears relevant to immunosuppression is the deletion rather than the preservation of lymphocytes; and while immunoblast transformation does occur in lymph nodes after ALS treatment, similar degrees of such transformation occur in animals given normal rabbit serum, indicating only that the constituents of both ALS and NRS may be immunogenic in mice, and the lymphoid tissue changes are those of an orthodox immune response to these substances.

Summary

The acute effects of antilymphocyte sera (ALS) were studied in CBA mice with respect to hematologic and histologic parameters, and by autoradiography of peripheral blood and lymphoid tissues in mice perfused intravenously with tritiated thymidine.

The ability of a single dose of antiserum to produce lymphopenia for longer than 48 h appeared to parallel its immunosuppressive potency as measured by prolongation of skin allograft survival. The magnitude and duration of the lymphopenia produced, however, did not necessarily correlate with the degree of immunosuppression achieved. In some animals, there was evidence suggesting that there had been a shift from predominantly longlived to predominantly newly-formed cells in the peripheral blood after ALS treatment.

A characteristic pattern of depletion of lymphocytes from lymphoid tissues seemed invariably associated with immunosuppression by ALS. This was sharply localized to lymph node paracortical areas and to splenic periarteriolar regions; the thymus usually showed little or no change even after repeated doses of ALS, despite the loss of cells from other lymphoid organs. Autoradiography of the depleted areas in animals perfused with tritiated thymidine disclosed a near-absence of long-lived small lymphocytes, and a heavy deposition of label within reticulum cells.

The relationship of the histological findings to some of the various mechanisms postulated to explain the mode of action of ALS are discussed. It is suggested that immunosuppression by ALS may involve a rapid and drastic depletion of the long-lived recirculating lymphocytes from the lymphoid tissues and the blood.

References

1. Billingham, R.E. and Medawar, P.B.: The technique of free skin grafting in mammals. J. exp. Biol. *28:* 385–402 (1951).
2. Cronkite, E.P.; Jansen, C.R.; Cottier, H.; Rai, K. and Sipe, C.R.: Lymphocyte production measured by extracorporeal irradiation, cannulation, and labelling techniques. Ann. N.Y. Acad. Sci. *113:* 566–577 (1964).
3. Denman, A.M. and Frenkel, E.P.: Mode of action of antilymphocyte globulin. II. Changes in the lymphoid cell population in rats treated with antilymphocyte globulin. Immunology *14:* 115–125 (1968).
4. Gray, J.G.; Monaco, A.P. and Russell, P.S.: Heterologous mouse antilymphocyte serum to prolong skin homografts. Surg. Forum *15:* 142–144 (1964).
5. Gowans, J.L. and Knight, E.J.: The route of recirculation of lymphocytes in the rat. Proc. roy. Soc. B *159:* 257–281 (1964).
6. Jooste, S.V.; Lance, E.M.; Levey, R.H.; Medawar, P.B.; Ruszkiewicz, M.; Sharman, R. and Taub, R.N.: Notes on the preparation and assay of antilymphocyte serum for use in mice. Immunology (in press).
7. Lance, E.M.: The effects of chronic ALS administration in mice. In: Advances in transplantation, pp. 107–116 (Eds.) J. Dausset, J. Hamburger and G. Mathé, Monksgaard (1967).
8. Levey, R.H. and Medawar, P.B.: Some experiments on the action of antilymphoid antisera. Ann. N.Y. Acad. Sci. *129:* 164–177 (1966).
9. Levey, R.H. and Medawar, P.B.: Further experiments on the action of anti-lymphocytic antiserum. Proc. nat. Acad. Sci., Wash. *58:* 470–477 (1967).
10. McGregor, D.D. and Gowans, J.L.: The antibody responses of rats depleted of lymphocytes by chronic drainage from the thoracic duct. J. exp. Med. *117:* 303–320 (1963).
11. McGregor, D.D. and Gowans, J.L.: Survival of homografts of skin in rats depleted of lymphocytes by chronic drainage from the thoracic duct. Lancet *i:* 629–632 (1964).
12. Monaco, A.P.; Wood, M.L.; Van der Werf, B.A. and Russell, P.S.: Effects of antilymphocyte serum in mice, dogs and man. In Antilymphocytic Serum, pp. 111–134. Ciba Foundation Study Group No. 29 (Eds.) G.E.W. Wolstenholme and M. O'Connor (Churchill, London 1967).
13. Parrott, D.M.V.: The response of draining lymph nodes to immunological stimulation in intact and thymectomized animals. J. clin. Path. (Suppl.) *20:* 456–465 (1967).
14. Parrott, D.M.V.; De Sousa, M.A.B. and East, J.: Thymus dependent areas in the lymphoid organs of neonatally thymectomized mice. J. exp. Med. *123:* 191–203 (1966).
15. Starzl, R.E.; Marchioro, T.L. and Iwasaki, Y.: Attributes of clinically used immunosuppressive drugs. Possible future uses of antilymphoid antisera. Fed. Proc. *26:* 944–952 (1967).
16. Taub, R.N. and Lance, E.M.: The histologic effects of heterologous antilymphocyte serum (ALS) in CBA mice. J. exp. Med. (in press).
17. Taub, R.N. and Lance, E.M.: Effects of heterologous antilymphocyte serum on the distribution of Cr-51 labelled lymph node cells in mice. Immunology *15:* 633 (1968).
18. Turk, J.L. and Willoughby, D.A.: Central and peripheral effects of antilymphocyte sera. Lancet *i:* 249–251 (1967).
19. Wigzell, H.: Quantitative titrations of mouse H-2 isoantibodies using Cr-51 labelled target cells. Transplantation *3:* 423–429 (1965).
20. Woodruff, M.F.A. and Anderson, N.F.: Effect of lymphocyte depletion by thoracic duct fistula and administration of antilymphocyte serum on the survival of skin homografts in rats. Nature (Lond.) *200:* 702 (1963).

Author's address: Dr. R.N. Taub, Mount Sinai Hospital, School of Medicine, 5th Avenue, *New York, N.Y. 10029* (USA).

Antibiotica et Chemotherapia, vol. 15, pp. 267–294 (Karger, Basel/New York 1969)

An Analysis of the Multiplicity of the Effects of Antilymphocyte Serum – A Comparison with the Action of Other Immunosuppressive Agents in the Cell-Mediated Immune Response and Non-Specific Inflammation

J. L. Turk and D. A. Willoughby

Institute of Dermatology and St. Bartholomew's Hospital, London

A. *Introduction—The Mechanism of Cell-Mediated Immune Reactions* (fig. 1)

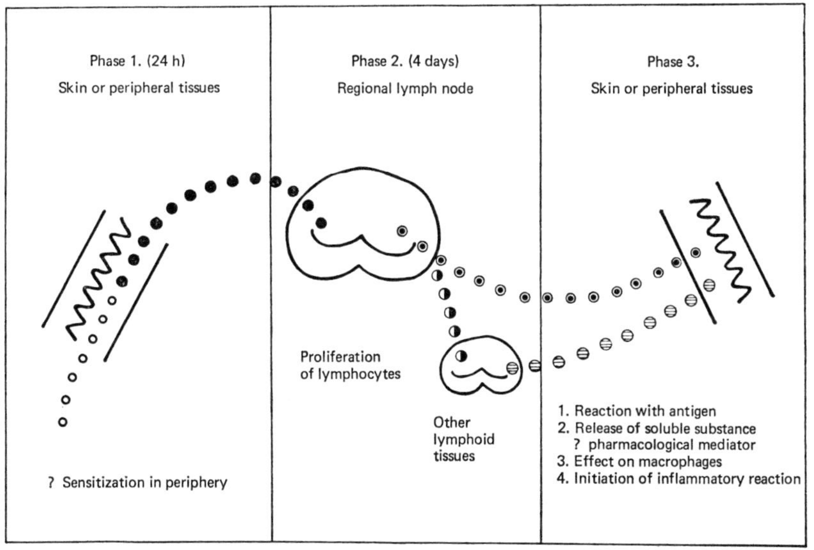

Fig. 1. The three stages of a cell-mediated immune reaction
○ ○ ○ ○   Unsensitized lymphocytes
● ● ◑ ◑   Sensitized lymphocytes
◉ ⊖ ⊖ ⬤   Immunologically reactive lymphocytes

Cell-mediated immune reactions involve three stages analogous to a reflex arc. There is first the process of antigenic recognition analogous to the afferent side of the nervous reflex arc. The second stage is one of cellular proliferation which occurs in the central lymphoid tissue. The third or efferent side of the sensitization arc involves the reaction of the specifically sensitized immunologically active cells with the target antigen. If the antigen is on the surface of an allogeneic cell as in the homograft reaction this will result in cell death. On the other hand if the reaction between antigen and specifically activated lymphocytes occurs in the region of macrophages, changes will occur on the surface of these cells which will result in the release of pharmacologically active agents and possibly enzymes. These in turn will produce vascular changes such as dilatation and increased permeability causing erythema, induration, haemorrhage and necrosis. There will also be changes in the physico-chemical nature of collagen in the skin resulting in induration.

The Afferent Side of the Sensitization Arc (fig. 2)

The differences between the cell-mediated immune response and humoral antibody production can be related directly to the means by which sensitization occurs. In a pure state of humoral antibody production, the antigen in its soluble form will drain down the lymphatics to the medulla where it will be taken up by the many

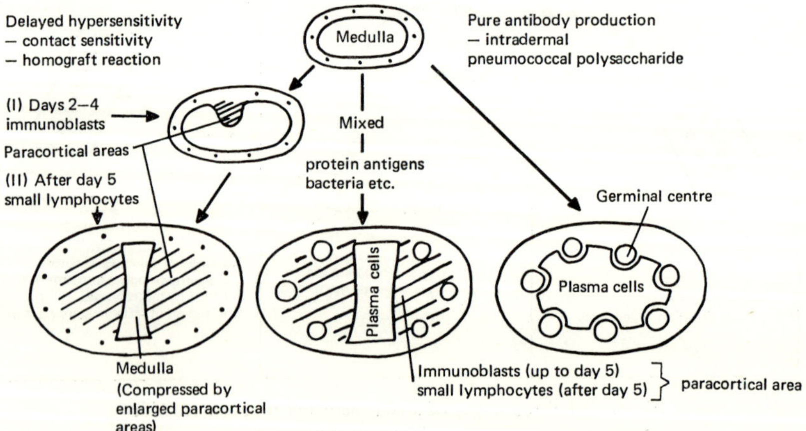

Fig. 2. Diagram of the primary response of a lymph node to antigenic stimulation.

macrophages which occur in this region of the lymph node. Macrophages have the property of processing soluble antigen so that it becomes extremely potent in sensitizing the cells which are the precursors of plasma cells, probably lymphocytes, occurring at the cortico-medullary junction. These cells are then stimulated to proliferate specifically into plasma cells both at the cortico-medullary junction and in the medullary cords. Plasma cells have their ribosomes, involved in protein synthesis, lying along the channels of the endoplasmic reticulum, which forms the mechanism for secretion of newly formed proteins into the extracellular fluids and thus down the efferent lymphatics into the blood stream. Some of this antibody tracks backwards into the cortex where it is trapped in the lymph follicles. This will then react with further antigen and cause antigen-antibody interaction to occur on the surface of macrophages in the lymph follicles. This process stimulates the adjacent cells within the lymph follicles to proliferate and eventually die forming what are known as "germinal centres". Germinal centres do not form as part of the cell-mediated immune response and are always associated with plasma cell proliferation and humoral antibody production.

The cell-mediated immune response, however, is a response to fixed antigen in the periphery, typical examples are skin homografts and the skin modified antigenically by a chemical sensitizing agent in contact sensitivity. Under these conditions the antigen is not draining down into the lymph node in large quantities. Most of the antigen remains fixed in the periphery. Small lymphocytes pass continuously through the peripheral tissues. Here they receive their antigenic stimulus. There is evidence that this could be by pinocytosis, as following stimulation there is an increased number of small lymphocytes containing lysosomes or phagosomes identified by their content of acid hydrolases, in the draining lymph nodes and an increased number of lysosomes in each cell. The stimulated lymphocytes then pass down into the area of the cortex of the lymph node between the lymph follicles. It is here they find the right milieu for proliferation. This area of the lymph node cortex which contains the mobile pool of immunologically active lymphocytes has been called the "paracortical area" of the lymph node. It is also known to depend on the integrity of the thymus in neonatal life. Following neonatal thymectomy lymphocytes cannot proliferate in this area and are in fact absent from it. Thus it has also been called the "thymus-dependent area" of the lymph node. The integrity of this area of the lymph node for true development of cell-mediated immune re sponses is confirmed by the fact that these responses cannot occur in an animal in which these areas have not developed as a result of neo natal thymectomy.

It takes five days from the first contact with a chemical sensitizing agent for an animal to become sensi tive. During the first four days there is a rapid increase in the size of the paracortical areas of the lymph node, which replace the whole node compressing the medulla into a very narrow chink. During this period the paracortical area contains up to 20 % of large pyroninophilic cells many of which can be seen in mitosis. These cells are lymphocytes transformed under antigenic stimulus and are dividing either into cells, which are indistinguishable under the light microscope from small lymphocytes, or into other similar large pyroninophilic cells. These large pyroninophilic cells have been termed "immunoblasts" [Turk, 1967a] as they are cells which are dividing under antigenic stimulus and are inhibited from dividing if the animal has been made specifically immunologically tolerant. With the use of radioactive tracers the progeny of these cells can be shown to be present in grafts during rejection or in mononuclear cell suspensions which will react with antigen and produce typical delayed hypersensitivity reactions in a non-sensitized host animal. There is no evidence yet that those cells which develop from cells dividing under an immunological stimulus in the draining lymph node are in fact the cells which react with antigen in the periphery. However, removal of the draining lymph node before the fourth day after sensitization, the day upon which the earliest signs of sensitivity are seen, is sufficient to block the development of sensitivity. After this it appears that immunologically active cells are already in the periphery able to react with antigen, and are distributed throughout the rest of the lymphoid system, so that the animal remains sensitive even if the draining lymph nodes are removed after this period.

Soluble antigen passes down to both homolateral and contralateral lymph nodes in not very different concentrations. Removal of the homolateral lymph nodes before the fourth day after sensitization blocks the development of sensitivity. Therefore the passage of soluble antigen to a lymph node is not sufficient to stimulate the cell-mediated immunological response and sensitization must be brought about by something draining preferentially to the homolateral lymph nodes. Lymphocytes would be expected to drain preferentially to the homolateral lymph nodes in far greater quantities than to the contralateral lymph node. Therefore it is most likely that these lymphocytes receive their antigenic stimulus in the periphery before they drain down to the homolateral lymph nodes [TURK, 1967b].

The Efferent Side of the Immunisation Arc

If the lymphocytes which react with antigen in the periphery contain a recognition factor, possibly analogous to part of an immunoglobulin molecule, which can react with antigen in the periphery, it is necessary to determine how and when such a peptide could be formed. The only cells which are making large amounts of protein during the sensitization process are the immunoblasts. Examination of the ultra-structure of these cells under the electron microscope show that they contain large numbers of ribosomes in their cytoplasm arranged in polyribosome clusters. This is in marked contrast to plasma cells where the ribosomes are arranged along an endoplasmic reticulum, the means whereby cells secrete proteins in the extracellular fluid. Immunoblasts are thus making large amounts of protein, but have no means of secreting it. It can be shown that immunoblasts are making large amounts of enzymes, such as those involved in the pentose shunt, which will be taking part in nucleic acid synthesis and replication. However, there are also cells intermediate between immunoblasts and lymphocytes in the lymph node, after sensitization has already developed, which contain many polyribosomes. It could be that immunoblasts and intermediate cells are also making peptide chains which form the recognition factors, which the latter cells, morphologically indistinguishable from small lymphocytes under the light microscope, can also produce in the periphery. Examination of protein synthesis by lymph nodes during and soon after sensitization, show that a new protein is being made. This protein appears to have a molecular weight of approximately 30,000 to 50,000 but this is present in such low concentration that it is difficult to characterise it any further [WILSON and TURK, 1968]. It is also known that lymph nodes and peripherally circulating lymphocytes from sensitized animals are making a substance which is released from the cell by antigen and can react with antigen outside the cell to produce an effect on the cell surface of macrophages *in vitro*.

Following the interaction between antigen and sensitized cells *in vivo* there follows what appears to be a typical inflammatory reaction which is characterised by increased vascular permeability to plasma proteins, swelling of collagen, massive infiltration with mainly mono-nuclear cells. These changes invariably follow a latent period which is due to the slow arrival of cells at the site. The reaction usually persists for about three to four days after its initiation. It has been found that these inflammatory changes do not appear to be mediated by the same pharmacological agents that participate in non-specific acute inflammation [Schild and Willoughby, 1967]. It is probable that a number of different pharmacological agents are involved, some of which are present in extracts of normal lymphoid and other tissues. These factors have been termed generically the "lymph node perme-ability factor". Membrane-free extracts of normal lymphoid tissue (lymph node permeability factor—LNPF) have been found to increase vascular permeability, cause leucocyte emigration and to be readily differentiated from histamine, 5-hydroxy-tryptamine, bradykinin, kal-likrein, and "globulin permeability factor" [Willoughby, Boughton and Schild, 1963].

A comparison of the effects of immunosuppressive drugs and anti-lymphocyte sera must take account of the fact that these two types of agents can have a central effect on the response of the central lymphoid tissue to antigenic stimulation and a peripheral effect on the ability of the body to produce an inflammatory response following the inter-action of sensitized cells or antibody with antigen in the periphery [Turk, 1964; Borel and Schwartz, 1964; Turk and Willoughby, 1967]. The central effects of these agents will be compared first of all. This will be followed by a comparison of the peripheral effect of drugs and antilymphocyte sera both on the specific cell-mediated immune reaction and on various non-specific inflammation reactions.

B. Central Effect of Immunosuppressive Treatment on Changes in
Lymphoid Tissue During the Development of Cell-Mediated Immunity

The effect of various drugs on the cellular events which occur during the induction of cell-mediated immunity has been reviewed previously [Turk, 1967c] and are summarized in figure 3. Most of the drugs studied appear to have a multiplicity of effects at different levels in the sensitization process. The effect of any one of these agents on the afferent arc can be at a number of different levels at the same time. These range from a direct effect on the turnover of normal lympho-cytes through the ability of the lymphocytes to be transformed as a

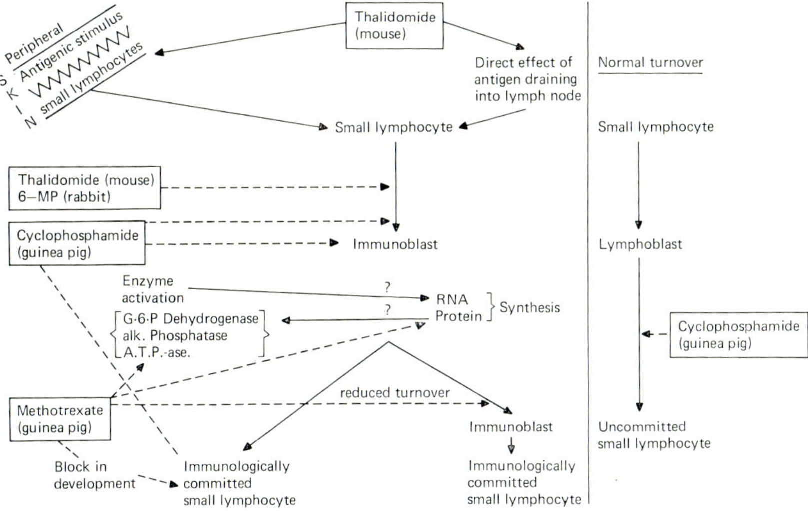

Fig. 3. Effect of immunosuppressive drugs on cell differentiation during the induction of delayed hypersensitivity (cell-mediated immunity).

result of the antigenic stimulus, to a failure in the increased output of small lymphocytes produced by the immunological response. These are the cells which are thought to react with antigen in the periphery to produce the immune response.

Cyclophosphamide can be shown to act centrally in the guinea pig by inhibiting the differentiation of lymphocytes into immunoblasts. Those few immunoblasts which develop are swollen and distorted, and up to five times normal size. This drug also has a marked anti-mitotic effect. 6-MP has also been shown to act on cell proliferation in the rabbit homograft reaction by blocking the differentiation of small lymphocytes into immunoblasts.

The effect of methotrexate, on cell-mediated immune sensitization in the guinea pig, was not found to be that which might be expected from the effect of this compound on other systems and in other species. No effect was found on the differentiation of small lymphocytes into immunoblasts as with the other drugs. Moreover, there was no block in the incorporation of thymidine by these cells which appeared to be synthesising DNA normally, even after six days drug treatment. However, there was some diminution in RNA and protein synthesis. There was also a marked diminution in enzyme activity in these cells. Whether the diminished protein synthesis was the cause of the decreased enzyme activity, or the decreased enzyme activity resulted in decreased RNA and protein synthesis is not known. Methotrexate also inhibited the division of immunoblasts into the new population of small lymphocytes which appeared in the draining lymph node on the fifth day after sensitization at the same time as the first signs of sensitivity could be found in the periphery.

Another compound which has recently been found to have an immunosuppressive effect on the homograft reaction in the mouse is thalidomide. It appears that this drug could act by blocking the afferent arc of sensitization in the periphery, as treatment of donor skin alone with thalidomide will significantly drop the number of immunoblasts appearing in the draining lymph node. For maximal effect however, both donor and recipient have to be treated with the drug.

One should offer a word of warning at this stage. Because a drug has a particular effect on a specific biological activity in one species, this does not mean that it will have the same effect in another species. Much confusion has been brought about in the past concerning the pharmacological action of drugs, by extrapolating the effect on one biological function in one species to explain the effect on the same or another biological function in a different species. However, one point appears clear and that is that the effect of immunosuppressive drugs in inhibiting the immune reaction *in vivo* cannot be explained by a single pharmacological action. The final effect is probably the result of the sum action of a number of different independent effects, many of which were not conceived by the chemists who first synthesised the drugs and suggested that they might have certain biological activities.

There is no doubt that certain agents such as thalidomide and antilymphocyte serum can act on lymphocytes in the periphery before they reach the paracortical area of the lymph node prior to cell proliferation. Martin and Miller [1967] have found that mouse thoracic duct lymphocytes incubated with antilymphocyte serum (ALS) are eliminated more rapidly from the circulation than those incubated with normal rabbit serum. These "damaged" cells appeared to be sequestrated in the liver as well as the spleen and lymph nodes. Moreover, it appears that the effect of ALS is directed more against the long-lived than short-lived small lymphocytes [Denman, Denman and Embling, 1968].

Lymphocytes treated *in vitro* with antilymphocyte serum (ALS) were examined in the Cambridge Stereoscan electron microscope

[CLARKE, SALISBURY and WILLOUGHBY, 1968]. Normal lymphocytes were found to have a smooth spherical surface. After treatment with ALS, the earliest changes seen after five minutes treatment consisted of roughening and pitting of the cell surface. Within fifteen minutes these changes were more severe and often only cellular debris could be found scattered among the agglutinated cells. Similar changes

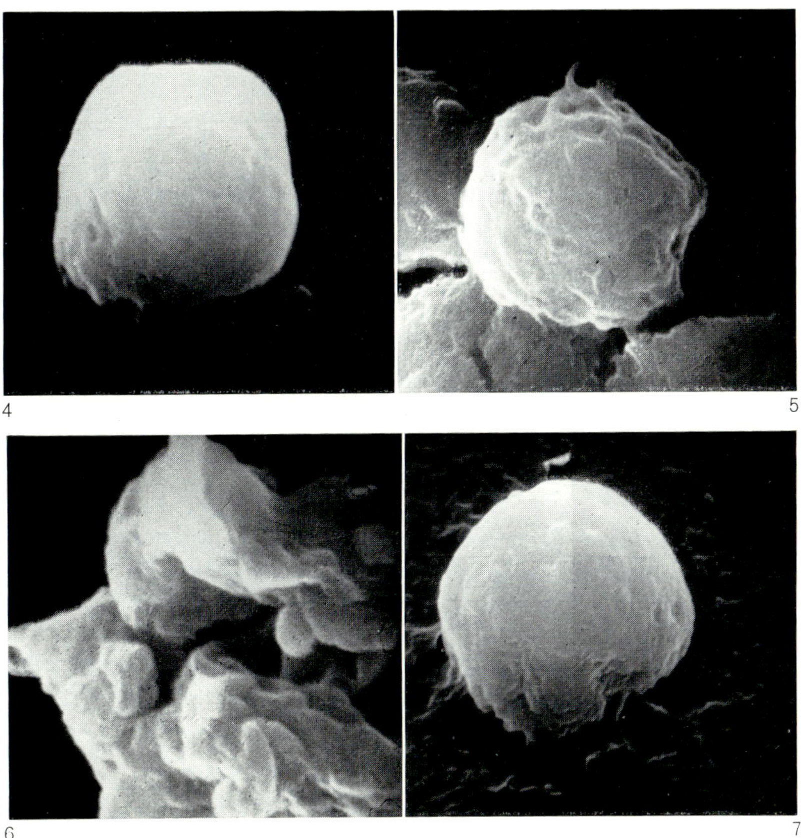

Fig. 4. Lymph node cell from rat sensitized to tuberculin, washed in Hank's solution. Stereoscan E.M. × 15,000.

Fig. 5. Lymph node cells from rat sensitized to tuberculin, incubated for 15 min in ALS then washed. Note the agglutination of cells. Stereoscan E.M. × 15,000.

Fig. 6. Lymph node cells from rat sensitized to tuberculin, incubated for 15 min in ALS, then washed in Hank's solution. Cellular destruction has occurred leaving cellular debris. Stereoscan E.M. × 15,000.

Fig. 7. Lymph node cell from rat sensitized to tuberculin, incubated for 15 min in antiserum against membrane free extracts of lymph nodes (anti-LNPF). Note minimal damage to cell surface. Stereoscan E.M. × 15,000.

were found to occur to lymphocytes following the injection of ALS *in vivo*. No such changes were found following the treatment of cells either *in vitro* or *in vivo* with antiserum prepared against membrane-free extracts of lymph nodes (Anti-LNPF) (figs. 4, 5, 6 and 7).

Following a previous observation [TURK and WILLOUGHBY, 1967] that antiserum prepared against guinea pig thymus cells had a damaging effect specifically on the thymus-dependent or paracortical area of the lymph node cortex (this is the area of the lymph node containing the mobile pool of small lymphocytes and which responds specifically in cell-mediated immune responses) it was important to compare this with what may be found using a serum prepared against lymph node cells derived from lymph nodes which were rich in both plasma cells and germinal centres using the method of immunisation described by LEVEY and MEDAWAR [1966], [TURK, WILLOUGHBY and STEVENS, 1968]. Figure 8 shows at low power that this serum had an identical effect to serum prepared against thymus cells. The auricular lymph node illustrated is one in which an attempt at stimulation of cell-mediated immunity has been made by the application of the chemical sensitizer oxazolone to the ear. However, there is also proliferation

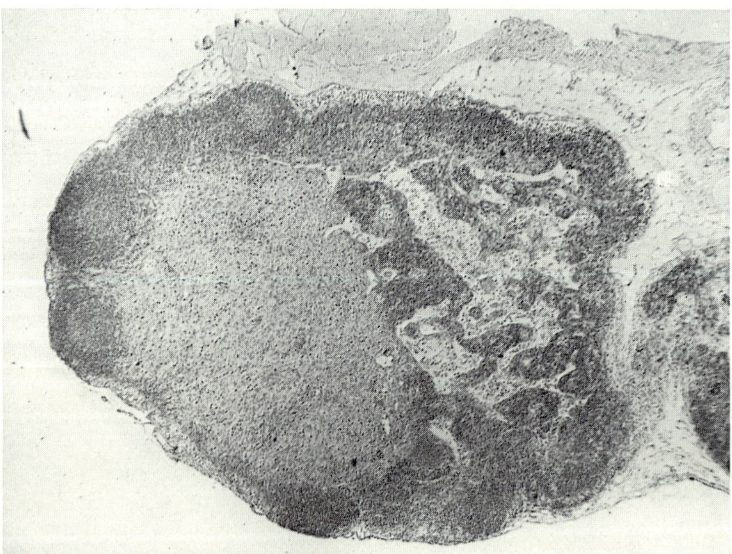

Fig. 8. Auricular lymph node from guinea pig draining area of application of oxazolone, four days previously; also treated for *six days* with anti-lymph node lymphocyte serum. *Note:* Fibrosis of paracortical area of lymph node. Sparing of germinal centres and medulla. Methyl green pyronin × 40.

of germinal centres and plasma cells in the medulla, due to the parenteral injections of the foreign serum. As with the antithymocyte serum the small lymphocytes of the paracortical area are absent and replaced by cells closely resembling fibroblasts (fig. 9). Cells resembling macrophages were seen in this area containing intracellular inclusions of nuclear material. Immunoblasts [TURK, 1967a] which normally occur in this area on the fourth day after application of oxazolone to the skin could still be seen but at the area of maximum concentration these were reduced to 50%, or less, of that found in lymph nodes from untreated animals. In striking contrast the germinal centres and plasma cells in the medulla were completely unaffected. It is of interest that there was a marked cut off between the area of fibrosis and the plasma cells in the medulla (fig. 10).

These results were found with a six-day course of antiserum. The same antiserum was given for three days only, starting one day after the application of oxazolone to the ear. In half the animals examined little effect could be demonstrated when the animals were killed 24 h after the last injection. In the other half, however, there was a similar depletion of lymphocytes from the paracortical areas as seen in animals

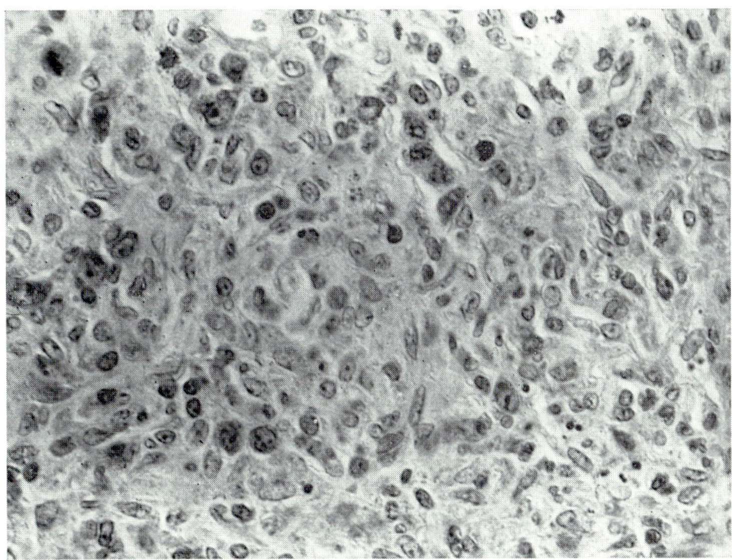

Fig. 9. High power of paracortical area from lymph node shown in figure 4 demonstrating pronounced depletion of small lymphocytes and immunoblasts, replacement by fibroblasts and nuclear debris in cells resembling macrophages. Methyl green pyronin × 450.

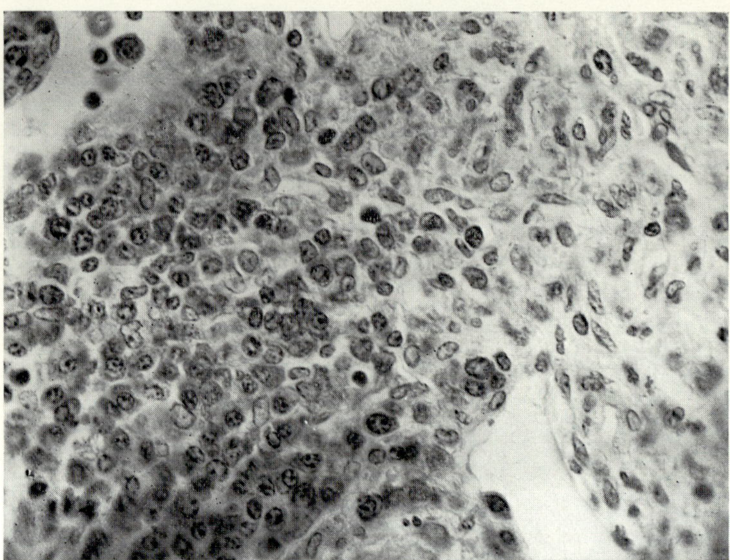

Fig. 10. High power of junction of paracortical area and plasma cells in medulla from lymph node shown in figure 4. Note complete lack of involvement of plasma cells in damage process. Methyl green pyronin × 450.

treated for six days. Also there was a similar sequestration of nuclear debris in macrophages. However, these nodes were different in that there was no reduction in the number of immunoblasts. To determine what part of the effect of ALS on lymph nodes was due to antibodies directed against antigens forming an integral part of the cell membrane, these results were compared with those produced by the antiserum against membrane-free extracts of lymph nodes (anti-LNPF serum). One ml anti-LNPF serum given daily for six days starting two days before sensitization, had no noticeable effect on the small lymphocytes of the paracortical area of the cortex of the lymph node, although there was an approximately 50 % reduction in the number of immunoblasts present in this area four days after sensitization, as compared with animals not treated with the antiserum.

One ml of antithymocyte serum (ATS) for six days was found to produce an 88 % drop in circulating lymphocytes, a similar course of antilymph node lymphocyte serum (ALS) produced a 92 % drop, whereas anti-LNPF produced only a 53 % drop. A six-day course of ATS and ALS produced a marked rise in circulating basophils, while anti-LNPF produced a rise in circulating eosinophils.

No changes in the thymus were found in any of the animals treated in this way. Both the spleens and mesenteric lymph nodes from guinea pigs treated with ATS and ALS showed depletion of the thymus-dependent or paracortical areas. However, those treated with anti-LNPF showed marked proliferation of all areas similar to that found following six daily intraperitoneal injections of one ml normal rabbit serum.

In our previous report [Turk and Willoughby, 1967] using antiserum prepared against thymus cells in a sensitizing course over a period of 28 days, it was found that this serum had a specific effect in suppressing small lymphocytes in the paracortical or "thymus-dependent area" of the lymph node [Oort and Turk, 1965; Parrott, de Sousa and East, 1966]. This was associated with a replacement of these cells in this area by cells morphologically resembling fibroblasts. The report of Levey and Medawar [1966] which was published shortly before suggested that the optimum time course for the production of antilymphocyte serum was in fact three weeks. Thus subsequent sera were prepared using the course of injections described by these authors. An identical effect on contact sensitivity and acute inflammation in the periphery and on lymph nodes, during the latent period between a first application of a contact agent and the resultant development of sensitivity, was found using sera prepared as in our original communication [Turk and Willoughby, 1967] and prepared according to the method of Levey and Medawar [1966]. The next question of interest was whether the specific effect on the thymus-dependent area of the lymph node was due to the fact that we were using sera prepared against lymphocytes derived solely from the thymus. In subsequent experiments rabbits were immunised with cells derived from the cervical and mesenteric lymph nodes. These tissues contain germinal centre and plasma cells as well as lymphocytes derived from the narrow compact cortex and the thymus-dependent area of the lymph node. Such a serum, it was thought, might affect the lymph node as a whole. However, it was found that this serum also has an effect specific to the "thymus-dependent area", identical with that produced by the antithymocyte serum. No effect was found on the germinal centres or sheets of plasma cells which occurred in the medullary cords of the lymph node in response to the parenteral injection of foreign serum. Antiserum prepared against membrane-free extracts of lymph nodes (anti-LNPF) had a central effect only in that it produced an approximately 50 % reduction in immunoblasts which were present in this area of the lymph node four days after application of oxazolone to the skin which it drained. A similar effect was found in three out of five guinea pigs treated with antiserum prepared against epidermal cells.

No change was found in the histological appearance of thymuses from guinea pigs treated with antilymphocyte serum prepared with thymus or lymph node cells, if the serum was first adsorbed with guinea pig red cells. If sera were not adsorbed, a severe haemolytic anaemia was seen accompanied by the circulation of numerous normoblasts. This was associated with marked wasting of the thymus, possibly due to a stress factor and similar to that produced by LANDY, SANDERSON, BERNSTEIN and LERNER [1965] by the injection of endotoxin into rabbits.

How the thymus-dependent areas of the lymph node are affected so specifically is very much a matter of speculation. It is known that lymphocytes, which pass through these areas continuously, are damaged in the periphery with the result that this area can rapidly become depleted. Moreover, macrophages are found in this area containing nuclear debris, suggesting that there is some sequestration of dead cells at this site. It is interesting that if the animals are given only a three-day course of antilymphocyte serum beginning the day after sensitization, there is no depletion of immunoblasts although in half the animals the small lymphocytes are already absent and replaced by fibroblast-like cells. This could indicate that lymphocytes which have already received a stimulus to differentiate, possibly from antigen in the periphery, are less affected by the antiserum than those which have not been stimulated in the periphery. This might suggest that the major effect of antilymphocyte serum was not on the process of peripheral sensitization [MEDAWAR, 1958] but possibly on unstimulated small lymphocytes and those derived from the division of already differentiated immunoblasts.

These findings indicate that a considerable amount of the effect of antilymphocyte serum in the guinea pig is directed against cells in the "thymus-dependent areas" of the lymph node involved in cell-mediated immunity. No changes were however found in the areas of the lymph node involved in the humoral antibody response. This was somewhat surprising as it has now been reported that under certain circumstances antilymphocyte serum can suppress the primary humoral antibody response to sheep erythrocytes and bovine albumin in rats [JAMES and ANDERSON, 1967; JAMES and JUBB, 1967]. Whereas some of the effects on cell-mediated immunity can be explained on the basis of the histological changes found in the central lymphoid tissue, these changes cannot yet account for the effect on humoral antibody production, and further information will have to be sought to explain these effects [TURK, WILLOUGHBY and STEVENS, 1968]. If it were to be postulated that ALS treatment in the adult had a similar effect to neonatal thymectomy, then the effect of ALS on antibody production could be explained as being on those "thymus-dependent" cells, involved in some way in the mechanism of humoral antibody formation.

C. Action of Drugs and Antilymphocyte Sera on Cell-Mediated Immune Reactions and Non-Specific Inflammation in Periphery

There is no doubt that certain immunosuppressive drugs can suppress the inflammatory aspects of both cell-mediated immune reactions and the Arthus reaction in the periphery. Cyclophosphamide has been found to reduce the ability of guinea pigs to manifest the inflammatory aspects of both the tuberculin reaction and contact sensitivity in the guinea pig [TURK, 1964]. 6-mercaptopurine (6 M-P) has been found to suppress the inflammatory aspects of the Arthus reaction in the rabbit without affecting the level of circulating antibody [BOREL and SCHWARTZ, 1964].

Table I compares the effects of cyclophosphamide, methotrexate, phytohaemagglutinin (PHA), 6 M-P, deep X-irradiation (650r), and ALS in suppressing various forms of non-specific inflammation in the rat.

There seems little doubt that ATS (antithymocyte serum) and ALS (antilymph node lymphocyte serum) injected intravenously just before the elicitation of the reaction are powerful agents capable of acting against the peripheral manifestations of the cell-mediated immune reaction and non-specific acute inflammatory reactions. It has been found that they will suppress the acute inflammation provoked by both thermal and chemical (turpentine intradermally and intrapleurally) injury (figs. 11 and 12). It is of interest however, that these sera fail to affect a classical model of chronic inflammation, namely the granuloma produced by inplantation of a cotton wool pellet. Their effect on acute inflammation seems to be more marked on acute vascular changes such as vasodilatation and altered vascular perme-

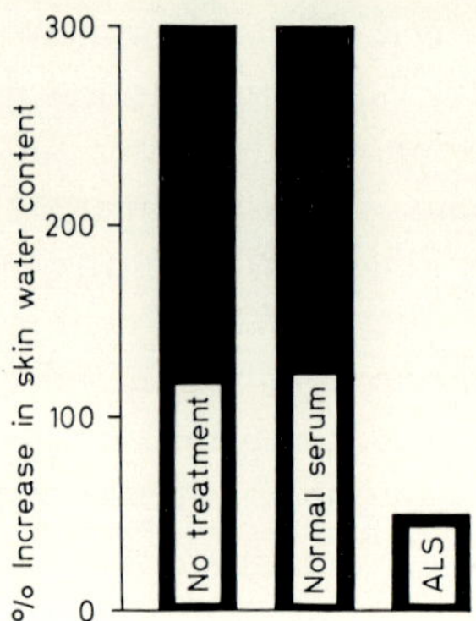

Fig. 11. Effect of anti-lymphocyte serum on oedema produced as a result of thermal injury to the skin in rats.

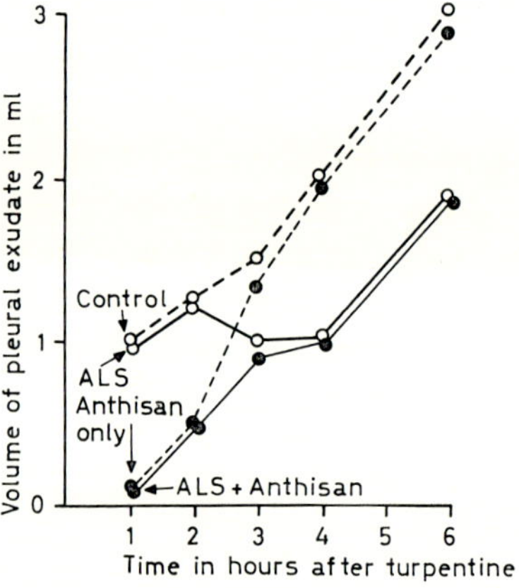

Fig. 12. A comparison of the effect of anti-lymphocyte serum (ALS) and anthisan on the volume of pleural exudate produced by the intrapleural injection of turpentine in the rat.

O --- O Control
O —— O ALS alone
● --- ● Anthisan alone
● —— ● ALS and Anthisan

ability to plasma proteins. Antiserum against membrane-free extracts of lymph nodes (Anti-LNPF) also possesses comparable activity to the antilymphocyte serum in its ability to suppress delayed hypersensitivity reactions [Schild and Willoughby, 1967], among them the tuberculin reaction, cutaneous hypersensitivity to DNCB [Willoughby, Walters and Spector, 1965], pertussis hypersensitivity [Willoughby, 1966] and experimental allergic thyroiditis in rats

[WILLOUGHBY and COOTE, 1966]. On the other hand there is a notable discrepancy between the ability of the anti-LNPF to suppress the acute inflammatory reaction when compared with ALS (fig. 13). This discrepancy could possibly indicate that there are two modes of action on the part of ATS and ALS in the periphery, whereas the anti-LNPF serum might be more specifically directed against mediators of the delayed hypersensitivity reaction.

Adrenalectomy in our hands failed to influence the anti-inflammatory activity of ALS which would seem to eliminate the possibility that this serum is acting via adrenal cortical or, in acute situations, adrenal medullary hormones.

The duration of action of ALS as an anti-inflammatory agent seems to be limited in time, and administration of the serum up to five hours in advance of the injurious stimulus would seem to be the limit of its duration of action. As its activity is most pronounced four hours after the stimulus it would seem that the action of the serum is limited to approximately nine hours.

The possibility that ALS was exerting its action on acute inflammation through cross-reaction with antigens on polymorphonuclear leucocytes has been excluded by adsorbing antithymocyte sera with polymorphonuclear leucocytes which failed to produce any loss of activity.

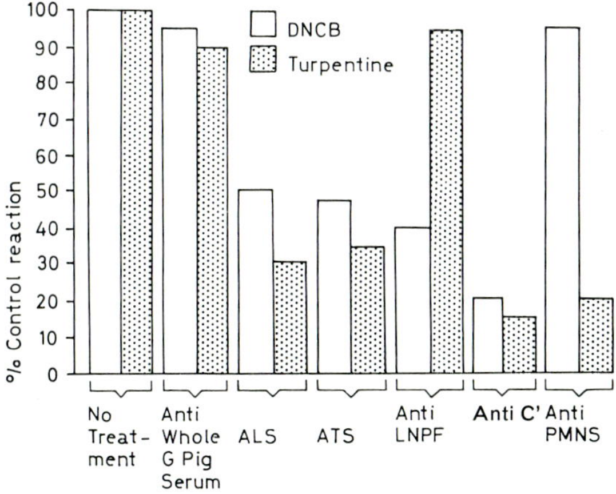

Fig. 13. Comparison of the effect of anti-whole guinea pig serum, anti-lymph node lymphocyte serum (ALS), anti-thymocyte serum (ATS), anti-lymph node permeability factor serum (anti-LNPF), anti-complement serum (anti-C') and anti-polymorphonuclear leucocyte serum (anti-PMNS) on contact sensitivity to DNCB and acute inflammation caused by the intradermal injection of turpentine, in the guinea pig.

The most likely explanation for the mode of action of anti-lymphocyte sera on acute inflammation appeared to be that it was acting on a pharmacologically vaso-active mediator. Attempts to identify this hypothetical mediator have failed. The serum does not antagonise any of the substances which are considered to be pharmacological mediators of the acute inflammatory response, among them, histamine, 5-HT, bradykinin, or RNA. These experiments also remove the possibility that ALS was acting in a nonspecific manner on blood vessels and preventing them from becoming permeable. Indeed, the turpentine-induced pleurisy experiments gave a clear indication that the serum was not acting by antagonising histamine (fig. 12). It has previously been shown [Spector and Willoughby, 1957] that histamine and 5-HT are both active only on the earliest phase of this inflammatory response. This early phase remained unaffected by the action of ALS whereas the later phase of the response was markedly reduced. It has been postulated by many authors that the important mediator of this phase is probably a vasoactive polypeptide resembling bradykinin [see reviews by Spector and Willoughby, 1963 and Wilhelm, 1962]. This was found to be unaffected by ALS. In addition the formation of a substance resembling bradykinin but of a higher molecular weight, described by Spector and Willoughby [1962] and postulated as a mediator, was also unaffected. It is of great interest that various substances believed to interfere with kinin formation and also to suppress the later period of exudate development are markedly potentiated by the action of antihistamine drugs. This has been interpreted in the past as evidence that kinin formation follows sequentially from histamine and 5-HT release. The failure of antihistamine drugs to potentiate the suppression of the exudate at four hours by ALS, suggests a different mechanism other than interference with kinin formation. Furthermore, this could be taken as highly presumptive evidence for a hitherto unsuspected mechanism involved in the inflammatory response. Possibly mediators operate in the rat in the following sequence (1) histamine, (2) 5-HT, (3) kinin activation, (4) something susceptible to ALS. One cannot overlook the possibility that the fourth step might involve complement and such a mediator as PF/P postulated by Davies and Lowe [1962]. The massive combination of ALS with lymphocytes might fix the available complement and serve as a means of temporarily exhausting the appropriate part of the complement system. A similar mechanism could explain the effect of antipolymorphonuclear serum on inflammation (fig. 13). This would also explain the greater efficacy of ALS and ATS as opposed to anti-LNPF in the acute inflammatory states. The failure of anti-whole guinea pig serum and anti-guinea pig LNPF to affect acute inflammation could be due to the fact that more complement is inactivated when the effect is on particulate antigens such as whole cells, rather than on soluble antigens. The anti-whole guinea pig serum used did not appear to contain significant amounts of antibody against complement components.

As can be seen in figure 13, the anti-inflammatory effects of antilymphocyte serum on both contact sensitivity and non-specific inflammation to turpentine can be reproduced by treatment of guinea pigs with antiserum containing antibodies against the third component of complement ($C'_3-/\beta_{1A}/\beta_{1C}$) (fig. 14). It was also found that treatment of guinea pigs with antilymphocyte serum dropped the levels of circulating complement by 80%. The role of complement in cell-mediated immune reactions has previously been emphasised by NEVEU and BIOZZI [1965] who found that decomplementation of rats by antigen/antibody complexes or aggregated human γ-globulins, so that the level of complement dropped by 90%, would completely suppress delayed cutaneous hypersensitivity reactions to picrylated egg albumen.

It seems highly likely that complement should be implicated in acute inflammatory reaction as within the components of complement are all the factors required to mediate an inflammatory response. These include histamine liberators and other permeability factors [OSLER, RANDALL, HILL and OVARY, 1959; DAVIES and LOWE, 1962]. Moreover, components five, six and seven have been shown to cause

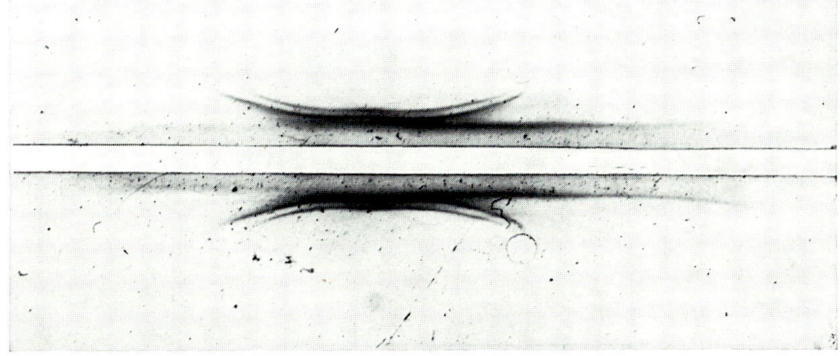

Fig. 14. Immunoelectrophoresis of normal guinea pig serum—anti-guinea pig complement (β_{1A}/β_{1C}) in centre well.

leucocyte emigration *in vivo* and *in vitro* [COCHRANE and WARD, 1965]. It seems likely therefore that following a non-specific injury to the tissue, there would be leakage of plasma proteins which would then become modified or aggregated and activate the complement system. This would then lead to the well recognised sequence of events which occur in acute inflammation—leucocyte emigration, histamine release, vasodilatation and increased vascular permeability. This concept gains further support when one considers the efficacy of the anti-malarial group of drugs in suppressing inflammation. These drugs have been shown to have anti-esterase activity [SPECTOR and WILLOUGHBY, 1960]. This could lead to a suppression of the first stage of complement activation.

It will be noticed from figure 13 that anti-polymorphonuclear serum suppresses acute inflammation whilst not affecting cell-mediated immune reactions in the periphery. Anti-polymorphonuclear serum given intravenously also caused a drop in the level of circulating complement, of the order of 60%. Whereas both antilymphocyte serum and anti-C'_3 serum produced a marked suppression in the cell-mediated immune response, no such suppression could be found with anti-polymorphonuclear serum. Although this finding has been well known since the work of INDERBITZIN [1956] this became somewhat surprising in view of the evidence for the possible role of complement in cell-mediated immune reactions and the observed fall in the level of complement following treatment of guinea pigs with antipoly-morphonuclear serum. These results could reflect either a quantitative difference in the degree of inactivation of complement by the different antisera or be due to a qualitative difference in the components of complement affected by treatment with the different antisera. It may also be that complement levels recover faster after treatment with antipolymorphonuclear serum than after antilymphocyte serum or anti-C'_3 serum and thus the effect of antipolymorphonuclear serum on complement may be sufficient to block complement activity in non-specific inflammation, but insufficient to affect complement activity in cell-mediated immune reactions. Moreover, antipolymorphonuclear serum affects the behaviour of circulating granulocytes and may interfere with the participation of their lysosomal enzymes in the inflammatory response. Thus the anti-inflammatory affect of antipolymorphonuclear serum may well be due to a summation of these two properties i. e. an indirect effect on circulating complement and a direct effect on circulating granulocytes.

Table I. Effect of immunosuppressive agents on non-specific inflammation
in the rat

Treatment	Thermal injury		Turpentine pleurisy		Chronic inflammation (cotton pellet implantation)
	Early	Late	Early	Late	
Cyclophosphamide 10 mg/kg for 3 days (I.P.)	+++	±	○	+±	+
Methotrexate 5 mg/kg for 3 days (I.P.)	++++	++	○	+++	+
Phytohaemagglutinin 2.5 ml/kg for 3 days (I.V.)	++	+	○	±	○
6 M-P 25 mg/kg for 3 days (orally)	+++	+±	○	++	+
DXR (650r)	++	+	++	+	+++
Anti-LNPF (1 ml I.V.)	○	○	○	○	○
ALS (1 ml I.V.)	+±	+	○	++	+

$$
\begin{aligned}
○ &= <10\% \text{ suppression} \\
+ &= 25\% \text{ suppression} \\
++ &= 50\% \text{ suppression} \\
+++ &= 75\% \text{ suppression} \\
++++ &= 100\% \text{ suppression}
\end{aligned}
$$

The specific peripheral effect of antilymphocyte serum on cell-mediated immune reactions can be investigated independently of the non-specific anti-inflammatory effect, by studying the effect of an antiserum prepared against membrane-free extracts of lymph nodes (Anti-LNPF) more thoroughly. So as to analyse the effect of this serum more deeply, the reactions studied were those in which sensitized cells together with antigen (tuberculin) were injected intradermally into normal unsensitized animals [TURK and POLÁK, 1968]. In this reaction (local passive transfer of tuberculin sensitivity) using histocompatible strain XIII guinea pigs, the effect of the serum on agents released by the sensitized cells after contact with antigen could be separated from an effect on agents released by the normal tissues of the recipient as a result of the immune reaction. The effect on local passive transfer of the tuberculin reaction in strain XIII guinea pigs was compared with the effect of the antiserum on the reaction caused by the intradermal injection of cells from Hartley strain guinea pigs into the strain XIII guinea pigs (Normal lymphocyte transfer reaction) [BRENT and MEDAWAR, 1963]. The effect of anti-LNPF injected intravenously just before transfer was compared with the effect of anti-polymorphonuclear serum (APNS) which will reduce the level of circulating polymorphs to the extent of abolishing the Arthus reaction [Humphrey, 1955]. The tuberculin transfer and the normal lymphocyte transfer can be analysed into four components— (1) erythema, due to dilatation of blood vessels; (2) haemorrhage, due to increased permeability of the vessel walls to red cells; and (3) induration or swelling. These three phenomena could be due to the release of pharmacological agents and the size of the reaction, the fourth component could be dependent on the degree to which these pharmacological agents spread in the region of the injection.

The erythema component of both the tuberculin transfer and the normal lymphocyte transfer is diminished by anti-LNPF to a far greater extent in one half of the recipients than in the other half (table II). Thus the effect of the antiserum is probably on a substance released by the tissues of the recipient animal rather than by the sensitized donor cells following contact with antigen. APNS however, diminished the erythema of the tuberculin transfer only and did not have any effect on this aspect of the normal lymphocyte transfer (tables III and V).

This failure of APNS to affect erythema in the normal lymphocyte transfer could be because this reaction is mainly cell-mediated, whereas the tuberculin transfer is more of a mixed humoral antibody and cell-mediated reaction. The effect of APNS on the tuberculin transfer was less and lasted for a shorter time (4 to 8 h) than the effect of anti-LNPF which lasted for 24 h. The effect of anti-LNPF was found to have worn off after 24 h and did not affect the tuberculin transfer or the normal lymphocyte transfer, 48 h after the intravenous injection

Table II. Effect of anti-LNPF on intensity of erythema
in local passive transfer reactions

Time (hours)	Controls	Treated	
		Group I	Group II
a) Tuberculin			
4	+	+	o
8	+±	+±	o
24	+±	++	o
48	++±	++±	++
b) Normal lymphocyte transfer			
4	++	+	o
8	+±	+	o
24	++	+	+±
48	+	±	+

Table III. Effect of anti-polymorphonuclear serum on intensity
of erythema in local passive transfer reactions

Time (hours)	Controls	Treated
	a) Tuberculin	
4	+	±
8	+±	+
24	+±	++
	b) Normal lymphocyte transfer	
4	++	++
8	+±	+±
24	+±	+±

Table IV. Effect of anti-LNPF and anti-polymorphonuclear serum on haemorrhages
in local passive transfer of tuberculin reaction

	Time after intradermal injection		
	4 h	8 h	24 h
Controls	6/12	7/12	2/12
Anti-LNPF Group I	0/10	0/10	3/10
Group II	0/10	0/10	0/10
Anti-polymorphonuclear Serum (APNS)	0/10	1/10	0/10

Note: Results expressed as proportion of reactions showing central haemorrhages.

Table V. Comparison of the effect of anti-LNPF and APNS
on local passive transfers

Anti-LNPF Time (hours)	Haemorrhage	Erythema	Induration
		a) Tuberculin	
4	↓	↓	↓
8	↓	↓	↓
24	↓	↓	↓
48		↔	↔
		b) NLT	
4		↓	↓
8		↓	↓
24		↔	↓
48		↔	↓
APNS		*a) Tuberculin*	
4	↓	↓	↓
8	↓	↓	↓
24	↓	↔	↓
		b) NLT	
4		↔	↓
8		↔	↓
24		↔	↓

of the serum and the intradermal transfer given simultaneously. Thus the effect of anti-LNPF on erythema appears independent of the effect of APNS on erythema. This would confirm the impression that anti-LNPF does not act on the erythema resulting from interactions involving humoral antibody. The presence of these two components is confirmed by the histological appearance of the reactions, following treatment with APNS, which abolishes the infiltration with polymorphs without affecting the mononuclear cell infiltrate.

Haemorrhage is not found in normal lymphocyte transfer reactions but occurs frequently in tuberculin transfers. It is blocked by both anti-LNPF and APNS and thus probably results from a combination of humoral antibody and cell-mediated immune mechanisms (table IV).

Induration is reduced by both anti-LNPF and APNS in both the tuberculin transfer and the normal lymphocyte transfers (table V). Induration is probably the result of the release of a different pharmacological agent from that causing erythema. This pharmacological agent could act by causing the accumulation of fluid between the fibrillar components within collagen fibres [Black, Humphrey and Niven, 1963].

The effect of these antisera on the size of the reactions is irregular. However, anti-LNPF causes a definite reduction in the size of the tuberculin transfer reaction 8 h after transfer in the more sensitive group of recipients (Group II). A more prolonged reduction in size of the normal lymphocyte transfer reaction can be produced by anti-LNPF. This can be detected in Group II recipients at both 4 and 8 h after transfer, but only at 8 h after transfer in Group I recipients. APNS had no effect on the size of the tuberculin transfers but reduced the size of the normal lymphocyte transfers. This effect could be explained, if APNS acted on a spreading factor which could play a greater part in the normal lymphocyte transfer than in the tuberculin transfer. The action of this particular substance would then appear to be blocked by APNS rather than by anti-LNPF.

These studies would, therefore, indicate that more than one pharmacological agent is released in cell-mediated immune reactions. At least one of these substances is released by the recipient's unsensitized tissues as a result of the interaction between the injected sensitized cells and antigens. Some recipients would appear to release more of this substance than others and thus be less sensitive than others to the effect of the intravenous injection of anti-LNPF. Certain components of the reaction produced by identical sensitized donor cells and antigen can be blocked more readily by anti-LNPF in some recipients than in others.

It is also evident that the reaction produced by the intradermal injection of cells from tuberculin-sensitive donors together with tuberculin is a mixed reaction due to the involvement of Arthus-like elements as well as cell-mediated immune mechanisms. The normal lymphocyte transfer reaction would not appear to involve Arthus-like phenomena to the same extent, and is a purer manifestation of cell-mediated immunity than the local passive transfer of the tuberculin reaction.

Summary

The multiplicity of effects of chemical immunosuppressive agents has been emphasised previously. It has been found that the immunosuppressive action of these agents in cell-mediated immune responses can be divided into a central effect on the afferent side of the sensitization arc and a peripheral effect on the reaction between the sensitized cells with antigen, and the pharmacological agents released as a result of this reaction. These compounds can also be shown to have a suppressive effect on non-specific inflammatory reactions, not necessarily induced by immunological reactions.

The effect of any one of these agents on the afferent arc can be at a number of levels at the same time. These range from a direct effect on the turnover of normal lymphocytes, through the ability of the lymphocyte to be transformed as a result of antigenic stimulus. Another effect that has been noticed has been a decreased enzyme activity and protein synthesis in the cells responding to the immunological stimulus.

As a result of this there is a failure in the increased output of small lymphocytes, produced by the immunological response, which are thought to be the cells that react with antigen in the periphery. Despite the widespread acceptance that chemical immuno-suppressive agents act simultaneously at different metabolic levels, it has recently been suggested that the immunosuppressive effect of antilymphocyte serum (ALS) might be explained on the basis of a relatively simple one point mode of action.

It became obvious in current studies that the action of ALS was comparable to that of other immunosuppressive agents in that a number of actions could be demonstrated at different levels of the sensitization arc (fig. 15). In addition ALS could be shown to have a marked non-specific anti-inflammatory action, independent of its specific effect on the efferent side of the sensitization arc. This is not to say that this agent does not have a direct effect on the mobile pool of lymphocytes in the periphery. With the use of three dimensional electron microscopy it has been possible to show gross distortion of the surface of lymphocytes following the administration of ALS both *in vivo* and *in vitro*. There is replacement of the paracortical areas of lymphoid tissue by reticulo-histiocytes as early as three days after the beginning of a course of ALS. There is also evidence of nuclear breakdown and phagocytosis in this area in more than one species. The action of ALS on the central lymphoid tissue is specific to those areas of the lymph node which is populated by the mobile pool of small lymphocytes and which is specifically involved in the cell-mediated immune response. No gross effects have yet been observed on plasma cells in the medulla and the germinal centres, which are considered to be the areas of lymphoid tissue concerned in the humoral antibody response.

The specific effect of ALS on peripheral manifestations of the cell-mediated immune response can be analysed by the use of antisera prepared against membrane-free extracts

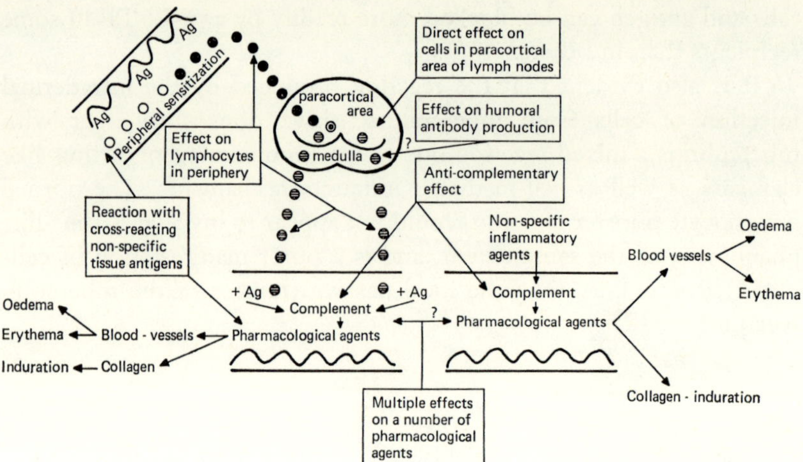

Fig. 15. Multiplicity of sites of action of antilymphocyte serum on specific cell-mediated immune reactions and non-specific inflammation.

of lymph nodes (anti-lymph node permeability factor—Anti-LNPF) which only acts on the specific immune reactions and not on non-specific inflammatory reactions in the periphery. The effects of this agent appear to be on more than one pharmacological substance released in the periphery. Evidence has been presented to show that the action of this serum is to a large extent on the release of pharmacological agents from normal unsensitized tissue rather than from sensitized cells reacting directly with antigen.

The non-specific anti-inflammatory effect of ALS cannot be attributed to its effect on permeability increasing substances such as histamine, 5 H-T, bradykinin etc. nor to a direct action of blood vessels which are still capable of responding to other permeability factors. ALS can, however, be shown to have marked anti-complement effects. Moreover, its peripheral action can be reproduced by anti-complement serum.

It has been suggested that both cell-mediated immune reactions and non-immune inflammatory responses may be mediated by components of complement. Thus it may be that some of the effects of ALS on the cell-mediated immune response in the periphery and the non-immune inflammatory response could be related to its ability to inactivate complement *in vivo*.

References

Black, S.; Humphrey, J.H. and Niven, J.: Inhibition of mantoux reaction by direct suggestion under hypnosis. Brit. med. J. *1:* 1649 (1963).

Borel, Y. and Schwartz, R.: Inhibition of immediate and delayed hypersensitivity in the rabbit by 6-mercaptopurine. J. Immunol. *92:* 754 (1964).

Brent, L. and Medawar, P.B.: Tissue transplantation: A new approach to the 'typing' problem. Brit. med. J. *2:* 269 (1963).

Clarke, J.A.; Salisbury, A.J. and Willoughby, D.A. The effects of various antisera on the surfaces of sensitized rat lymph node cells. J. Path. Bact. *96:* 235 (1968).

COCHRANE, C.G. and WARD, P.A.: The role of complement in lesions induced by immunologic reactions. IVth International Symposium on Immunopathology, p. 433 (Eds.) P. GRABAR and P.A. MIESCHER (Schwabe and Co., Basel/Stuttgart 1966).

DAVIES, G.E. and LOWE, J.S.: Further studies on a permeability factor released from guinea-pig serum by antigen-antibody precipitates: Relationship to serum complement. Int. Arch. Allergy *20:* 235 (1962).

DENMAN, A.M.; DENMAN, E.J. and EMBLING, P.H.: Changes in the life-span of circulating small lymphocytes in mice after treatment with antilymphocyte globulin. Lancet *i:* 321 (1968).

HUMPHREY, J.H.: The mechanism of Arthus reactions. II. The role of polymorphonuclear leucocytes and platelets in reversed passive reactions in the guinea pig. Brit. J. exp. Path. *36:* 283 (1955).

INDERBITZIN, T.: The relationship of lymphocytes, delayed cutaneous allergic reactions and histamine. Int. Arch. Allergy *8:* 150 (1956).

JAMES, K. and ANDERSON, N.F.: Effect of anti-rat lymphocyte antibody on humora antibody formation. Nature *213:* 1195 (1967).

JAMES, K. and JUBB, V.S.: Effect of anti-rat lymphocyte antibody on humoral antibody formation. Nature *215:* 367 (1967).

LANDY, M.; SANDERSON, R.P.; BERNSTEIN, M.T. and LERNER, E.M.: Involvement of thymus in immune response of rabbits to somatic polysaccharides of gram negative bacteria. Science *147:* 1591 (1965).

LEVEY, R.H. and MEDAWAR, P.B.: Nature and mode of action of antilymphocyte antiserum. Proc. nat. Acad. Sci. *56:* 1130 (1966).

MARTIN, W.J. and MILLER, J.F.A.P.: Site of action of antilymphocyte globulin. Lancet *ii:* 1285 (1967).

MEDAWAR, P.B.: The Croonian Lecture. The homograft reaction. Proc. roy. Soc. B. *149:* 145 (1958).

NEVEU, T. and BIOZZI, G.: The effect of decomplementation on delayed-type hypersensitive reactions to a conjugated antigen in rats. Immunology *9:* 303 (1965).

OORT, J. and TURK, J.L.: A histological and autoradiographic study of lymph nodes during the development of contact sensitivity in the guinea pig. Brit. J. exp. Path. *46:* 147 (1965).

OSLER, A.G.; RANDALL, H.G.; HILL, B.M. and OVARY, Z.: Studies on the mechanism of hypersensitivity phenomena. III. The participation of complement in the formation of anaphylatoxin. J. exp. Med. *110:* 311 (1959).

PARROTT, D.M.V.; DE SOUSA, M.B. and EAST, J.: Thymus-dependent areas in the lymphoid organs of neonatally thymectomized mice. J. exp. Med. *123:* 191 (1966).

SCHILD, H.O. and WILLOUGHBY, D.A.: Possible pharmacological mediators of delayed hypersensitivity. Brit. med. Bull. *23:* 46 (1967).

SPECTOR, W.G. and WILLOUGHBY, D.A.: Histamine and 5 Hydroxy-tryptamine in acute experimental pleurisy. J. Path. Bact. *74:* 57 (1957).

SPECTOR, W.G. and WILLOUGHBY, D.A.: The suppression by anti-esterases of increased capillary permeability in acute inflammation. J. Path. Bact. *79:* 21 (1960).

SPECTOR, W.G. and WILLOUGHBY, D.A.: The activation of slow contracting substances, and their relation to the vascular changes of inflammation in the rat. J. Path. Bact. *84:* 391 (1962).

SPECTOR, W.G. and WILLOUGHBY, D.A.: The inflammatory response. Bact. Revs. *27:* 117 (1963).

TURK, J.L.: Studies on the mechanism of action of methotrexate and cyclophosphamide on contact sensitivity in the guinea pig. Int. Arch. Allergy *24:* 191 (1964).

TURK, J.L.: Cytology of the induction of hypersensitivity. Brit. med. Bull. *23:* 3 (1967a).

TURK, J.L.: Response of lymphocytes to antigen. Transplantation *5:* 952 (1967b).

Turk, J. L.: The effect of immunosuppressive drugs on cellular changes after antigenic stimulation. Immunity, Cancer and Chemotherapy, p. 1. (Ed.) Enrico Mihich (Academic Press N.Y. and London, 1967c).

Turk, J. L. and Willoughby, D.A.: Central and peripheral effects of antilymphocyte sera. Lancet *i:* 249 (1967).

Turk, J. L. and Polák, L.: A comparison of the effect of anti-lymph node serum and antigranulocyte serum on local passive transfer of the tuberculin reaction and the normal lymphocyte transfer reaction. Int. Arch. Allergy *34:* 105 (1968).

Turk, J. L.; Willoughby, D.A. and Stevens, J.E.: An analysis of the effect of some types of antilymphocyte sera on contact hypersensitivity and certain models of inflammation. Immunology *14:* 683 (1968).

Wilhelm, D.C.: The mediation of increased vascular permeability in inflammation. Pharmacol. Rev. *14:* 251 (1962).

Willoughby, D.A.: The mechanism of cutaneous hypersensitivity in the rat and its suppression by immunological methods. J. Path. Bact. *92:* 1391 (1966).

Willoughby, D.A.; Boughton, B. and Schild, H.O.: A factor capable of increasing vascular permeability present in lymph node cells: A possible mediator of the delayed reaction. Immunology *6:* 484 (1963).

Willoughby, D.A. and Coote, E.: The lymph node permeability factor a possible mediator of experimental allergic thyroiditis in the rat. J. Path. Bact. *92:* 28 (1966).

Willoughby, D.A.; Walters, M.N.I. and Spector, W.G.: Lymph node permeability factor in the dinitrochlorobenzene skin hypersensitivity reaction in guinea pigs. Immunology *8:* 578 (1965).

Wilson, A.B. and Turk, J.L.: Protein synthesis in lymph nodes during the development of contact sensitivity in the guinea pig. Immunochemistry *5:* 33 (1968).

Authors' addresses: Dr. J.L. Turk, Department of Immunology, Institute of Dermatology, St. John's Hospital for Diseases of the Skin, Homerton Grove, *London* and Dr. D.A. Willoughby, Department of Pathology, St. Bartholomews Hospital Medical College, *London* (England).

Antibiotica et Chemotherapia, vol. 15, pp. 295–309 (Karger, Basel/New York 1969)

Cytotoxicity of Lymphocytes and its Suppression

G. Holm and P. Perlmann

Wenner-Gren Institute for Experimental Biology, Stockholm

Lymphocytes are assumed to participate in the tissue damage associated with transplantation reactions, autoimmune diseases and delayed hypersensitivity reactions. This assumption is based on histological observations of the diseased organs [26] and is further supported by the development of tissue lesions in healthy animals after the transfer of lymphoid cells from immune donors [3]. The cytotoxic potential of lymphoid cells has been documented by *in vitro* experiments in which lymphocytes are incubated with tissue culture cells. This approach was first exploited by Govaerts in 1960, who showed that lymphocytes from dogs, sensitized by kidney transplantation, destroyed tissue culture cells explanted from the remaining kidney of the transplant donor [6]. Since then, it has been shown by many authors that lymphocytes, sensitized by transplantation or autoimmunization, damage tissue culture cells containing the sensitizing antigens. Moreover, under certain conditions, lymphocytes from unsensitized donors also destroy cells in tissue culture. At present, one can distinguish three different experimental situations in which lymphocytes destroy other cell types *in vitro*.

Cytotoxicity of Stimulated Lymphocytes

Unsensitized lymphocytes damage red cells or tissue culture cells in the presence of phytohaemagglutinin (PHA) [17, 19, 22]. After incubation for 1–24 h cell damage can be measured quantitatively as the release of radioactivity from target cells labelled with ^{51}Cr-chromate. Labelled Chang cells spontaneously release some radioactivity into the medium. Human lymphocytes added in 5- to 25-fold excess did not significantly increase this release. However, in the presence of PHA, lymphocytes damaged the target cells already within 1–3 h [13].

PHA agglutinates lymphocytes and target cells, and also stimulates the lymphocytes. Both factors are important for the cytotoxic reaction [14]. Thus, cell damage did not occur in experiments in which target cells and PHA-stimulated lymphocytes were separated by a cell-impermeable membrane [17]. Extracts of PHA-stimulated lymphocytes were not cytotoxic [12]. A close correlation was also noted between the cytotoxicity of human lymphocytes and their RNA and DNA synthesis at different concentrations of PHA [14]. The importance of lymphocyte stimulation was further emphasized by the observations that human lymphocytes stimulated by non-agglutinating agents such as Staphylococcal filtrate or by antigens, unrelated to target cell antigens were strongly cytotoxic without the aid of PHA [14].

Cytotoxic Action of Lymphocytes, Unsensitized to Target Cell Antigens, in the Presence of Antibodies to Target Cell Antigens

Tissue culture cells or chicken erythrocytes are damaged by normal lymphocytes in the presence of certain heat-inactivated antisera against antigens which are part of the target cells. This was studied with PPD as the antigen. Chicken erythrocytes were coated with PPD by the tannic acid method and labelled with ^{51}Cr-chromate. The PPD-coated cells were damaged when incubated for 20 h with heat-inactivated serum from guinea pigs vaccinated with BCG and spleen cells from unsensitized guinea pigs [21]. PPD-coated erythrocytes, first treated with immune serum and then washed, were also lysed when exposed to normal spleen cells. The active gammaglobulin of the immune serum could also be adsorbed onto non-immune spleen cells which thereby became cytotoxic to PPD-coated target cells. The reaction was immunologically specific.

A similar interaction has been observed between lymphocytes and immune serum against Chang cell antigens. A hyperimmune serum was produced in rabbits by injection of Chang cells in Freund's complete adjuvant. ^{51}Cr-labelled Chang cells were treated with the heat-inactivated antiserum for 30 min at 37°C and then washed. The treated cells were incubated with an excess of purified human blood lymphocytes (>99% small lymphocytes). The incubation medium consisted of Parker 199 with 5% heat-inactivated foetal calf serum. After incubation, cell damage was determined as the percentage of isotope released from the Chang cells into the medium [13]. A typical experiment is illustrated in figure 1. Chang cells, treated with anti-

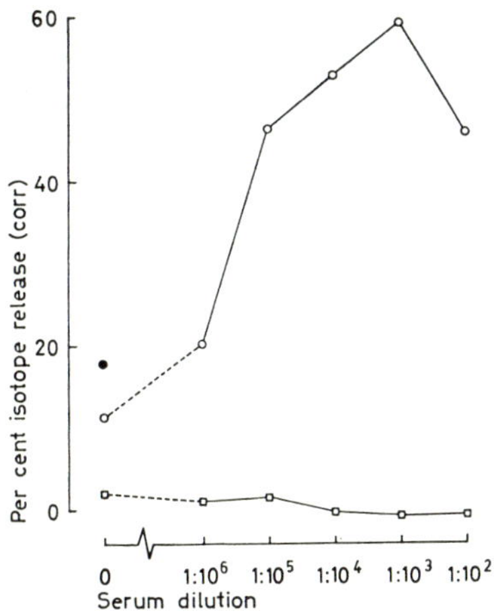

Fig. 1. Cytotoxicity of normal lymphocytes against target cells treated with antiserum. Chang cells labelled with ^{51}Cr-chromate were incubated for 30 min with heat-inactivated rabbit anti-Chang serum diluted as indicated on the abscissa. After washing, 5×10^4 Chang cells were either incubated alone (squares) or with 1.25×10^6 human lymphocytes in the presence of PHA (filled circle) or without PHA (open circles). After 20 h incubation cell damage was determined as the isotope released into the medium which was expressed as a percentage of the total radioactivity in the tube. This percentage was corrected for the spontaneous release of isotope from Chang cells (26.4%) (= corrected isotope release).

serum diluted up to 10^6 times, were damaged in the presence of lymphocytes. It should be noted that PHA was not required. When applied to Chang cells under similar conditions in the presence of 20% fresh guinea pig serum but in the absence of lymphocytes, cytotoxic effects were only noted with the antiserum diluted less than 100 times. The Chang cells were also damaged by lymphocytes and high concentrations of rabbit antisera against other tissues of human origin. The cytotoxic titers of these sera did not exceed 1:1000. Even normal rabbit sera in the presence of lymphocytes diluted 1:5–1:10 sometimes had this effect, probably reflecting the action of heterophilic antibodies.

Cytotoxicity of Lymphocytes from Donors Sensitized to Target Cell Antigens

Lymphoid cells from donors sensitized by transplantation or auto-immunization destroy tissue culture target cells containing the sensitizing antigens which usually are part of the target cell surface. However, red cells coated with the antigen may also serve as target cells in such experiments [21]. Thus, lymphoid cells from guinea pigs sensitized to PPD damage chicken erythrocytes coated with PPD. Red cells, only treated with tannic acid, are not affected. Serum from the sensitized spleen cell donor is also cytotoxic to PPD coated erythrocytes in the presence of lymphoid cells from an unsensitized donor (see above).

Some Common Features

The cytotoxic action of lymphocytes exhibited under the different conditions described above has some general characteristics in common. Thus, in all reactions cell damage is an effect of living lymphocytes. Extracts of lymphocytes or killed lymphocytes are inactive. In all these models, cell damage develops without addition of complement to the incubation mixture. The kinetics of the lymphocyte mediated cytotoxic reactions is different from that of cytotoxic antibodies and complement. It is usually a slow process which develops during 24–48 h incubation. However, by means of sensitive methods, lymphocyte mediated cell damage is revealed within 3–6 h [13].

Until recently, histoincompatibility between lymphocytes and target cells has been regarded as a prerequisite for target cell damage by PHA stimulated normal lymphocytes. However, lymphocyte induced cell damage has now also been demonstrated in truly autologous situations. Thus, fowl erythrocytes are lysed by PHA-stimulated blood lymphocytes from the same animal [22]. Highly purified human blood lymphocytes destroy autologous fibroblast or thyroid cells in the presence of PHA [1]. Mouse cells in tissue culture usually are not destroyed by syngenic lymphoid cells, but allogenic lymphoid cells produce a more pronounced cell injury [19]. Histoincompatibility between lymphocytes and target cells thus increases the effectiveness of the PHA induced cytotoxic reactions in some systems. Lymphocytes from autoimmune donors also damage syngenic or autologous target cells containing the sensitizing antigens [8, 27]. Moreover, the cytotoxic action of normal lymphocytes and antibodies to target cell antigens is exerted against autologous target cells [21].

The effector cell in the cytotoxic reactions is thought to be the small lymphocyte. Lymphocyte preparations contaminated with less than one granulocyte or monocyte per 500 lymphocytes are highly cytotoxic in all models discussed above. However, this does not exclude that other cells such as monocytes or macrophages possess cytotoxic activity as well. Thymocytes, malignant lymphoid cells and non-lymphoid cells do not damage target cells in the presence of PHA, nor in the presence of antibodies to the target cells [9, 11, 16, 21].

An interesting common feature in all these models is the aggregation of lymphocytes to target cells. This step precedes cell damage. Rosenau and Moon first described how sensitized lymphocytes accumulated around the target cells in tissue culture and later damaged them [25]. Essentially the same microscopical picture is seen in mixtures of unsensitized lymphocytes and tissue culture cells incubated with PHA [17]. Unsensitized lymphocytes aggregate in a similar manner to target cells coated with antibodies. In contrast, mixed agglutination is not apparent in cultures containing target cells and lymphocytes stimulated by various non-agglutinating agents. Yet, such lymphocytes damage the target cells [14]. Hence, aggregation of lymphocytes to target cells is favourable but is not an absolute requirement for cytotoxicity.

Inhibition of the Cytotoxic Action of Lymphocytes

1. Antimetabolites. Available data indicate that dead lymphocytes or extracts of lymphocytes are inactive in the cytotoxic reaction [12]. This implies that the lymphocytes participate actively in the cytotoxic reaction. It was assumed that the application of specific metabolic inhibition would throw some light on the nature of the lymphocyte activities involved. A completely passive function of the lymphocytes should not be inhibited by such means.

The cytotoxic action of PHA-stimulated normal human lymphocytes against Chang cells is a rapid process, which can be measured by means of the sensitive ^{51}Cr-technique already within 1–3 h. It is independent of PHA-induced DNA synthesis and cell division in the lymphocytes, which are late events in the stimulatory process. The cytotoxic action of PHA-stimulated cells was not suppressed when

Table I. The effect of antimetabolites on the cytotoxic action
of unsensitized human lymphocytes

Antimetabolite	Conditions	Inhibition of cytotoxicity	Effect on lymphocyte metabolism
Cyclophosphamide	100 μg/ml, present	—	Inhibition of
Imuran	100 μg/ml, present	±	mitosis and
Actinomycin D	10 μg/ml, pretreatment	±	nucleic acid synthesis
Puromycin	25 μg/ml, present	—	Inhibition of
Parafluorophenylalanine	500 μg/ml, present	—	protein synthesis
Hydrocortisone	100 μg/ml, present	±	
Heat	43–45° C, pretreatment for 1 h	+	
Iodoacetate	10^{-3}–10^{-2}M, pretreatment	+	Inhibition of glycolysis
Antimycin A	10^{-4}M, pretreatment	+	Inhibition of
2,4-dinitrophenol	10^{-3}–10^{-2}M, present	+	respiration

From HOLM and PERLMANN [15].

RNA synthesis or protein synthesis were completely inhibited by actinomycin D, or puromycin, respectively (table I). However, antimetabolites which block energy supply in the lymphocytes (antimycin A, 2,4-dinitrophenol, iodoacetate) completely abolish their cytotoxic activity. Cytotoxicity is inhibited under conditions where the lymphocytes did not stain with trypan blue [10]. However, antimycin A and iodoacetate are irreversibly bound to the lymphocytes and the inhibited lymphocytes are damaged during prolonged incubation. In contrast, dinitrophenol is reversibly bound to the cells. Lymphocytes, which had been treated with dinitrophenol for 3 h, could be restimulated by PHA to RNA synthesis after washing [15]. Hence, the complete inhibition by these antimetabolites of the early phase of cytotoxicity was not due to their causing death of the lymphocytes.

These results suggest that the cytotoxic action of lymphocytes is an energy requiring process which is independent of continuous protein synthesis. The nature of this activity is unknown. It may include activation or demasking of surface receptors or enzymes, which are necessary for the ensuing damage of the target cells. Preliminary studies by light and electron microscopy indicate that the motility of stimulated lymphocytes may be *one* important and energy requiring factor in the cytotoxic reaction [1].

The PHA-induced cytotoxic action of human lymphocytes is completely suppressed by salazosulfapyridine [15]. The action of this substance on the metabolism of the lymphocytes is not known. However, studies of the kinetics of this inhibition suggested that cytotoxicity is due to some changes induced in the lymphocytes by PHA within 30 min. It may be assumed that this early activation of the lymphocytes would lead to morphological transformation and other signs of lymphocyte stimulation during prolonged incubation. This is in accordance with the observation that PHA induces alterations in the DNA-histone complex of lymphocytes within 30 min [18, 24]. Although the lymphocytes may be activated to a cytotoxic response by several means, these stimulating processes will not always lead to blastoid transformation. Therefore, we prefer to use the term "activation" instead of "stimulation" in order to describe the process connected with the cytotoxic activity of these cells.

Preliminary experiments suggest that the antibody mediated cytotoxicity of unsensitized lymphocytes described in the previous section is also inhibited by antimycin A. Similarly, the cytotoxicity of lymphoid cells from PPD-sensitized donors against PPD-coated erythrocytes is also blocked by this agent (unpublished observations).

Sensitized lymphocytes have antibody-like receptors on their surface which enable them to recognize target cells containing the sensitizing antigen [21]. Provided that these antibodies are continuously synthesized by cells in the cytotoxic lymphocyte population, it should be possible in these systems to suppress cytotoxicity with antimetabolites which block protein or RNA synthesis. Actually, Brunner *et al.* recently showed that actinomycin D or cyclohexemide partially inhibited the cytotoxic action of mouse lymphoid cells, sensitized against allogenic target cells [4]. When sensitized lymphocytes were treated with trypsin and then with cyclohexemide their cytotoxicity was completely abolished [Brunner, personal communication].

2. Antisera to target cell antigens. The cytotoxic action of sensitized lymphocytes is prevented by antibodies to the sensitizing antigen on the target cells. This has been shown by E. Möller [20] and later by Brunner *et al.* [4] using different methods for the quantitation of cell damage. Mouse target cells, treated with anti-H-2 serum, were not damaged by lymphoid cells from allogenic mice, sensitized to the same H-2 antigens. The inhibition of cell damage was immunologically specific.

A nephrotic syndrome connected with a state of autoimmunity to kidney antigens can be induced in rats by repeated injections of homologous kidney extract in Freund's complete adjuvant. Lymphoid cells from these rats damaged allogenic or syngenic kidney cells in tissue culture [7, 8]. When the kidney target cells were pretreated with serum from diseased rats, cell damage by sensitized cells was prevented. In contrast, this treatment potentiated the cytotoxic action of control lymphoid cells from normal rats or from rats sensitized with adjuvant only.

The most likely explanation of these results is, that the added antibodies block the receptor site for the attachment of the sensitized lymphocytes. In this way the aggregation between lymphocytes and target cells is prevented. This step is probably necessary for the activation of a cell damaging response in the lymphocytes (see below). It should be noted, however, that antisera to target cells sometimes also potentiate the cytotoxic action of lymphoid cells, sensitized to the same cells [8]. This is reminiscent of the cytotoxicity of unsensitized lymphocytes against antibody-coated target cells. It may be concluded that cell damage is the result of complicated synergistic and antagonistic interactions between antibodies on the lymphocytes and antibodies on the target cells. I may also be assumed that the class and type of antibody produced in immune animals will determine the outcome of the interaction between humoral antibodies, lymphocytes and other cells.

3. Antibodies to lymphocyte antigens. Aggregation between lymphocytes and target cells is characteristic for the cytotoxic reaction. In those instances where cell damage develops without obvious cell aggregation direct contact between lymphocytes and target cells is probably required [14]. Evidently, the cytotoxic reaction is dependent on surface structures of the lymphocytes, serving as receptors for recognition, activation and effectuation of cell damage. Antibodies to lymphocyte surface antigens can therefore be expected to block the cytotoxic response.

Anti-lymphocyte sera (ALS) were produced in rabbits by intramuscular injections of human thoracic duct or blood lymphocytes. The incorporation of ^{14}C-thymidine into lymphocytes, cultivated for three days with heat-inactivated ALS, diluted 1:10, was equal to that of PHA-stimulated lymphocytes. When lymphocytes were pretreated for 30 min with ALS 1:10 and then washed, DNA synthesis in them was only slightly stimulated.

In the presence of complement, the ALS diluted 1:10, was toxic to lymphocytes. The leucoagglutinating titres of these antisera were 1:200. In the following, the effects of ALS treatment on the cytotoxic activity of lymphocytes will be described.

The test system consisted of Chang cells from suspension cultures and human blood lymphocytes. The Chang cells were labelled with ^{51}Cr-chromate and washed. 0.5 to 1×10^5 labelled cells were added to roller tubes. The lymphocytes were isolated from venous blood. Granulocytes and monocytes were completely removed by passage through a nylon wool column. The erythrocytes were then lysed by treatment with hypotonic sodium chloride. The purified lymphocyte suspension was added to the tubes at a lymphocyte Chang cell ratio of 25:1. After incubation the release of isotope from the Chang cells was determined as usual. [For further details of the methods see reference 13.]

Addition to the incubation mixture of heat-inactivated ALS, diluted 1:20–1:50, completely suppressed the PHA-induced cytotoxicity (table II). The lymphocytes were not killed by treatment with ALS. The number of lymphocytes which did not stain with trypan blue was approximately the same in tubes with and without ALS.

Table II. The effect of ALS on the PHA-induced cytotoxicity
of human lymphocytes

Additions to the incubation mixture	% isotope release (corr.)	
	PHA present	No PHA
No addition	25.0	1.5
ALS diluted 1:10	6.2	–2.5[1]
ALS diluted 1:50	10.4	1.0

Time of incubation 20 h Spontaneous isotope release 40.1 %.
[1] Lower than spontaneous release.

When present in the incubation mixture ALS always suppressed cytotoxicity. However, the PHA induced cytotoxicity was sometimes also inhibited when lymphocytes were first pretreated with ALS (table III). 15×10^6 lymphocytes in 3 ml medium, containing the desired dilution of ALS, were incubated at 37°C for 30–45 min. Control lymphocytes were treated in the same way with heat-inactivated normal rabbit serum (NRS). The cells were then washed and added to labelled Chang cells.

Table III. The effect of ALS on cytotoxicity and aggregation
of lymphocytes

Treatment of lymphocytes	% isotope release (corr.)	Aggregation	
		Mixed	Only lymphocytes
NRS	2.9	0	0
NRS + PHA	15.9	+++	+
ALS	1.0	+	+++
ALS + PHA	2.5	++	+++

The lymphocytes were pretreated for 30 min with serum, diluted 1:10. They were then washed and added to labelled Chang cells. Mixed aggregation between lymphocytes and target cells as well as pure lymphocytic aggregation was evaluated under the microscope. Time of incubation 20 h. Spontaneous isotope release 29.2%.

Microscopic observations of the cultures revealed that ALS changes the pattern of aggregation between lymphocytes and target cells. In the experiment of table III, the mixed aggregation between lymphocytes and Chang cells was roughly scored. Mixed aggregation was predominant in tubes with PHA and lymphocytes where the target cells were damaged. In tubes containing ALS the lymphocytes aggregated mainly to each other but mixed aggregates were also present. Since ALS changes the pattern of aggregation between lymphocytes and target cells this could be assumed to contribute to the inhibition of cell damage. However, in other experiments ALS prevented PHA-induced cytotoxicity in spite of a strong mixed aggregation, more intense than that caused by PHA alone.

The concentrations of ALS which inhibited cytotoxicity, strongly stimulated the lymphocytes to transformation and DNA synthesis. It will be recalled that lymphocytes, stimulated by other means, damage target cells without the aid of PHA [14]. The inability of ALS-treated lymphocytes to damage target cells is the first example of a situation where stimulated lymphocytes are not cytotoxic.

The action of ALS on the cytotoxicity of normal human lymphocytes against Chang cells treated with antiserum was also studied. Chang cells were treated with the proper dilution of anti-Chang cell serum for 30 min and washed. The lymphocytes were incubated for 30 min with the diluted ALS as described above. As seen in figure 2, Chang cells treated with antiserum diluted 1,000 times were damaged by lymphocytes treated by NRS. Treatment of the lymphocytes with ALS, diluted 25 times completely suppressed their cytotoxic action.

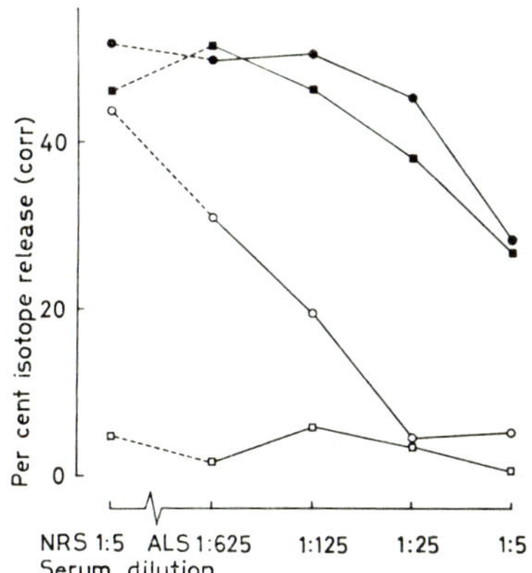

Fig. 2. Inhibition by ALS of lymphocyte-induced cell damage. Chang cells were treated with anti-Chang cell serum (circles) or normal rabbit serum (NRS) (squares) diluted 1:1000. Lymphocytes were treated for 30 min with heat-inactivated NRS or ALS diluted as indicated on the abscissa and were then added to the Chang cells with PHA (filled symbols) or without PHA (open symbols). Cell damage was determined as described in figure 1. Time of incubation 20 h. Spontaneous isotope release 25.4 %.

In contrast, in this experiment, PHA-induced cell damage was only partially depressed by the highest concentrations of ALS. Microscopic observations revealed again that ALS prevented the aggregation between lymphocytes and antibody coated Chang cells. The aggregates between lymphocytes and antibody coated target cells were more easily disintegrated by shaking than those induced by PHA. This suggests that the stronger binding between the cells, the more ALS is needed to block the aggregation. This is also brought out by experiments, where Chang cells were first treated with different concentrations of anti-Chang cell serum and were then exposed to ALS-treated lymphocytes. The higher the antibody concentration on the target cells, the more anti-lymphocyte antibodies were needed to block cell damage. ALS diluted 3,000 times, inhibited the cell damage, mediated by anti-Chang serum diluted 10,000 times. This concentration of ALS was far beyond that which agglutinates or stimulates lymphocytes.

ALS is a mixture of antibodies to several kinds of human antigens, including serum proteins. At present, it is not known, whether the inhibition of cytotoxicity by ALS is due to blocking of one type of lymphocyte receptors, or if it represents an additive effect of antibodies against different antigens. Experiments are in progress to test antisera against different antigens on the surface of lymphocytes. Preliminary results indicate that some complement factors such as C'3 and C'8 may be involved in the lymphocyte mediated cytotoxic reaction [23]. Antibodies to IgG also suppress the reaction. Hence, several structures on the lymphocytes might be involved in the damaging reaction. Some of them may serve as receptors for contact and stimulation, while others may represent effectors of the lytic reaction.

Concluding Discussion

This review has touched upon two major aspects of the cytotoxicity of lymphocytes: the contact between lymphocytes and target cells, and the activation (or stimulation) of the lymphocytes. Evidently, both factors are necessary for the PHA-induced cytotoxic action of unsensitized lymphocytes. Are both also required for the cell damage induced by lymphocytes under the other conditions discussed in this paper? Table IV summarizes some of the data which may have

Table IV. Contact between lymphocytes and target cells, activation of lymphocytes and cell damage

Target cells incubated with	Contact	Activation	Cell damage
I. *Lymphocytes not sensitized to target cell antigens*			
No additions	+	— [1]	— [1]
PHA or other stimulants added	+	+	+
PHA and ALS added	—	+	—
PHA and antimycin A added	+	—	—
II. *Lymphocytes not sensitized to target cell antigens + antibodies to target cell antigens*			
No additions	+	+?	+
ALS added	—	+	—
Antimycin A added	+	—	—
III. *Lymphocytes sensitized to target cell antigen*			
No additions	+	+?	+
Antiserum to the sensitizing target cell antigens added	—	—?	—
Antimycin A added	+	—	—

[1] See however ref. 5.

bearing on this question. In general, cell damage only occurs, where activated lymphocytes are brought into close contact with target cells. *Unsensitized* lymphocytes usually do not kill allogenic target cells during short incubations. They are probably not activated. However, during long periods of incubation, the target cells are often damaged. In such cultures, Ginsburg and Sachs found transformed lymphocytes [5]. Thus, prolonged contact with foreign cells seems to stimulate the lymphocytes and this may lead to cell damage. The state of activation of sensitized lymphocytes in contact with target cells is not known. This is also true for *unsensitized lymphocytes incubated with antibody-coated target cells*. However, Hirschhorn and others have shown that lymphocytes can be stimulated by antigen-antibody complexes [2]. Such complexes are present on the cell surface in these incubation mixtures and may activate the lymphocytes.

The inhibitory effect of ALS is probably due to a blockade of lymphocyte receptors which mediate the contact with the target cells regardless whether antibodies are present or not. The fact that lymphocytes which have been strongly stimulated by ALS, are not cytotoxic to target cells, suggests that the inhibitory action of ALS does not reflect an inhibition of activation. In contrast, antimycin A probably prevents the activation of the lymphocytes without affecting their aggregation to the target cells.

Contact between lymphocytes and target cells may have a twofold function in the cytotoxic reaction. In some situations it is probably necessary for the activation of the lymphocytes. In addition, contact is probably always needed for the effectuation of cell damage. As already pointed out, lymphocytes can be activated and become cytotoxic by other means than direct contact with target cells. These findings, as well as those regarding the inhibition, achieved with ALS, support the notion that the process of activation is distinct from the cytotoxic effector mechanism. The common denominator in the three models of lymphocyte mediated cytotoxicity discussed here may actually lay in the effector mechanism. In contrast, the steps leading to activation seem to be different in these three models.

References

1. Biberfeld, P.; Holm, G. and Perlmann, P.: Data to be published.
2. Block-Shtacher, N.; Hirschhorn, K. and Uhr, J.W.: Stimulation of non-immunized human lymphocytes by antigen-antibody complexes. Proc. 3rd Ann. leucocyte Conf. (Iowa City, 1967).

3. BLOOM, B.R. and CHASE, M.W.: Transfer of delayed-type hypersensitivity. A critical review and experimental study in the guinea pig. Progr. Allergy *10:* 151 (1967).

4. BRUNNER, K.T.; MAUEL, J.; CEROTTINI, J.-C. and CHAPUIS, B.: Quantitative assay of the lytic action of immune lymphoid cells on ^{51}Cr-labelled allogeneic target cells *in vitro;* inhibition by isoantibody and by drugs. Immunology *14:* 181 (1968).

5. GINSBURG, H. and SACHS, L.: Destruction of mouse and rat embryo cells in tissue culture by lymph node cells from unsensitized rats. J. comp. Physiol. *66:* 199 (1965).

6. GOVAERTS, A.: Cellular antibodies in kidney transplantation. J. Immunol. *85:* 516 (1960).

7. HOLM, G.: *In vitro* cytotoxic effects of lymphoid cells from rats with experimental autoimmune nephrosis. Clin. exp. Immunol. *1:* 45 (1966).

8. HOLM, G.: Studies on the *in vitro* cytotoxicity of lymphoid cells. (Thesis, Stockholm 1967.)

9. HOLM, G.: The *in vitro* cytotoxicity of human lymphocytes: Comparison with other cells. Exp. Cell Res. *48:* 327 (1967).

10. HOLM, G.: The *in vitro* cytotoxicity of human lymphocytes: The effect of metabolic inhibitors. Exp. Cell Res. *48:* 334 (1967).

11. HOLM, G.: Lack of cytotoxicity by human thymocytes *in vitro*. Scand. J. Haemat. *4:* 230 (1967).

12. HOLM, G. and PERLMANN, P.: Phytohaemagglutinin-induced cytotoxic action of unsensitized immunologically competent cells on allogeneic and xenogeneic tissue culture cells. Nature (Lond.) *207:* 818 (1965).

13. HOLM, G. and PERLMANN, P.: Quantitative studies on phytohaemagglutinin-induced cytotoxicity by human lymphocytes against homologous cells in tissue culture. Immunology *12:* 525 (1967).

14. HOLM, G. and PERLMANN, P.: Cytotoxic potential of stimulated human lymphocytes. J. exp. Med. *125:* 721 (1967).

15. HOLM, G. and PERLMANN, P.: The effect of antimetabolites on the cytotoxicity by human lymphocytes. In: Advance in transplantation, p. 155. (Eds.) J. DAUSSET, J. HAMBURGER and G. Mathé (Munksgaard, Copenhagen 1968).

16. HOLM, G.; PERLMANN, P. and JOHANSSON, B.: Impaired phytohaemagglutinin-induced cytotoxicity *in vitro* of lymphocytes from patients with Hodgkin's disease or chronic lymphatic leucaemia. Clin. exp. Immunol. *2:* 351 (1967).

17. HOLM, G.; PERLMANN, P. and WERNER, B.: Phytohaemagglutinin-induced cytotoxic action of normal lymphoid cells on cells in tissue culture. Nature (Lond.) *203:* 841 (1964).

18. KILLANDER, D. and RIGLER, R.: Initial changes of deoxyribonucleoprotein and synthesis of nucleic acid in phytohaemagglutinin-stimulated human leucocytes *in vitro*. Exp. Cell Res. *39:* 701 (1965).

19. MÖLLER, E.: Contact-induced cytotoxicity by lymphoid cells containing foreign isoantigens. Science *147:* 873 (1965).

20. MÖLLER, E.: Antagonistic effects of humoral isoantibodies on the *in vitro* cytotoxicity of immune lymphoid cells. J. exp. Med. *122:* 11 (1965).

21. PERLMANN, P. and HOLM, G.: Studies on the mechanism of lymphocyte cytotoxicity. In: Mechanisms of inflammation induced by immune reactions, p. 325 (Eds.) P.A. MIESCHER and P. GRABAR (Schwabe, Basel 1968).

22. PERLMANN, P.; PERLMANN, H. and HOLM, G.: Cytotoxic action of stimulated lymphocytes on allogenic and autologous erythrocytes. Science *160:* 306 (1968).

23. PERLMANN, P.; PERLMANN, H.; MÜLLER-EBERHARD, H. and MANNI, J.: Cytotoxicity of leukocytes, triggered by target cell bound complement. Science (submitted for publication).

24. Pogo, B.G.T.; Allfrey, V.G. and Mirsky, A.E.: RNA synthesis and histone acetylation during the course of gene activation in lymphocytes. Proc. nat. Acad. Sci. *55*: 805 (1966).
25. Rosenau, W.: Interaction of lymphoid cells with target cells in tissue culture. In: Cellbound antibodies, p. 75 (Eds.) B. Amos and H. Koprowski (Wistar Institute Press, Philadelphia 1963).
26. Waksman, B.H.: Tissue damage in the "delayed" (cellular) type of hypersensitivity. In: Mechanisms of cell and tissue damage produced by immune reactions, p. 146 (Eds.) P. Grabar and P. Miescher (Schwabe, Basel 1962).
27. Watson, D.W.; Quigley, A. and Bolt, R.J.: Effect of lymphocytes from patients with ulcerative colitis on human adult colon epithelial cells. Gastroenterology *51*: 985 (1966).

Authors' address: Dr. G. Holm and Prof. Dr. P. Perlmann, University of Stockholm, The Wenner-Gren Institute, *S-11345 Stockholm* (Sweden).

Antibiotica et Chemotherapia, vol. 15, pp. 310–327 (Karger, Basel/New York 1969)

Experimental Observations Bearing on the Clinical Use of ALS

E. M. LANCE[1]

National Institute for Medical Research, London

Introduction

The importance of antilymphocyte serum (ALS) lies in its potential for clinical use. However, it may prove difficult if not impossible to establish the principles in man to guide this application. Therefore in this paper I will draw upon our experience in animal studies to draw analogies which may be pertinent. No attempt will be made to review the work at other laboratories, but many of the ideas and supporting data will have been contributed by my colleagues at Mill Hill: Sir PETER MEDAWAR, ROBERT TAUB, RAPHAEL LEVEY, SOMARIE JOOSTE and MARIAN RUSZKIEWICZ.

A. Methods of Raising ALS

1. Schedule of Immunization

The schedules proposed and adopted by different laboratories fall into two groups: those favoring a brief course of injections of antigen (two- or three-pulse serum) and those who prefer repeated dosage over a long period of time (hyperimmune serum). While the routine method employed for raising ALS at our laboratory is the two-pulse method [11] we have had experience with both [4]. The two-pulse method has much to commend it. A consistently active serum is

[1] Supported by Training Grant TI AM 5414 from the National Institute for Arthritis and Metabolism, U.S.P.H.S., National Institutes of Health.

reliably produced. Such sera double or treble the survival of A strain skin grafts on CBA mice when tested in our standard assay system [4]. Furthermore these sera may be given to animals by the subcutaneous route without prior absorption and are non-toxic. The major drawback to this method is that the yield of serum per animal is limited since there is no opportunity for serial bleeding. Although most of our experience has been with rabbit anti-mouse or anti-guinea pig serum raised in this way, we have recently found this method applicable to the production of goat and rabbit anti-monkey serum.

Hyperimmunization has the practical advantage of increasing the yield per animal and the theoretical advantage of raising the titre of antibody by repeated boosting. In our hands this latter possibility has not been always realized. We have often found that repeated administration of antigen is associated with a decline in potency. Whether this observation results from the elaboration of interfering antibodies or through the progressive preoccupation of the immunized animal with irrelevant antigens the practical result is the same. Another drawback to hyperimmunization is the concomitant rise in titre of toxic antibodies, e.g. those directed against erythrocytes, so that after four doses of antigen the serum obtained is lethal upon injection and must be absorbed prior to use.

Little systematic investigation of the merits of these two schedules has been applied thus far by those who have prepared and used anti-human lymphocyte serum, largely through lack of an adequate assay. Most reports have dealt with sera prepared by hyperimmunization which routinely require absorption prior to use [2, 24]. Another objection to serum raised in this manner has been pain at the injection site. In this regard it is of interest to note that Shorter *et al.* have found that anti-human lymphocyte serum raised according to the two-pulse method is active *in vivo* and does not cause pain upon injection [18].

We should like briefly to mention our findings concerning the incorporation of adjuvants into the immunizing inoculum. Sera raised using either Arquad or aluminium phosphate as adjuvants have been potent but extremely toxic. These sera all require extensive absorption with both erythrocytes and tissue brei to render them suitable for administration and some batches cannot be rid of all toxic products even after absorption. Injections of unabsorbed whole serum raised with adjuvants have given rise to a variety of lesions in recipients which we have never observed after ALS raised in our routine fashion. These include massive depletion of the lymph nodes, thymus and spleen of lymphocytes probably as a secondary manifestation of stress, gross intravascular hemolysis, focal necrosis of the liver and kidney, and the presence of antibodies to mouse serum proteins. We therefore urge caution in incorporating adjuvants in regimens for raising anti-human ALS.

2. Choice of Species

Antibody molecules produced by one species vary considerably in the efficiency with which they interact with the complement of different species [1]. For instance, ALS raised in chickens or ducks to mouse lymphocytes have high agglutinin titres and are cytotoxic *in vitro* to mouse lymphocytes when the complement source is avian (fig. 1). The efficiency with which these antisera kill lymphocytes falls off when rabbit complement is substituted and even further with guinea pig complement. When mouse complement is used there is no demonstrable cytotoxic effect and avian antilymphocytic sera do not prolong the survival of skin homografts in mice. If, as we believe, effective interaction between antibody, lymphocyte and complement is necessary to achieve an immunosuppressive effect *in vivo*, then surely this must be a consideration in choosing appropriate animals in which to raise anti-human ALS.

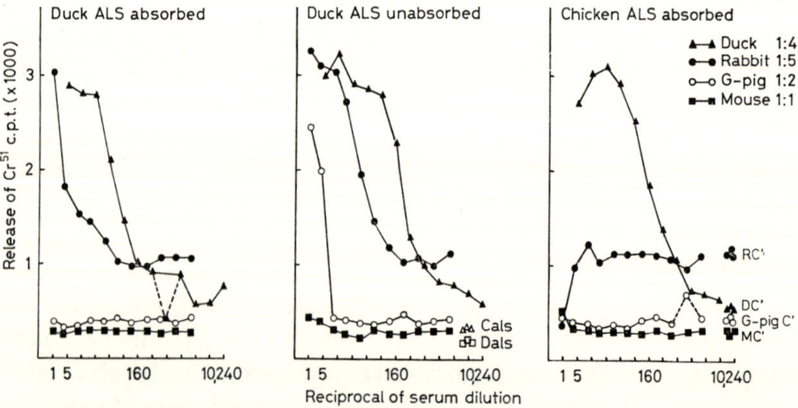

Fig. 1. Showing the influence of complement source on the *in vitro* cytotoxicity of avian ALS on mouse lymphocytes. High titres are found when avian complement is used. Rabbit and guinea pig complement are less effective and there is no demonstrable cytotoxicity with mouse complement.

Another consideration is that the half-life of globulins from one species varies to a great extent depending upon the choice of recipient. Spiegelberg and Weigle [19] have summarized the evidence on this point and have pointed out, for example, that mouse IgG has a half-life of 4.0 days in the mouse, but only 1.5 days when injected into rabbits. It would be an obvious advantage to use animals for immunization whose antibody molecules enjoyed a relatively long half-life in man.

A point of theoretical interest at this time stems from the observation of Taub and Ruszkiewicz [23] who have shown by differential absorption studies that different species may give rise to antibodies directed against different antigenic lymphocyte constituents. This raises the possibility that mixtures of two different heterologous antibody populations may be more effective than the use of either alone.

B. Purification Procedures

The need for purification stems from the desire to be able to administer the minimum of foreign protein containing the maximum of active components. There is now general agreement that the antibodies responsible for the immunosuppressive action of ALS are of IgG specificity [3, 5]. Surely then the minimum requirement in purifying ALS for human use would be the separation of IgG molecules from all other serum components. This procedure would considerably reduce the hazard of serum sickness and anaphylaxis as many immunogenic and extraneous serum protein components would be removed. An additional benefit would be the removal of those noxious antibodies which are of IgM specificity. However, within the IgG fraction there may still remain antibodies irrelevant to the action of ALS but which are potentially toxic. Those components directed against erythrocytes, platelets and serum proteins are examples in point. These can and should be removed by absorption prior to clinical use. Additional absorption procedures may be dictated by the clinical circumstances. For instance in the use of ALS to promote the survival of renal homografts it may be desirable to absorb further antisera with renal tissue. Absorption procedures have certain drawbacks however. They are time-consuming, expensive, may not be entirely efficient, and are apt to be associated with some loss of potency.

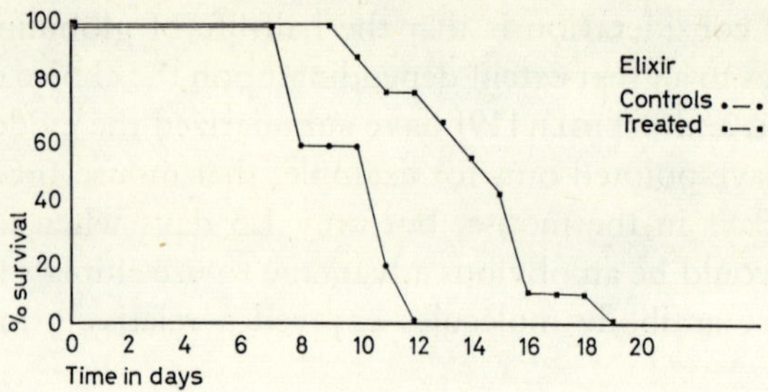

Fig. 2. Weanling CBA mice received A strain skin grafts. One group was treated by the subcutaneous injection of 40 μg of ALS IgG molecules which had been absorbed onto and then eluted from mouse lymphocyte membranes. The control group received no injection. The treatment with the purified preparation clearly prolongs the survival of skin homografts across H-2 barriers.

Another approach to this problem might be through the enrichment of specific antibodies by the absorption of ALS IgG onto lymphocyte preparations and the subsequent elution of lymphocyte-specific antibodies. We have shown that it is possible to carry out such procedures by absorbing rabbit antimouse lymphocyte IgG onto mouse lymphocyte membrane and subsequently eluting the antibody at acid pH. The resulting eluate retains the ability to prolong the survival of skin homografts in microgram quantities (fig. 2). We feel, however, that this protocol is more suitable for experimental investigation than clinical application because it is relatively inefficient, impractical on a large scale and because some denaturation of antibody seems to be a necessary concomitant.

Thus far we have dealt with purification possibilities in which the antiserum was subjected to manipulations. I should like now to consider the alternate possibility, namely purification of the antigen used to raise ALS. As a first principle the source of lymphocytes should be as homogeneous as possible. Thoracic duct cells and thymocytes constitute a relatively pure lymphocyte population whereas peripheral blood, lymph nodes, and spleen are relatively heterogeneous with respect to cell type and ideally should not be used for immunization without a preliminary separation step. Having obtained a relatively pure population of lymphocytes can further fractionation procedures improve the quality of the antiserum raised? An ideal material for immunization should have at least the following three properties: (1) it should induce the formation of antibodies potent *in vivo;* (2) repeated immunizations should not lead to a fall off in this activity;

(3) the antiserum raised should be non-toxic. One approach has been the fractionation of lymphocytes making use of the differential solubility of their constituents in salts of varying concentrations [11]. The "crude insoluble" fraction produced by this method contains the bulk of membrane antigens and was the most efficient in raising a potent ALS. However, repeated immunization with this product had two undesirable effects: decline in potency and a rise in titre of haemagglutinins. Another approach has been to fractionate lymphocytes into relatively pure preparations of their subcellular components [Lance, Ford and Ruszkiewicz, 1968[1]]. Mouse thymocytes were fractionated by differential centrifugation and the use of gradients on two separate occasions to yield supernatant, "microsome-membrane", "mitochondrial", and "nuclear" fractions in the first instance and "membrane", "microsome", and "mitochondrial" fractions in the second. These fractions were then injected into rabbits intravenously and sera obtained after two, three and four serial immunizations. The resulting sera were tested by assaying their ability to protect skin homografts, the ability to kill target lymphocytes *in vitro,* and in some instances the titre of haemagglutinins was determined. In addition an *in vivo* toxicity test was performed on the sera produced after the fourth antigen dosage. The results may be summarized as follows (table I). All fractions were capable of eliciting antisera which could

Table I. The potency of sera raised with thymocyte subcellular fractions

Thymocyte fraction	Serum obtained after		
	2 injections	3 injections	4 injections
Supernatant	13.4±1.0[1] (160)[2]	13.8±1.8 (100)	13.7±1.2 (640)
Membrane	22.5±3.7 (6400)	28.1±4.6 (3800)	23.7±4.3 (3840)
Microsome	19.6±3.3 (3200)	14.6±2.0 (2560)	22.5±5.1 (1600)
Mitochondria	19.8±4.6 (3200)	17.0±4.2 (2560)	16.8±2.0 (2140)
Nuclear	21.3±3.7 (5120)	18.7±1.9 (500)	13.8±2.8 (400)

[1] M.E.L. (mean expectation of life) based in all assays on groups of 7–10 CBA male mice bearing A strain tail skin grafts.

[2] Cytotoxic titre expressed as the reciprocal of that dilution which causes half maximal liberation of Cr^{51} from the labelled lymphocytes.

---

[1] Immunology 1968 (in press).

extend the survival of skin homografts. Sera raised with some fractions (principally the nuclear one) showed progressive fall off in activity with repeated immunization, whereas others (mitochondrial) were associated with a rising titre of haemagglutinins and toxicity *in vivo*. The membrane fraction was the most consistently effective in raising a potent ALS, in maintaining potency with repeated immunization, and in producing a non-toxic product. Extrapolation of these findings to man suggests that membrane preparations of lymphocytes might be helpful in solving some of the problems attendant on raising ALS. The potential advantages would be a product which could be prepared in bulk and conveniently stored. Animals could be repeatedly immunized without fear of loss in potency or excessive toxicity, and the need for absorption could be reduced. It remains to be seen whether these findings are applicable to the human situation, but the principle of antigen purification seems to demand further consideration.

C. *Assays of Potency*

One of the most pressing problems confronting those who would apply ALS clinically is the search for a suitable and reliable assay of potency. We routinely assay anti-mouse lymphocyte serum by its ability to prolong the survival of skin homografts in a standardized system. The advantage of this assay is that it measures directly the property of ALS in which we are interested, but is unfortunately not applicable in man. In the search for a substitute we have attempted to appraise the potency of horse anti-human ALS by adminstering standard doses to rhesus monkeys bearing skin homografts (table II). At the present time we feel that this method offers a rough estimate of toxicity and can be used to rank the potency of a series of different antisera but does not provide sufficiently quantitative data to rely upon solely.

Various *in vitro* tests have been evaluated. Lymphocyte agglutination titres are not entirely satisfactory because they measure a perhaps necessary but not sufficient property of ALS. For example, duck and chicken ALS as well as F(ab)2 and 19S antibodies will agglutinate lymphocytes but are ineffective *in vivo*.

Tests based upon the measurement of lymphocyte activation are subject to the same criticism. There is no confirmation that this property is related to the *in vivo* immunosuppression achieved by

Table II. The use of rhesus monkeys to assay the potency and toxicity
of horse anti-human ALS

	Dosage and schedule	Mean survival of first set homografts	Toxicity
Pool 1	5 ml/kg day 0 2.5 ml/kg t.i.w.	11 days minimal activity	None observed
Pool 2	40 mg IgG/kg every other day beginning –3	Over 15 days quite active	None observed
Pool 3	5 ml/kg day 0 2.5 ml/kg t.i.w.	7 days inactive	3 of 5 animals died. Injections painful
Two-pulse ALS	100 mg IgG/kg day 0 then 50 mg/kg t.i.w.	8 days inactive	None observed

Note: Some animals in pools 1 and 3, and two-pulse group had a second rhesus skin homograft placed after rejection of the first. In all these cases there was definite prolongation over that of control grafts which are rejected between seven to nine days.

ALS, and furthermore the test is non-specific in the sense that anti-allotype antibody [17] and F(ab)2 [26] can activate lymphocytes strongly but do not produce immunosuppression.

The cytotoxic test has not thus far been an accurate predictive tool. While all sera tested which are active *in vivo* have been cytotoxic *in vitro* the converse is not always true. We are, however, predisposed towards this test because of our belief that ALS achieves its immunosuppressive effect largely through the destruction of lymphocytes. Some of the possible sources of error have already been alluded to. Tests on whole sera are apt to be misleading since 19S antibody will contribute to the cytotoxic titre (fig. 3) but not to the prolongation of homograft survival [3, 5]. Furthermore 7S antibody may contain components directed towards irrelevant antigens. Antibodies against erythrocytes or H-2 antigens are cytotoxic *in vitro* but when injected into the whole animal are ineffective presumably because the great bulk of tissue other than lymphocytes which possess these antigens absorb them. Another consideration mentioned above is the error which may be introduced by not using complement obtained from the intended host. We would therefore suggest that the value of the cytotoxic test could be enhanced if only fully absorbed IgG antibodies were tested against lymphocytes and complement of the species of the intended recipient.

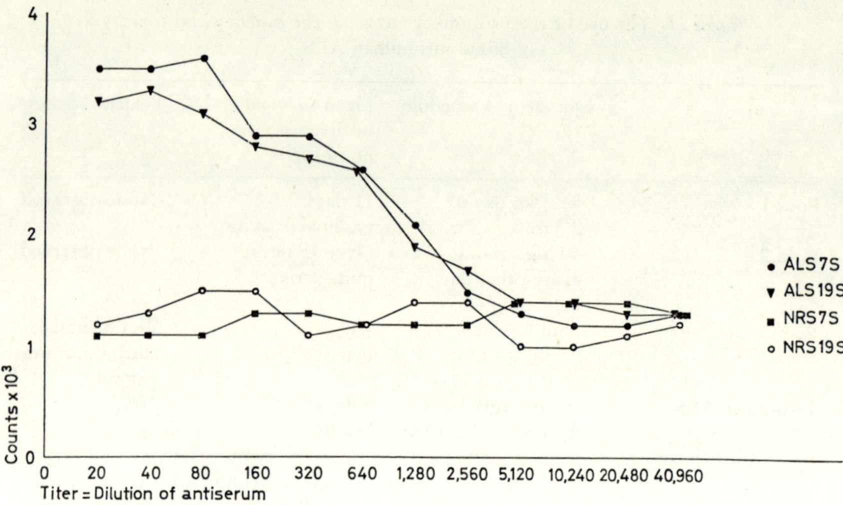

Fig. 3. A comparison of the *in vitro* cytotoxicity of 19S and 7S fractions which had been prepared by chromatography of whole ALS on G-200 and subsequently restored to original serum concentration. Controls are similar fractions of NRS. Both fractions from NRS are inactive whereas both fractions from ALS are equally and highly active.

In mice it is possible to perform an *in vivo* lymphocyte toxicity test. The scheme involves the intravenous injection of syngeneic lymphocytes which have been labelled with radioactive chromium into mice which have received a prior subcutaneous injection of ALS. Under normal circumstances lymphocytes will migrate largely to the lymph nodes and spleen but when preinjected with an active antiserum (whole or IgG) then a substantial portion of the injected cells is diverted away from these organs (presumably because they have been killed) and the label is largely recovered in the liver [22]. The advantages of this technique are that non-immunosuppressive fractions, i.e. F(ab)2 or 19S antibody, do not manifest this *in vivo* property (table III), and 7S antibodies directed towards irrelevant antigens are screened out by the body prior to the cell injection. Therefore one can measure the ability of pertinent antibodies to kill lymphocytes *in vivo*. This test could be adapted for man in the following way (fig. 4). Lymphocytes from the prospective ALS recipient could be obtained from an aliquot of peripheral blood and labelled with radioactive chromium *in vitro*. These cells would then be reinjected intravenously several hours after administration of a test dose of ALS. The relative uptake of label in the liver and spleen could be determined by cumulative scanning of these organs with external scintillation detectors. The ratio between

Table III. Lymphocyte migration in pretreated recipients

Pretreatment	Localization (%) in	
	Lymph nodes	Liver
Untreated control	11.5	9
ALS 7S day −1	4.6	26
ALS 7S day −2	8.0	20
ALS 19S day −1	11.0	20
ALS F(ab)2 day −1	14.0	11

Groups of CBA mice received an intravenous injection of Cr⁵¹ labelled syngeneic ymph node lymphocytes either 24 h or 48 h after subcutaneous injection of ALS 7S, 19S, or F(ab)2. The serum injections were adjusted to represent that amount of protein corresponding to the original serum content of 0.5 ml.

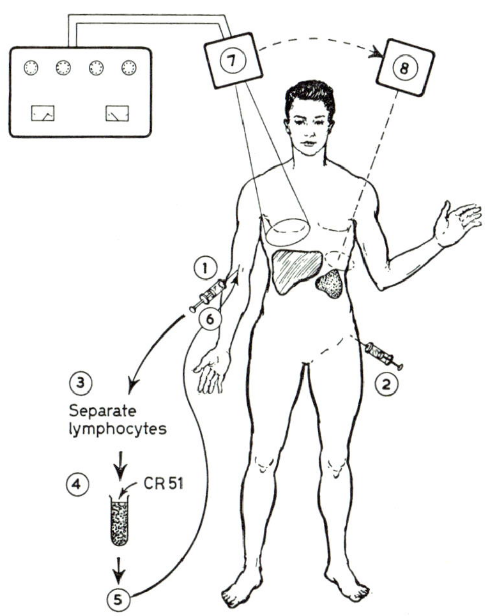

Fig. 4. Proposal for a hypothetical test for ALS potency in man. – 1. An aliquot of blood is withdrawn by venapuncture and the lymphocytes separated from other elements. – 2. The test dose of ALS is injected intramuscularly. – 3. The separated lymphocytes are labelled *in vitro* with Cr⁵¹ (4 and 5) and reinjected intravenously (6). – 7. und 8. The relative distribution of the injected labelled lymphocytes between the liver and spleen are compared by cumulative scanning with an external detector over these two organs.

the counts in these two organs would be a measure of the number of labelled cells which have been killed and presumably would reflect proportionately the effect on the pool of recirculating lymphocytes.

D. Natural History of the Pertinent Antibodies

1. The Short-Lived Effect of a Single Dose

Three lines of evidence strongly suggest that the effect of a single dose of ALS is short-lived. Pichylmayer [16] and Taub and Ruszkie-wicz [23] have followed the disappearance of cytotoxic antibodies from the sera of injected animals. Both studies have shown that after a single injection there is a rapid fall in titre so that within a few hours after injection no activity can be detected. The pattern of decay depends to some extent upon the route of injection (intravenously administered ALS decays more rapidly than an equal dose given subcutaneously).

A second observation is that whereas a single dose of ALS given just prior to the injection of syngeneic lymphocytes can prevent their migration to lymphoid tissue, this effect is also rapidly lost. Table III shows that a single injection of ALS IgG still diverts lymphoid cells from lymph nodes 24 h later but that this effect is largely gone at 48 h.

More direct evidence on this point comes from the study of the fate of specific eluted antibody (fig. 5). Serial counts of the whole

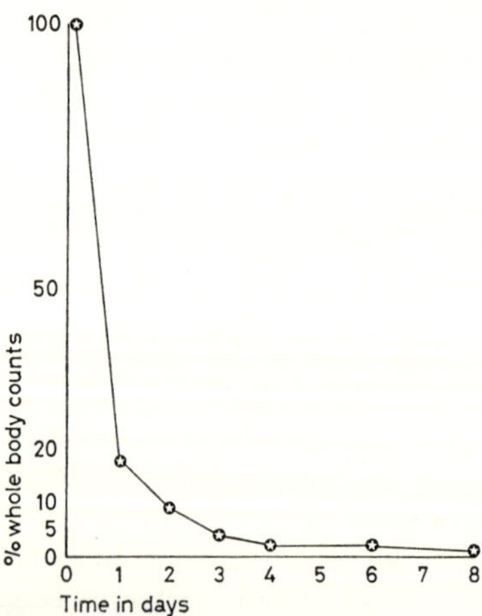

Fig. 5. The rate of clearance of ALS IgG molecules absorbed onto and eluted from lymphocyte membrane from the whole body. Six mice received an aliquot of ^{131}I labelled eluate and the radioactivity was assayed by placing mice individually into the cone of an external scintillation detector. The relative percentages of retention with time were calculated by defining the radioactivity present one hour after injection as 100 % and comparing subsequent values with that figure after appropriate correction for decay.

body and serum of animals receiving injections of radioactively tagged eluted antibody show that both the disappearance from the serum and the elimination from the body are extremely rapid. Roughly 80% of the molecules are eliminated from the body in the first 24 h, and the half-life of the remaining fraction is about one day.

2. The Failure to Penetrate Significantly Central Lymphoid Tissue

Levey and Medawar were the first to point out the selective effect of ALS on peripheral as contrasted with central lymphoid tissue [13]. This conclusion was drawn from the observations that ALS was largely ineffective in overcoming the immunization caused by the prior injection of lymphoid cells as contrasted to that aroused by a skin graft, and by the finding that inhibition of the lymphocyte transfer reaction was much more difficult to achieve by pretreating the lymphocyte donor than by treatment of the recipient. Histological evidence also suggests that ALS is less effective in reaching central sites [6]. The lymph nodes and spleens of mice treated with repetitive doses of ALS over months still show preservation or even hyperplasia of cortical and medullary elements in lymph nodes and retention of numerous lymphocytes in the periphery of the follicles of the spleen. Furthermore, the thymus appears quite normal.

More direct evidence on this point is the observation that ALS given after the injection of chromium-labelled lymphocytes does not efficiently leach out these cells once they have migrated to lymphoid organs [22]. Moreover, studies with labelled specific eluate antibody have shown that only a minute proportion localizes within lymphoid organs and is rapidly cleared from these sites as well (fig. 6).

3. The Discriminate Effect on Cell-Mediated Immunity

Although ALS can be used to suppress immune reactions mediated by circulating antibody as well as those mediated by cells yet a fair amount of evidence suggests that it is much more efficient against the latter [6, 8]. Whereas ALS inhibits both first and second set skin homograft rejection [11], the secondary response to protein, bacterial or particulate antigens is suppressed feebly even in large doses [5, 14]. A program of ALS administration which will abolish memory of a previous sensitization to transplantation antigens will not prevent a secondary response to BSA [7].

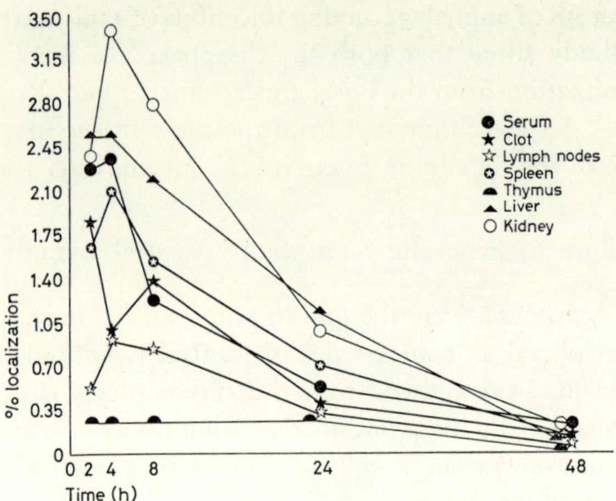

Fig. 6. Format similar to that in figure 5, except that groups of two mice were sacrificed at the indicated time intervals and the distribution of the radioactive label with time in the various organs was calculated by comparison with a standard representing the amount injected. The highest amounts are found in the kidney, liver and serum whereas the thymus and lymph nodes take up little of the eluted antibody. These levels are considerably below that found for IgG from normal rabbit serum at any time and decay rapidly from these low levels to minimal amounts within 48 h.

We have previously shown that it is possible to treat mice chronically with ALS at dosage levels which completely inhibit cell-mediated immune transactions but leave the animals almost normally responsive with respect to the elaboration of humoral antibodies [6].

4. The Mode of Action of ALS

The above observations have led to a proposed mechanism of action for ALS [6]. According to this hypothesis ALS exerts a cytotoxic effect selectively on the population of recirculating lymphocytes which by virtue of their life-cycle are obliged to enter the blood stream where they are exposed to high concentrations of antibody. Because (in mice) of the rapid turnover of the recirculating pool, high antibody titres would not have to be long maintained before drastic reduction of this population of lymphocytes would occur. The relatively slow rate of regeneration of these long-lived cells implies that the immuno-suppressive effect would long outlast the metabolic life-span of ALS in the host.

If this proposed mechanism of action be true then there are important implications for clinical application. The timing and dosage of ALS in man must be linked with a knowledge of the turnover of the pool of long-lived recirculating lymphocytes and a regimen of administration selected most appropriate to ablate this population of cells.

E. Immunogenicity of ALS IgG

We have already mentioned the desirability of removing serum proteins other than IgG from any preparation intended for clinical use. Since animals treated with ALS retain the capacity to elaborate humoral antibodies in response to protein antigens, chronic treatment with whole serum is associated with the development of serum sickness, anaphylaxis and with time the development of "complex" nephritis [6]. Use of IgG preparations would be expected to reduce this hazard but unfortunately not entirely eliminate it. Whereas IgG from normal rabbits is non-immunogenic in mice, IgG prepared from ALS is highly immunogenic [9]. This has several undesirable consequences: it recreates the hazards associated with the administration of whole serum and furthermore may render subsequent ALS IgG doses less effective as immune clearance will reduce the effective dose delivered. We have suggested that these problems might be overcome by the induction of paralysis to IgG by the injection of normal unimmunized IgG prior to ALS treatment. Such a regimen induces a state of paralysis with respect to subsequent ALS IgG and does not impair (in fact the contrary may be true) the immunosuppressive effect [5]. This principle was established in mice using rabbit IgG, but we have recently shown that the same is true in rhesus monkeys with respect to horse IgG (fig. 7). There is no reason to think that the same principles will not also apply to man.

F. ALS and the Induction of Tolerance

The ultimate goal in clinical transplantation is to be able to induce a state of tolerance in the recipient specific for donor antigens. Monaco *et al.* [15] have already shown that this circumstance can be achieved in mice through the combination of thymectomy, ALS and the injection of large amounts of donor antigen in the form of lymphoid cells. Lance and Medawar [10] have found that it is possible to achieve the same result when ALS is used as the only immunosup-

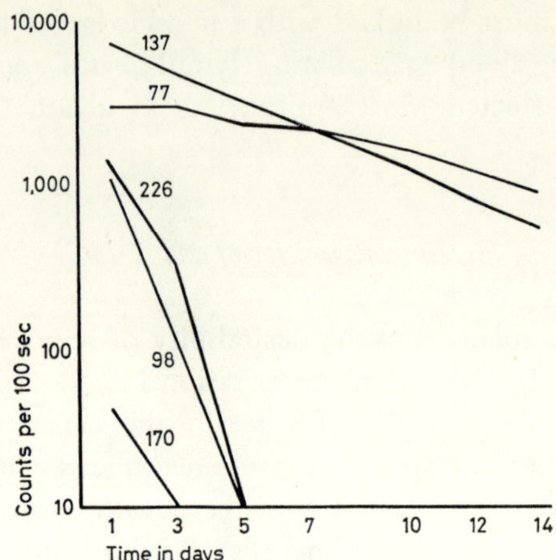

Fig. 7. The rate of elimination of a test dose of ^{131}I labelled equine IgG (EGG) from the blood of rhesus monkeys which had been treated as follows: 137 no pretreatment; 98, 226, 170 all had received multiple injections of horse anti-human ALS prior to the test dose of ^{131}I EGG; 77 two weeks prior to the course of injections of horse anti-human ALS as above this monkey received an intravenous injection of normal horse IgG which had been centrifuged at 60,000 g av. just before administration. Animals 226, 98 and 170 have elimination patterns characteristic of a secondary response, whereas animals 77 and 137 show no evidence of an immune reaction at all. Therefore ALS IgG is immunogenic for monkeys, whereas non-immune IgG is not. Furthermore, pretreatment with normal IgG induces a state of paralysis to IgG.

pressive agent. In a typical experiment CBA mice receive A strain skin grafts accompanied by a series of closely spaced injections of ALS. Several days after the last ALS injection a single pulse of antigen in the form of lymphoid cells is injected intravenously. Control animals are treated identically with the omission of the cell injection. The degree to which the skin grafts on the animals receiving cells survive longer than those borne by control animals is a reflection of the extent of tolerance which has been induced. The results thus far may be summarized as follows. When the antigenic differences between donor and host involve the H-2 locus, the pretreatment schedule of ALS must be on a par with that required to completely inactivate cell-mediated reactivity or to abolish memory of a prior sensitization (i.e. total dose of about 1.5 ml). The duration of the tolerant state is proportional over a wide range with the dose of the tolerance-conferring cell inoculum. Some effect is detectable with as little as 1×10^6 cells and that conferred by 100×10^6 cells may last hundreds of days or in fact throughout the lifetime of the recipient.

The unreactive state extends to both cell-mediated and humoral systems, i.e. there is no detectable serum antibody response to donor antigens, and splenic cells from these animals do not cause graft-versus-host disease when injected into newborn hybrids possessing donor antigens. The unreactive state is specific for donor antigens and does not depend upon continued generalized immunosuppression. Third party skin grafts applied together with the test skin graft are rejected long before any reaction to the test skin graft can be detected and, furthermore splenic cells from recipients cause a vigurous graft-versus-host response in newborn hybrids of a third strain, while at the same time they fail to do so in hybrids of the strain of the cell donor.

The tolerant state is associated with but not necessarily dependent upon a state of lymphoid chimerism and has this far required the injection of viable cells. Preliminary evidence suggests that cells receiving lethal irradiation *in vitro* may also be effective. Lastly, although the principles have been worked out in mice, we have recently been able to reproduce this finding in a monkey, and there is no reason to think that it cannot be reproduced in man.

G. *ALS and Heterografts*

The observation that ALS will prolong the life of heterografts has been previously reported [11, 14]. Extension of these observations [Lance and Medawar, 1968[1]] has shown that it is possible to maintain heterografts in mice for prolonged periods of time by the continued administration of small weekly doses (2 × 0.25 ml) of ALS. Wide species differences have been studied and donor skin has been obtained from rats, guinea pigs, rabbits and man. For example, human skin grafts have been maintained on mice for over two months without gross or microscopic evidence of rejection. It has been possible also to achieve prolonged survival of second set heterografts (guinea pig to mouse) with ALS. We are not aware of any previous success in this rather demanding situation achieved by any other means.

The relevance of these findings to clinical transplantation is the demonstration that ALS can effectively overcome antigenic differences far greater than those ordinarily encountered in human homotransplantation. This property may lessen the dependency on close matching by tissue typing and broaden thereby the pool of permissible

---

[1] Lancet *i:* 1174 (1968).

donors without jeopardizing the end result. Some indication that this may be true is contained in Starzl's finding [20, 21] that since the incorporation of ALS into the regimen of immunosuppression the survival of well matched and poorly matched renal grafts has not differed.

H. Summary

Nothing we know about ALS excludes its use in man. On the contrary, guided by the experience of animal experimentation it seems reasonable to expect that a product of high potency and specificity can be produced which can be rendered non-toxic. Extraction of the IgG fraction and its administration into pre-paralysed recipients should eliminate the hazards of host reaction to foreign protein. An assay of potency based upon testing the lymphocytotoxic properties of ALS *in vitro* or *in vivo* seems within reach. A schedule of administration based upon a knowledge of the natural history of the relevant antibody molecule and the population of recirculating lymphocytes in man should enhance its effectiveness. The remarkable ability of ALS to promote survival of tissues transplanted across great antigenic differences should broaden the selection of donor organs for grafting and finally it seems possible that ALS will be useful in achieving the goal of tolerance induction in man.

Acknowledgements

The author would like to acknowledge the assistance of Miss S. Carswell in the preparation of this manuscript, and to thank Dr. N.A. Mitchison for making the facilities of his department available to me. I have already indicated my debt to my colleagues

References

1. Cushing, J.E., Jr.: A comparative study of complement. II. The interaction of components of different species. J. Immunol. *50:* 75–89 (1945).
2. Iwasaki, Y.; Porter, K.A.; Amend, J.R.; Marchioro, T.L.; Zühlke, V. and Starzl, T.E.: The preparation and testing of horse antidog and antihuman antilymphoid plasma or serum and its protein fractions. Surg. Gynec. Obstet. *124:* 1–24 (1967).
3. James, K. and Medawar, P.B.: Characterization of antilymphocytic antibody. Nature (Lond.) *214:* 1052–1053 (1967).
4. Jooste, S.; Lance, E.M.; Levey, R.H.; Medawar, P.B.; Sharman, R. and Taub, R.N.: Notes on the preparation and assay of antilymphocytic serum for use in mice. Immunology (In press 1968).
5. Lance, E.M.: The nature and scope of action of antilymphocytic serum. In Symposium on Cell Bound Immunity with Special Reference to Antilymphocytic Serum and the Immunotherapy of Cancer. Les Conq. et Colloq. de l'Université de Liège *43:* 103–116 (1967).
6. Lance, E.M.: The effects of chronic ALS administration in mice. In Advances in Transplantation, pp. 107–116 (Eds.) J. Dausset, J. Hamburger and G. Mathé (Munksgaard, 1968).
7. Lance, E.M.: Erasure of immunological memory with ALS. Nature (Lond.) *217:* 557–558 (1968).

8. Lance, E.M. and Batchelor, J.R.: Discriminate suppression by heterologous antisera of cell mediated immune responses. Transplantation 6: 490–491 (1968).

9. Lance, E.M. and Dresser, D.W.: Antigenicity in mice of antilymphocyte gamma globulin. Nature (Lond.) 215: 488–490 (1967).

10. Lance, E.M. and Medawar, P.B.: The use of antilymphocytic serum to induce transplantation tolerance in the mouse. Proc. Roy. Soc. B (In press 1969).

11. Levey, R.H. and Medawar, P.B.: Some experiments on the action of antilymphoid antisera. Ann. N.Y. Acad. Sci. 129: 164–177 (1966).

12. Levey, R.H. and Medawar, P.B.: Nature and mode of action of antilymphocytic antiserum. Proc. nat. Acad. Sci., Wash. 56: 1130–1137 (1966).

13. Levey, R.H. and Medawar, P.B.: Further experiments on the action of antilymphocytic antiserum. Proc. nat. Acad. Sci., Wash. 58: 470–477 (1967).

14. Monaco, A.P.; Wood, M.L.; Gray, J.G. and Russell, P.S.: Studies on heterologous antilymphocytic serum in mice. J. Immunol. 96: 229 (1966).

15. Monaco, A.P.; Wood, M.L. and Russell, P.S.: Studies on heterologous antilymphocyte serum in mice. III. Immunologic tolerance and chimerism produced across the H-2 locus with adult thymectomy and antilymphocytic serum. Ann. N.Y. Acad. Sci. 129: 190–210 (1966).

16. Pichylmayr, R.; Brendel, W.; Mikaeloff, B.; Wiebecke, J.P.; Rassat, J.P.; Pichylmayr, I.; Bomel, J.; Fateh-Moghadam, A.; St. Thierfelder; Messmer, K.; Descotes, J. and Knedel, M.: Survival of renal and liver homografts in dogs treated with heterologous antilymphocyte serum. In: Advances in Transplantation, pp. 147–154 (Eds.) J. Dausset, J. Hamburger and G. Mathé (Munksgaard, 1968).

17. Sell, S. and Gell, P.G.H.: Studies on rabbit lymphocytes in vitro. I. Stimulation of blast transformation with an antiallotype serum. J. exp. Med. 122: 423–440 (1965).

18. Shorter, R.G.; Spencer, R.J. and Hallenbeck, G.A.: Antilymphoid sera in clinical renal allotransplantation. J. amer. med. Ass. 202: 285–286 (1967).

19. Spiegelberg, H.L. and Weigle, W.O.: The catabolism of homologous and heterologous 7S gamma globulin fragments. J. exp. Med. 121: 323–338 (1965).

20. Starzl, T.E.; Marchioro, T.L.; Porter, K.A.; Iwasaki, Y. and Cerilli, G.J.: The use of heterologous agents in canine renal and liver homotransplantation and in human renal homotransplantation. Surg. Gynec. Obstet. 124: 301–318 (1967).

21. Starzl, T.E.; Porter, K.A.; Iwasaki, Y.; Marchioro, T.L. and Kashiwagi, N.: The use of heterologous antilymphocyte globulin in human renal transplantation. In: Antilymphocyte Serum. Ciba Foundation Study Group, No. 29, pp. 4–34 (J. and A. Churchill, London 1967).

22. Taub, R.N. and Lance, E.M.: Effects of heterologous antilymphocyte serum on the distribution of Cr-51 labelled lymph node cells in mice. Immunology (In press 1968).

23. Taub, R.N. and Ruszkiewicz, M.: Unpublished observations (1968).

24. Traeger, J.; Carraz, M.; Fries, D.; Brochier, J.; Triau, R. and Plan, R.: Preparations, properties and assay for standardization and titration of horse antihuman lymphocyte serum. Xth Int. Congr. Microbiol. Stand. Prague 1967 (Karger, Basel/New York, in press).

25. Traeger, J.; Perrin, J.; Fries, D.; Saubier, E.; Carraz, M.; Bonnet, P.; Archimbaud, J.P.; Bernhardt, J.P.; Brochier, J.; Beteul, H.; Veysseyre, C.; Bryon, P.A.; Prevot, J.; Jouvenceau, A.; Banssillon, V.; Zech, P. et Rollet, A.: Utilization chez l'homme d'une globuline antilymphocytaire: resultats clinique en transplantation rénale. Lyon méd. 5: 307–369 (1968).

26. Woodruff, M.F.A.; Reid, B.L. and James, K.: The effect of antilymphocytic antibody and antibody fragments on human lymphocytes in vitro. Nature (Lond.) 215: 591–594 (1967).

Author's address: Dr. E.M. Lance, 535 East 10th St. New York, N.Y. (USA).

Antibiotica et Chemotherapia, vol. 15, pp. 328–348 (Karger, Basel/New York 1969)

Studies on Heterologous Antilymphocyte Serum in Mice. IV. Modifications in the Effects of Antilymphocyte Serum Produced by Prior Adult Thymectomy.

A. P. MONACO, DOMINIQUE J. FRANCO and MARY L. WOOD

Department of Surgery, Harvard Medical School and the
Transplantation Division, Sears Surgical Laboratory, Boston City Hospital, Boston

Introduction

Previous studies in our laboratory [10, 18] demonstrated that rabbits immunized with mouse lymphoid cells produced an anti-serum which agglutinated and killed mouse lymphocytes *in vitro*. A small amount of rabbit anti-mouse lymphocyte serum (henceforth RAMLS) given to mice resulted in peripheral lymphopenia and tissue lymphocyte depletion for a finite period during which time there was depression of the first- and second-set allograft rejection responses as well as the xenograft rejection reaction. The primary humoral antibody response to sheep erythrocytes was moderately depressed but the secondary humoral response to this antigen was unaffected at doses of RAMLS which prolonged even second-set allografts across H-2 histocompatibility differences. After this finite period spontaneous restoration in the capacity to reject skin allografts and xenografts and to form humoral antibody occurred. Restoration of immune capacity correlated to some extent with the beginning of histological repopulation of peripheral lymphoid tissues.

Initial attempts at repeated and chronic administration of RAMLS over several months resulted in lymphoid atrophy and even areas of necrosis in lymph nodes [10]. Such attempts were made with admittedly toxic sera. Mice frequently wasted and died even with perfect H-2 allografts in place. Subsequently it was demonstrated [19] that adult-thymectomized mice (age 8–10 weeks) given small amounts of

RAMLS for seven days showed lymphopenia and lymphocyte depletion which lasted much longer in normal or shamthymectomized mice given similar amounts of RAMLS. Inhibition of the primary hemagglutinin response to sheep erythrocytes persisted much longer in the RAMLS-treated, thymectomized groups. Furthermore, repeat challenge with sheep erythrocytes in these latter animals showed depression of the secondary hemagglutinin response, an effect that was not achieved in mice given only serum. There was striking inability of treated animals to reject skin allografts, many grafts remaining in perfect condition 50–100 days longer on RAMLS-treated, thymectomized mice than on those normal mice given only serum. This prolonged period of time during which RAMLS-treated, adult-thymectomized mice were incapable or rejecting skin allografts was subsequently utilized for the establishment of a specific state of immunological tolerance and stable chimerism across the H-2 locus [20].

This paper reviews the various modifications in the effects of RAMLS when administration of this remarkable biological reagent is preceded by adult thymectomy. Attention has been paid not only to actual alterations achieved by superimposing adult thymectomy, but also to elucidation of the specific experimental circumstances under which removal of the adult thymus gland has an effect.

Much of the material described has been previously published in whole or in part [19, 20, 22, 27]. Newer areas of investigation are designated and elaborated in more detail. The data thus far permit conclusions about the mechanism of action of RAMLS and support certain concepts of the mechanism of function of the adult thymus.

Materials and Methods

Animals, skin grafts, adult thymectomy, cell suspensions, serological and *hematological observations,* and various other procedures were performed as previously described [10, 18, 19].

Preparation of antilymphocyte sera: Several types of antilymphocyte sera were prepared. Saline suspensions of A/Jax lymph node cells were emulsified in complete Freund's adjuvant (Difco) and injected into the footpads of groups of white New Zealand rabbits (100×10^6 cells/rabbit). After three weeks, rabbits received three consecutive daily intravenous booster injections of saline suspended cells (100×10^6 cells/injection) and were bled a week later. This serum prepared by primary immunization of rabbits with lymph node lymphocytes in adjuvant was the standard antilymphocyte serum used in previous [10, 18, 19] as well as the following experiments. When used alone in an experiment it is designated *RAMLS,* whereas if used with one of the other types of serum described below it is designated *RAMLS-LN-ADJ.* The lymphagglutinin titer of *RAMLS-LN-ADJ* was $^1/_{256}$. For the other sera below the titer of agglutination to lymph node lymphocytes is stated in parenthesis. An antilymphocyte serum against adult A/Jax thymocytes was raised in a similar manner using exactly the same cell doses and immunization schedules. This serum was designated *RAMLS-THY-ADJ* ($^1/_{128}$). Furthermore, antilymphocyte serum was prepared against A/Jax lymph node lymphocytes or adult A/Jax thymocytes by the schedule outlined by Levey and Medawar [13]. Rabbits received 1×10^9 lymph node lymphocytes or adult (eight week old) thymocytes intravenously followed two weeks later by a second intravenous injection of 1×10^9 lymphocytes or thymocytes. Rabbits were then bled one week later. Serum prepared by intravenous immunizations with lymphocytes was termed *RAMLS-LN-IV* ($^1/_{64}$) and that with thymocytes, *RAMLS-THY-IV* ($^1/_{32}$). Three or four rabbits were used to prepare each type of serum. After bleeding each serum type was pooled, heated to 56°C for 30 min to decomplement, and stored at –20°C after Merthiolate (E. Lilly Co.) 1:10 000, had been added.

Preparation of cell-free transplantation antigens. Cell-free transplantation antigen was prepared from C57BL/6 and C3H/He mouse spleens by the sucrose method described by Monaco *et al.* [21].

Determination of H-2 specific hemagglutinating antibody. Mice were bled from the ventral tail vein at appropriate intervals. The clots were allowed to separate at room temperature and then permitted to retract in the cold (4°C) overnight. All sera were separated, heated to 56°C for 30 min, and stored at –20°C until used. H-2 specific hemagglutinins to A/Jax erythrocytes were determined utilizing a modification of the method of Stimpling [25]. In brief, mouse erythrocytes were collected in Gibson's solution (ventral tail vein bleeding) and then washed four times in phosphate buffered saline. A 2% solution of erythrocytes in buffered saline was prepared. A 1 to 10 dilution of the appropriate test serum in polyvinylpyrrolidine (PVP), was made in the first tube, followed by doubling dilutions in PVP. 0.1 ml of the appropriate erythrocyte suspension was added and the tubes allowed to incubate at room temperature for 2 h. The tubes were then centrifuged (1000 g, 30 sec) and 0.5 ml normal saline added gently to each tube so as not to disturb the pellicle. The saline was then gently flushed over the pellicle. With strongly positive sera the pellicle could be lifted off the base of the tube intact as a thick agglutinated clump. Disruption of the clump to smaller fragments signified lesser degrees of agglutination. Separate controls were always performed using normal, non-immune mouse sera and isogeneic erythrocytes.

Results

1. Character and rate of allograft rejection in RAMLS-treated normal and adult-thymectomized mice. Previous studies demonstrated that normal adult A/Jax mice given *RAMLS-LN-ADJ* (0.25 ml × 7) rejected C57BL/6 skin grafts in 20–25 days (median survival time, M.S.T., for first-set C57BL/6 → A/Jax allografts = 9.8 ± 0.2 days) and C3H/He allografts in 26–32 days (M.S.T., C3H/He → A/Jax = 10.2 ± 0.3 days). Prolonged survival of these skin allografts was always accompanied by luxuriant hair growth. When immune competence returned and rejection began, edema, scab formation, and ulceration proceeded rapidly to complete rejection, leaving a disc of dry eschar with total necrosis in 48 h or less. So rapid is the tempo of rejection, once started, that perfect grafts with luxuriant hair coats were frequently completely rejected without alopecia, or swelling, the hair strands remaining in the rejected skin. Such grafts could at first be considered normal on cursory examination until palpation revealed the disc of dry eschar underneath. In contrast, not only is survival drastically prolonged by adult thymectomy prior to *RAMLS-LN-ADJ* administration, but the rate of rejection once begun was markedly attenuated. In the C57BL/6 → A/Jax combination, thymectomized mice frequently showed perfect grafts for 50–75 days, and with the C3H/He → A/Jax strains, perfect grafts lasted 100–150 days. Rejection began very slowly with progressive alopecia and insidious gradual contraction, frequently with no obvious edema or scab eschar formation. This indolent type of rejection was similar to that seen by MILLER *et al.* [16] in neonatally thymectomized mice which had survived wasting disease and had eventually rejected long-term, surviving skin allografts.

2. Effect of adult-thymectomy with various doses of antilymphocyte serum. Normal adult mice given lethal, whole-body irradiation are protected from lethal irradiation effects by infusions of isogeneic bone marrow cells and these mice readily recover their immune capacity in 4–10 weeks. Adult-thymectomized mice given lethal, whole-body irradiation are protected from irradiation effects by isogeneic bone marrow and readily recover immune responses when given infusions of isogeneic spleen or lymph node cells. In contrast, adult mice which are thymectomized, whole-body, lethally irradiated, and given bone marrow infusions, although protected from radiation effects, fail to recover their immune responses [3]. The recovery of immune responses after total body irradiation and bone-marrow therapy is therefore thymus dependent. It was originally felt that any potentiation of the effect of *RAMLS-LN-ADJ* by adult thymectomy was dependent upon total or near total transient ablation of the lymphoid system similar to that achieved by whole-body irradiation. Exactly the opposite has proven to be true. In our initial studies (fig. 1a) taken from Monaco *et al.* [22], groups of 14–26 normal or adult-

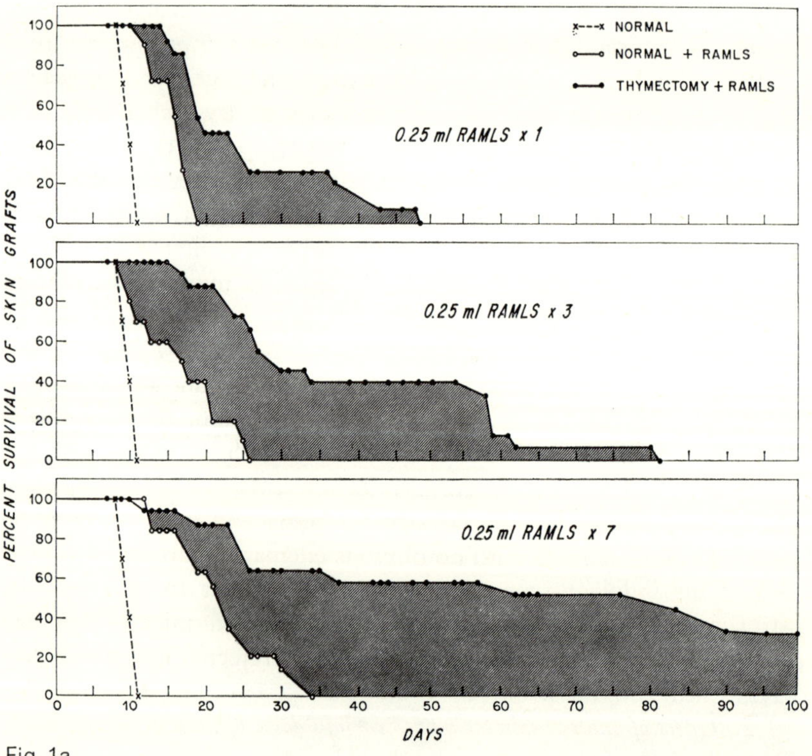

Fig. 1a

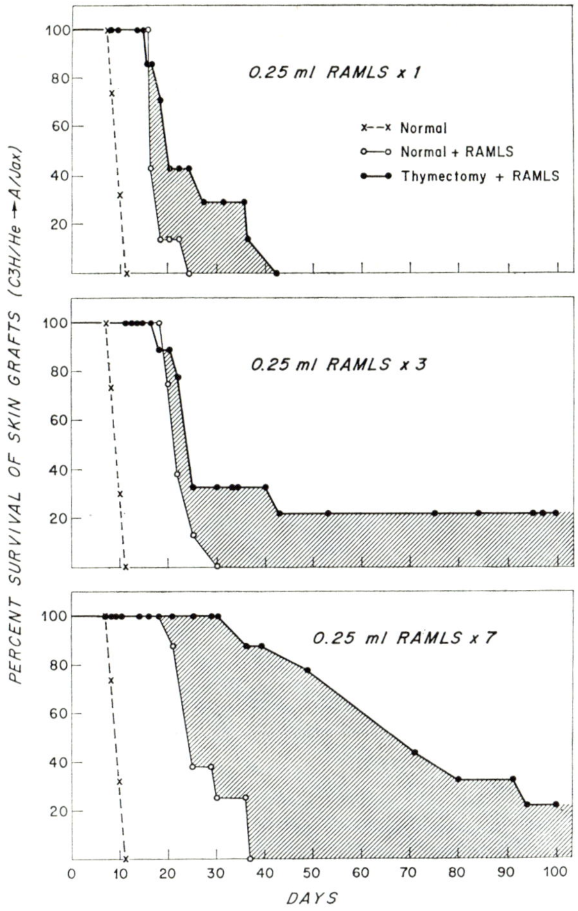

Fig. 1b

Fig. 1. Survival of skin allografts in normal and adult-thymectomized mice given various doses of RAMLS (see text). – a) C57BL/6 → A/Jax combination; b) C3H/He → A/Jax combination.

thymectomized A/Jax mice were given one, three or seven consecutive injections of 0.25 ml *RAMLS-LN-ADJ* intraperitoneally and grafted with C57BL/6 skin. Graft survival was dramatically longer in all thymectomized groups when contrasted to the normal group given the same amount of serum. This experiment was recently repeated utilizing the C3H/He → A/Jax combination (fig. 1b). It is noteworthy in both experiments that increases in antilymphocyte dosage produced only slight to moderate increases in augmented allograft survival in normal mice. Increased allograft survival was not directly proportional to increases in RAMLS dosage. This was particularly true with the C57BL/6 → A/Jax combination. In contrast, the amount of augmented survival resulting from adult thymectomy increased dramatically with increasing doses of *RAMLS-LN-ADJ*. Groups of mice given one or three injections of *RAMLS-LN-ADJ* exhibited essentially the same degree and duration of lymphopenia whether thymectomized or non-thymectomized. Thymectomized mice given seven injections of RAMLS had a longer duration of lymphopenia than their non-thymectomized counterparts, but the lymphopenic period of the thymectomized group was much shorter than the period of augmented allograft survival. Most important, however, was the fact that adult thymectomy potentiated a rather small dose of *RAMLS-LN-ADJ,* which in itself produced only slight immunosuppression as measured by the limited prolongation of allograft survival seen in normal animals.

3. *Significance of the type of antilymphocyte serum used and the timing of serum administration.* Levey and Medawar [12] failed to observe the potentiation of antilymphocyte serum by prior adult thymectomy in the mouse. In their experiments, intravenously prepared antithymocyte serum was given on day two and five after grafting of normal and adult-thymectomized mice. Failure to achieve the adult-thymectomy effect may have been secondary to the type of serum used or to the timing of its administration in relation to thymectomy or grafting or both. To investigate these possibilities different types of sera were administered to normal or adult-thymectomized mice either before or after grafting. Groups of normal or adult-thymectomized A/Jax mice were given 0.25 ml *RAMLS-LN-ADJ* or *RAMLS-LN-IV* $\times$ 6 and were then grafted with C57BL/6 skin. Figure 2a shows that the effect of *RAMLS-LN-ADJ* was markedly potentiated by adult-

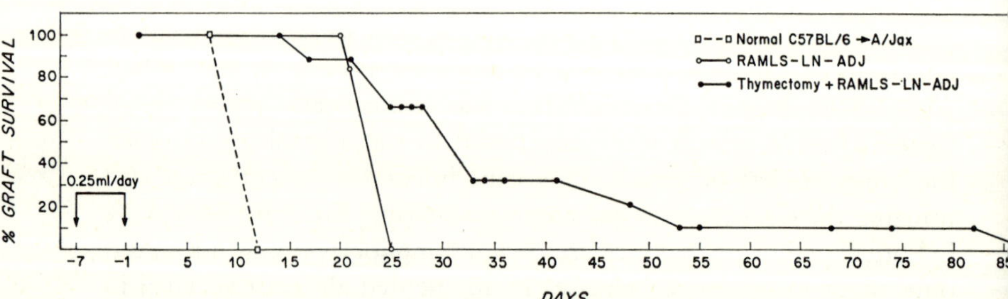

Fig. 2a

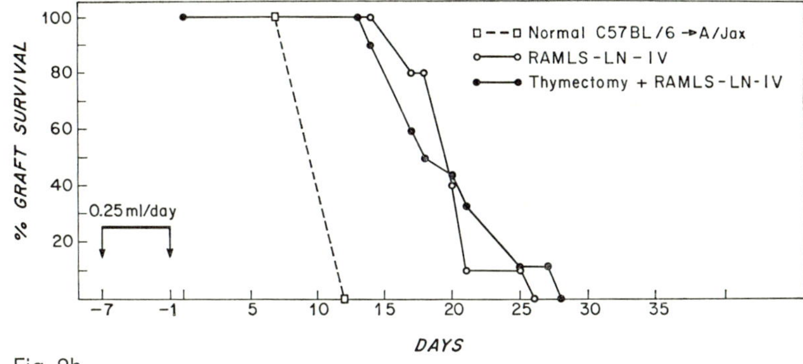

Fig. 2b

Fig. 2. a) Survival of C57BL/6 skin allografts on normal or adult-thymectomized mice given 0.25 ml × 6 RAMLS-LN-ADJ prior to grafting (15–30 mice/group); b) Survival of C57BL/6 skin allografts on similar groups of A/Jax mice given RAMLS-LN-IV.

thymectomy. In contrast, *RAMLS-LN-IV* had a little if any augmented survival secondary to adult thymectomy (fig. 2b). Furthermore, the degree of prolongation of skin allografts in normal mice was better with the adjuvant prepared serum (M.S.T. = 23.2 days) as opposed to the intravenous serum (M.S.T. = 18.0 days). In a second experiment, normal or adult-thymectomized A/Jax mice were grafted with C57BL/6 skin and given 0.5 ml *RAMLS-LN-ADJ* on days two and five. Figure 3 shows that adult-thymectomy potentiated the adjuvant prepared serum even when administered under this post-grafting schedule, although the potentiation was less dramatic than when *RAMLS-LN-ADJ* was given prior to grafting (fig. 1a). Thus,

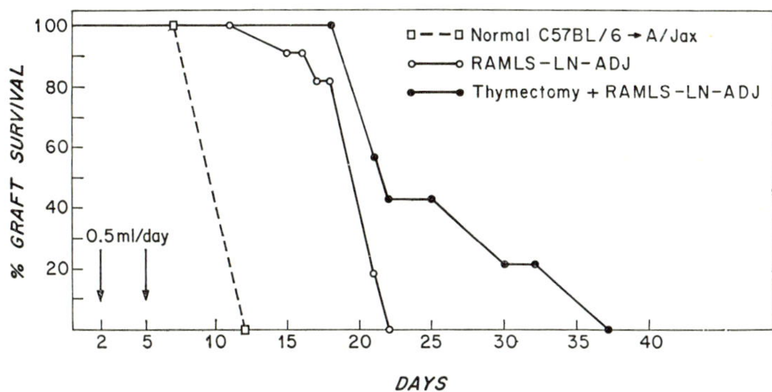

Fig. 3. Survival of C57BL/6 skin allografts on normal or adult-thymectomized mice given 0.5 ml RAMLS-LN-ADJ on day 2 and 5 post grafting.

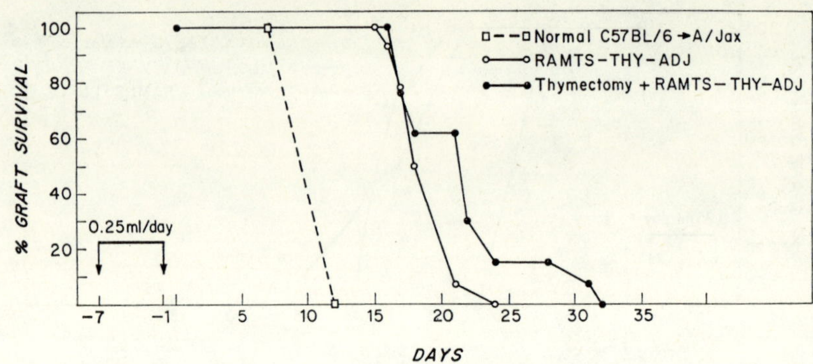

Fig. 4. Survival of C57BL/6 skin allografts on normal or adult-thymectomized A/Jax mice given 0.25 ml × 6 RAMLS-THY-ADJ prior to grafting.

adjuvant prepared antilymphocyte serum given after grafting can be potentiated by prior adult thymectomy, although the best effect is seen when the serum is given prior to grafting. *RAMLS-THY-ADJ* was given (0.25 ml × 6) to normal and adult-thymectomized A/Jax mice who were then grafted with C57BL/6 skin. Figure 4 shows that modest but significant augmented prolongation of allograft survival was achieved in the thymectomy group, although not nearly as prolonged as with *RAMLS-LN-ADJ* administration by this schedule. Finally, 0.5 ml *RAMLS-THY-IV* was given to similar groups of A/Jax mice on days two and five post grafting with C57BL/6 skin. Figure 5 shows that only modest prolongation of allograft survival was achieved with this serum in the normal group and no additional survival was produced by prior adult thymectomy. The results of

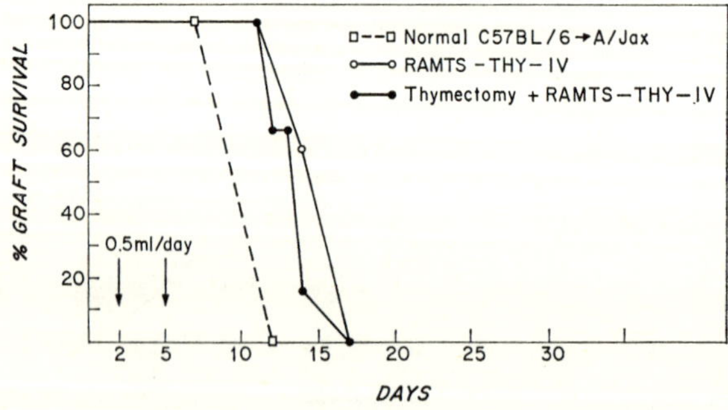

Fig. 5. Survival of C57BL/6 skin allografts on normal or adult-thymectomized A/Jax mice given 0.5 ml RAMLS-THY-IV on days 2 and 5 post grafting.

these relatively limited experiments suggest that antilymphocyte sera prepared by intravenous immunization of rabbits with adult thymocytes or lymphocytes are not potentiated by adult thymectomy, whereas adjuvant prepared sera are readily potentiated. When the adjuvant method is used, serum made with lymph node cell lymphocytes seem to be more effective than serum made to thymocytes, as judged by degree of allograft prolongation achieved in normal adult animals. The former type of serum was also more dramatically potentiated. Finally, the effect of adjuvant prepared serum was more readily augmented by adult-thymectomy when serum was administered before grafting than after grafting.

4. Degree of allograft immunity induced in normal or adult-thymectomized, RAMLS-treated mice which have rejected test allografts. The immunological consequences of eventual rejection of skin allografts which have enjoyed prolonged survival under RAMLS treatment are altered by prior adult thymectomy. This was shown by regrafting normal or adult-thymectomized mice which had rejected test skin allografts after periods of prolonged survival. In table I taken from MONACO *et al.* [22] normal or adult-thymectomized A/Jax mice were given 1, 3 or 7 0.25 ml injections of *RAMLS-LN-ADJ*, and were then grafted with C57BL/6 skin. All thymectomy groups showed more prolonged survival than their normal counterparts (i.e. see fig. 1a). At day 50, all normal and thymectomized mice which had already rejected their test grafts were regrafted with C57BL/6 skin. Table I shows that thymectomized, *RAMLS-LN-ADJ*-treated mice showed less evidence of allograft immunity induced by rejection of the first graft than mice given RAMLS alone, even though the former had more recently

Table I. Condition of second C57BL/6 grafts (day 6 postoperative) on normal and thymectomized A/Jax mice previously given various doses of RAMLS and previously grafted with first-set C57BL/6 skin

	No. of RAMLS injections (0.25 ml)	Percentage of second C57BL/6 graft surviving on day 6
Normal	1	0, 0, 0, 0, 0, 0
Thymectomized		100, 75, 100, 100, 100, 100, 75, 60, 60
Normal	3	10, 0, 0, 0, 80
Thymectomized		50, 80, 80, 100, 100, 30
Normal	7	0, 0, 10, 10, 25, 40
Thymectomized		100, 100, 100, 100, 100, 100, 100

rejected their first-set test grafts and would have been expected to evince more evidence of immunity on these grounds alone.

5. Effect of adult thymectomy in facilitating induction of specific immunologic tolerance after RAMLS-treatment. Many adult-thymectomized mice given RAMLS showed persistent inability to reject third-party skin grafts over 100 days later, at a time when the original test skin grafts were still in place [17]. Thus, the long-term immunological deficit induced by thymectomy and RAMLS is therefore, non-specific. The period of immune incompetence associated with lymphocyte depletion after RAMLS was analogous to the limited responsiveness of the developing immune system during the neonatal period. These observations prompted attempts to induce tolerance and chimerism by appropriate cell infusions after RAMLS treatment. Normal and adult-thymectomized mice were given 0.25 ml. *RAMLS-LN-ADJ* for one week and were then intravenously infused with suspensions of allogeneic lymphoid cells followed by appropriate test skin grafts. Initially, (A/Jax $\times$ C57BL/6) F_1 hybrid cells were infused and only slightly prolonged survival of test grafts beyond that seen with RAMLS and thymectomy alone was achieved. Mice given only serum were sensitized by the cell infusions. In contrast adult-thymectomized mice given RAMLS not only were not sensitized but half of mice given 150×10^6 cells and all the mice given 300×10^6 cells were lymphoid cell chimeras at day 100 in spite of the absence of skin graft tolerance [22]. When the C3H/He $\rightarrow$ A/Jax combination was

Table II. Effect of infusion of (A/Jax $\times$ C3H/He) F_1 habrid lymphoid cells on graft survival in groups of normal, RAMLS-treated, and RAMLS-treated, adult-thymectomized A/Jax mice

	Group	No. of Mice	Days of graft survival						
			7	8–13	14–26	27–40	41–80	81–>100	100
No cells	Normal	24		24					
	RAMLS	24			24				
	RAMLS + thymectomy	18						18	
Cell treatment:	Normal	20	20						
300×10^6	RAMLS	36	21	7	4	4			
	RAMLS + thymectomy	26[1]						4	22

[1] 26/26 animals tested were chimeras at day 100.

used successful tolerance was achieved [20, 22]. Serum-treated, thymectomized mice given 300×10^6 (A/Jax $\times$ C3H/He) F_1 hybrid cells showed prolonged survival of 26/26 grafts (table II, taken from MONACO *et al.* [22]). Four of 26 grafts were rejected at between 80–100 days, but 22/26 survived longer than 100 days. Of 22 grafts, 10 showed evidence of chronic rejection and 12 were in perfect condition. None of the normal or serum-treated mice given cells were chimeras at day 100, whereas all cell-infused, serum-treated, thymectomized mice were chimeras, even those which rejected grafts from day 80 to 100. Chimeric mice which rejected first grafts by day 100 rejected second C3H/He grafts in normal, first-set fashion. Mice showing chronic rejection at day 100 rejected second grafts of the same genotype in prolonged fashion, whereas animals with perfect grafts at day 100 accepted second C3H/He grafts without any evidence of rejection for another 100 days. These latter chimeric mice rejected third-party C57BL/6 grafts in normal fashion, however, while retaining perfect C3H/He grafts. Finally, re-equipment of chimeras with normal A/Jax lymph node cells abolished the chimeric state and resulted in rejection of long-standing first and second C3H/He grafts. Thus, RAMLS in combination with adult thymectomy was used to induce classical tolerance in respect to allograft immunity as elaborated by BILLINGHAM, BRENT and MEDAWAR [2].

Recently, we have attempted to induce chimerism in adult-thymectomized, *RAMLS-LN-ADJ*-treated A/Jax mice with infusion of homozygous allogeneic C3H/He or C57BL/6 cells. As expected, severe graft-versus-host reactions occurred after infusions of 50×10^6 cells or greater. Infusions of 25×10^6 cells produced no graft-versus-host reactions but no tolerance as well [17]. Subsequently, ABBOTT *et al.* [1] in our laboratory have attempted to induce tolerance in this system utilizing cell-free transplantation antigen. Normal, serum-treated (0.25 ml *RAMLS-LN-ADJ* $\times$ 6), and adult-thymectomized, serum-treated A/Jax mice were given a single spleen equivalent of C57BL/6 splenic antigen intravenously prior to grafting and one intravenous plus two intraperitoneal doses of one spleen equivalent per injection each week after grafting until rejection was completed. Figure 6 shows that cell-free antigen alone neither sensitized nor prolonged skin graft survival in normal A/Jax mice; a finding previously noted when this amount of antigen is given [21]. Cell-free antigen in combination with *RAMLS-LN-ADJ* produced the same survival as *RAMLS-LN-ADJ* alone, which was not as long as serum plus thymectomy

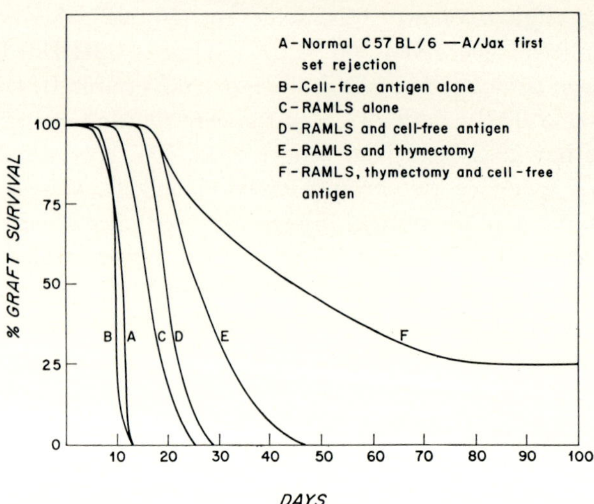

Fig. 6. Survival of C57BL/6 skin allografts in various groups of normal, serum-treated, and adult-thymectomized, serum-treated A/Jax mice given cell-free transplantation antigen (see text). Groups A-E (30–55 mice/group), Group F (16 mice).

without antigen. However, serum after adult thymectomy in combination with cell-free antigen, achieved markedly prolonged survival in 4/16 animals. This effect was not achieved with 3rd party allogeneic (C3H/He) antigen or isogeneic (A/Jax) antigen. These mice had normal lymphocyte counts at 100 days, and rejected 3rd party (C3H/He) grafts in somewhat prolonged fashion [11–15] but did not reject second C57BL/6 skin grafts for upwards of 40 days. These limited experiments suggest that adult thymectomy and RAMLS may permit induction of tolerance with non-replicating histocompatibility antigens. More experiments along these lines are indicated.

6. Growth of human normal and neoplastic xenografts. The pronounced cellular immune deficit induced by adult-thymectomy and *RAMLS-LN-ADJ* treatment has permitted relatively long-term growth of human normal and neoplastic cells in mice treated in this manner. RAMLS and thymectomy has permitted growth of human skin, ovary, and adrenal in A/Jax mice for periods of 30–50 days (fig. 7). Likewise, human carcinomas, lymphomas, and sarcomas have been grown for similar periods of time (fig. 8). Interestingly, no metastatic lesions have been noted from growth of malignant human xenografts in these mice. Use of RAMLS alone produced some growth of human xenografts, but not as effectively as when combined with thymectomy.

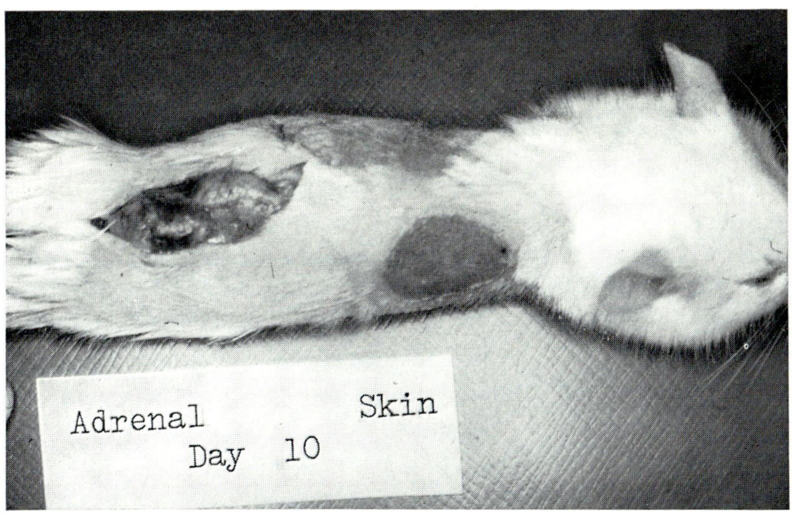

Fig. 7. An adult-thymectomized A/Jax mouse which received 0.25 ml × 6 RAMLS bearing a human adrenal xenograft and human skin xenograft on day 10. These grafts persisted for over 40 days.

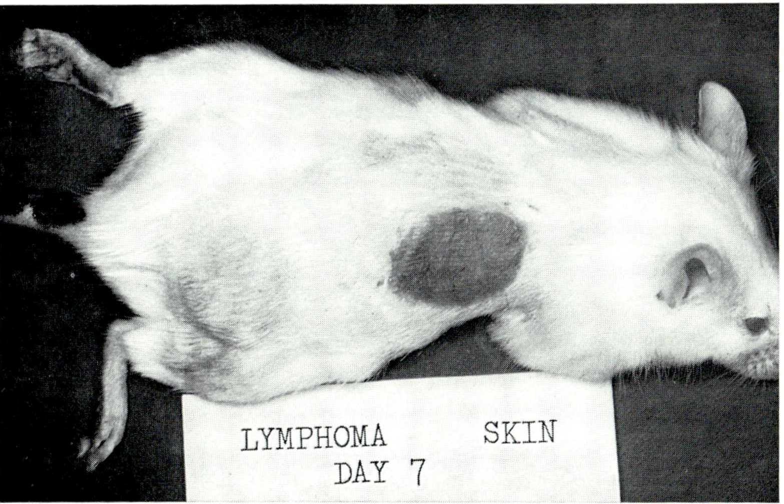

Fig. 8. An adult-thymectomized A/Jax mouse which received 0.25 ml × 6 RAMLS bearing a human lymphoma xenograft and human skin xenograft on day 7. These grafts persisted for over 40 days.

7. Effect of adult thymectomy and RAMLS on the H-2 specific antibody response to skin allografts. RAMLS-treated, adult-thymectomized mice may bear allogeneic skin grafts across H-2 histocompatibility differences for 100–200 days. These mice are frequently very healthy suggesting that their humoral antibody formation mechanism is intact. Furthermore, it is known that the amount of serum which prolongs second-set skin allografts frequently fails to decrease a secondary humoral antibody response to another antigen such as sheep erythrocytes [18]. This has lead to the conclusion that RAMLS has a preferential effect for depressing cellular immunity rather than humoral antibody formation [11]. To investigate this possibility we have studied the effect of RAMLS with and without thymectomy on the H-2 specific response to skin allografts. Thus, cellular and humoral immunities to the same antigen could be compared. Figure 9a shows that C57BL/6 mice reject A/Jax skin grafts in 9–11 days. H-2 specific anti-A/Jax hemagglutinins are detectable by day 15, increase to peak titers ($^1/_{320}$–$^1/_{640}$) by days 20 to 30 and remain elevated for several weeks; when *RAMLS-LN-ADJ* is given (0.25 ml × 6) before (fig. 9b) or after (fig. 9c) grafting there is prolongation of A/Jax skin allograft survival. It can be seen that there is a delay in the appearance of H-2 antibody consistent with the short term prolongation of A/Jax allograft survival. Studies were then performed to determine if long term surviving skin allografts after RAMLS treatment evoke an H-2 antibody response prior to or after rejection. C57BL/6 mice were thymectomized as adults, given 0.25 ml *RAMLS-LN-ADJ* × 6, and grafted with A/Jax skin. Groups of 10 mice

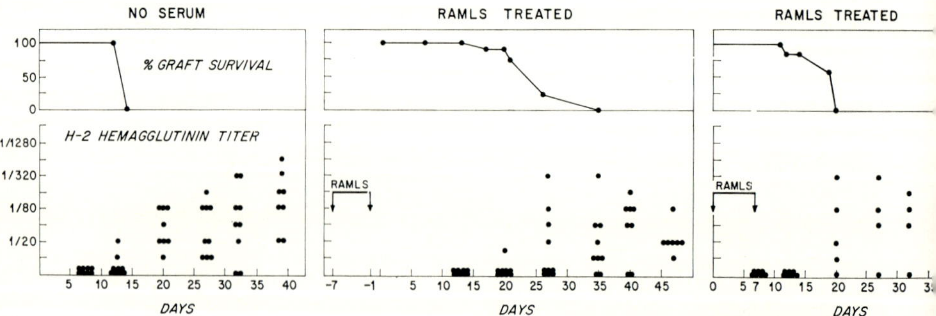

Fig. 9. Survival of A/Jax skin allografts and appearance of H-2 specific anti-A/Jax hemagglutinin antibody in groups of normal (a) C57BL/6 mice and in C57BL/6 mice given 0.25 ml RAMLS i.p. × 6 (b) before or (c) after skin allografting. Fifteen to 30 mice/group.

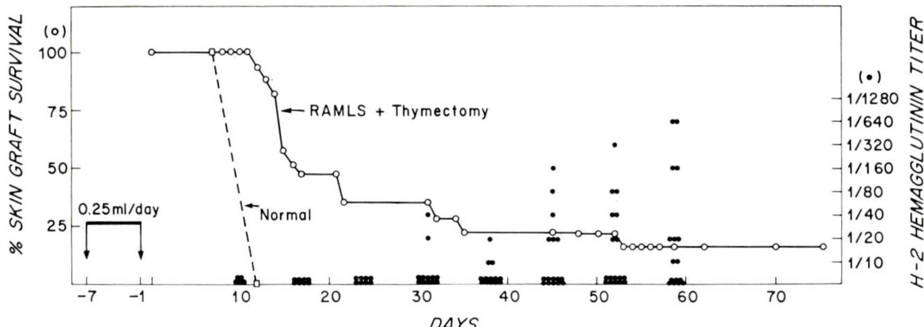

Fig. 10. Survival of A/Jax skin allografts and appearance of H-2 hemagglutinin antibody in adult-thymectomized C57BL/6 mice given 0.25 ml RAMLS i.p. prior to grafting. (Normal = normal first-set A/Jax → C57BL/6 skin graft rejection response).

were bled on alternate weeks and the anti-A/Jax erythrocyte titers correlated with the status of the graft. Figure 10 shows the survival curve of the test skin allografts and the antibody titers of the weekly bleedings of the individual mice. In general, titers were not detectable in mice until two to three weeks after they had rejected grafts. This is much better expressed in figure 11 where the period during which graft rejection occurred is plotted against the time period for detection of antibody. Antibody never appeared before rejection; the longer the graft remained unrejected the longer was the interval post rejection before antibody appeared. Mice which had not rejected grafts

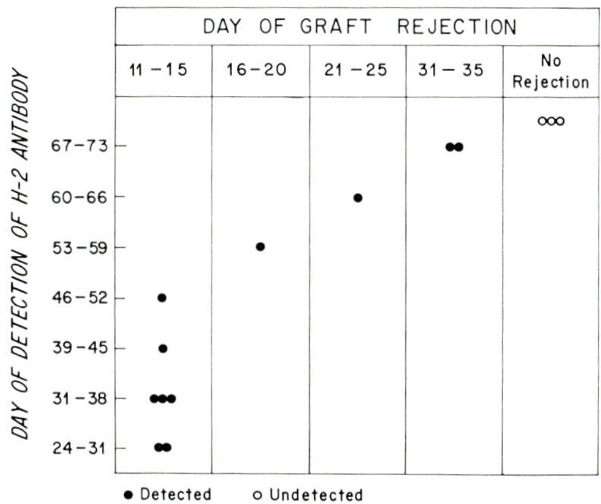

Fig. 11. Correlation of the time period during which H-2 specific hemagglutinin antibodies were detected with the day of A/Jax allograft rejection by adult-thymectomized C57BL/6 mice given 0.25 ml RAMLS i.p. × 6 prior to grafting (see text).

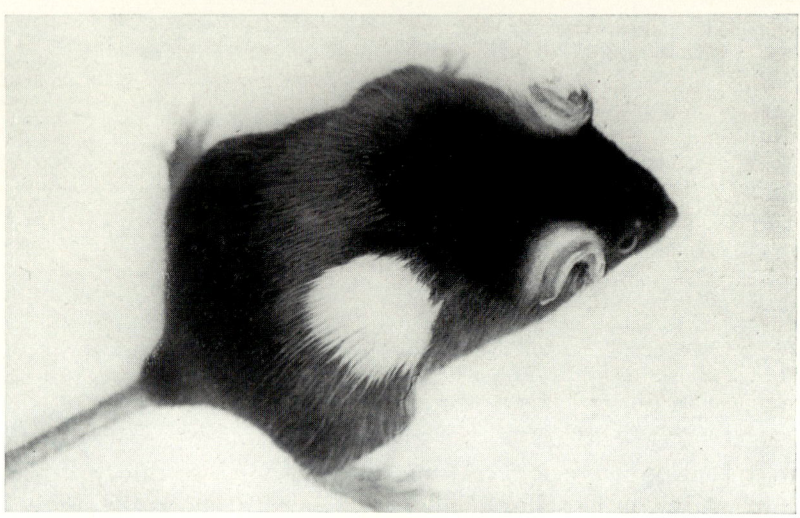

Fig. 12. An adult-thymectomized C57BL/6 mouse who had received 0.25 ml RAMLS i.p. × 6 prior to receiving an A/Jax skin allograft. The graft is in perfect conditions 75 days later. Repeated bleedings failed to reveal any H-2 specific antibody production in this mouse up to this time.

by day 75 (fig. 12) still showed no detectable antibody levels. These experiments show that both modalities of the immune response, i.e. cellular and humoral, directed against H-2 antigens are inhibited by RAMLS. The possibility that long-term unrejected allografts surviving after RAMLS might do so with the production of detectable titers of H-2 specific antibody was not substantiated.

Discussion

A number of theories of antilymphocyte serum action have been proposed. Generalized cytotoxicity to lymphoid cells was suggested by Gray *et al.* [10] because of obvious evidence of cell death in lymphoid organs after RAMLS treatment. Lack of correlation of immunosuppressive effect with degree and duration of lymphopenia prompted the idea of blocking the recognition of antigen, so-called lymphocyte "blindfolding". The fact that lymphoid cells exposed to antilymphocyte serum showed persistent immunological incapacity after presumed cell-replication was against this latter idea. The observation of Gräsbeck *et al.* [9] that antilymphocyte serum stimulated blast cell transformation of lymphocytes *in vitro* and the finding of lymphoid organ hyperplasia after initial antilymphocyte serum treatment suggested that the serum acted by "sterile activation" of lymphocytes to induce some type of transformation into blast cells without specific immunological obligation [12]. Currently there is good evidence that antilymphocyte serum does not cause blast cell transformation *in vivo* [6].

MARTIN and MILLER [14] recently showed that thoracic duct lymphocytes exposed to antilymphocyte serum *in vitro* failed to return on intravenous reinfusion to the lymphoid organs, but were eliminated from the circulation. Yet, mice given serum *in vivo* showed no diminution in output of thoracic duct lymphocytes. They suggested that antilymphocyte serum might eliminate a class of circulating lymphocytes but this effect was masked by over production of some other lymphoid cells which spilled out into the circulation. Thoracic duct small lymphocytes have a long life span, are immunologically competent, and may be thymus derived [15]. These authors suggested that lymphocytes produced or stimulated in lymph nodes after antilymphocyte serum may be a different cell class, not thymus-dependent, and lacking immunological competence. They further reasoned that failure of cells remaining in antilymphocyte serum treated animals to perform graft-versus-host reactions did not absolutely mean inactivation of immunologically competent cells had taken place but rather that a shift in cell population occurred. They felt that the prime effect of antilymphocyte serum was the elimination of thymus dependent cells.

Support for this idea has been found in histological studies. PARROTT *et al.* [24] showed that the mid-and deep areas of the cortex of the lymph node the so-called paracortical area—are severely depleted in neonatally thymectomized mice. Furthermore, this is the area in which immunoblasts appear in response to a regionally applied skin grafts on contact sensitizing chemicals [26]. TURK and WILLOUGHBY [27] recently showed that antithymocyte serum produced marked depletion of small lymphocytes in the paracortical areas of the node, where these cells were replaced by fibroblasts. No depletion of lymphocytes from the lymph follicles occurred and plasma cells were seen normally in the medulla. They concluded that the action of antilymphocyte serum was directed at the thymus-dependent areas of the lymph nodes.

Further evidence that immunosuppression secondary to antilymphocyte serum is derived from a shift in cell populations was offered by DENMAN *et al.* [5] who found that the blood and lymphoid organs of antiserum treated mice were depleted of long-lived small lymphocytes, following which these areas became populated with short-lived small lymphocytes. This change in composition of the circulating small lymphocyte population which was observed in intact animals and mice thymectomized as adults, was not reflected in peripheral lymphocyte counts. They suggested that excessive production of short-lived lymphocytes at the expense of the long-lived variety after antilymphocyte serum would explain the prolonged immunosuppressive effects achieved by this agent.

The remarkable capacity of adult thymectomy to potentiate antilymphocyte serum is quite consistent with these two recent observations. A strong case can be made to support the concept that the recirculating pool of lymphocytes is thymus derived. Recent evidence by DAVIES *et al.* [4] clearly demonstrates the fact that peripheral lymphocytes may be of thymus origin.

Although we have shown above that both cellular and humoral immune responses to skin allografts are depressed by antilymphocyte serum, there is substantial evidence that antilymphocyte serum is particularly effective against cellular immunities. Thus, the effect of 600r whole-body irradiation in prolonging A strain to CBA strain mouse skin allografts can be easily matched by 0.25 ml of potent antilymphocyte serum, yet this amount of irradiation produces prolonged and severe damage to humoral antibody production (see LEVEY and MEDAWAR [11] for references). The fact that adult-thymectomy has been shown above to potentiate a very small dose of RAMLS suggests that the unusual effectiveness of antilymphocyte serum in inhibiting the allograft reaction may be due to its unique specificity for the thymus-dependent, small lymphocyte. The ability of adult thymectomy to potentiate antilymphocyte serum-induced depression of the antibody response to sheep erythrocytes and to inhibit the degree of allograft immunity engendered by rejection of grafts after serum treatment, is consistent with the demonstrated participation of small lymphocytes in antibody formation and in maintenance of immunologic memory [7, 8].

Failure of certain antilymphocyte sera to be potentiated by adult-thymectomy is difficult to explain. The data presented indicate that adjuvant sera prepared against lymphocytes or thymocytes are potentiated by adult thymectomy but intravenously prepared sera of either type are clearly not. There is evidence that thymic control of thymus-dependent cells may be exerted through a humoral factor [23]. Adjuvant prepared sera may contain antibody against this presumed thymic factor or hormone which might not be present in intravenously prepared sera in view of the frequent need for adjuvant to stimulate antibody to trace amounts of antigen. Use of adjuvant sera may destroy or inactivate peripherally fixed thymic hormone which, in the face of thymectomy, would leave no source of thymic humoral factor for contribution to restoration of immune competence. Thymectomy in the presence of intravenous serum would not inhibit the restorative process, since peripherally fixed thymic factor would be operative. This possibility is clearly dependent on the fact that the presumed thymic factor does act on peripheral lymphoid tissues, an assumption which seems reasonable from the studies in which thymic function is restored by thymic tissue in Millipore chambers [23].

Summary

Thymectomy of adult mice prior to the administration of antilymphocyte sera prepared by methods of immunization utilizing adjuvant, markedly potentiates the immunosuppressive properties of these sera.

References

1. ABBOTT, W.M.; MONACO, A.P. and RUSSELL, P.S.: Antilymphocyte serum and cell-free antigen loading. Transplantation (accepted for publication).
2. BILLINGHAM, R.E.; BRENT, L. and MEDAWAR P.B.: Quantitative studies in tissue transplantation immunity. III. Actively acquired tolerance. Phil. Trans. B *239:* 357–414 (1956).
3. CROSS, A.M.; LEUCHARS, E. and MILLER, J.F.A.P.: Studies in the recovery of the immune response in irradiated mice thymectomized in adult life. J. exp. Med. *119:* 837 (1964).
4. DAVIES, A.J.S.; FESTERNSTEIN, H.; LEUCHARS, E.; WALLES, V.J. and DOENHOFF, M.J.A.: Thymic origin for some peripheral blood lymphocytes. Lancet *i:* 183–184 (1968).
5. DENMAN, A.M.; DENMAN, E.J. and EMBLING, P.H.: Changes in the life-span of circulating small lymphocytes in mice after treatment with antilymphocyte globulin. Lancet *i:* 321–325 (1968).
6. DENMAN, A.M. and FRENKEL, E.P.: Immunology *14:* 107–115 (1968).
7. GOWANS, J.L.: Immunobiology of the small lymphocyte. Hospital Practice *3:* 34–46 (1968).
8. GOWANS, J.L.: The role of lymphocytes in the destruction of homografts. Brit. med. Bull. *21:* 106–110 (1965).
9. GRÄSBECK, R.; NORDMAN, C.T. and CHAPELLE, A. DE LA: Mitogenic action of anti-leucocyte immune serum on peripheral leucocytes *in vitro*. Lancet *ii:* 385–387 (1963).

10. Gray, J.G.; Monaco, A.P.; Wood, Mary L. and Russell, P.S.: Studies on heterologous antilymphocyte serum in mice I. *In vitro* and *in vivo* properties. J. Immunol. *96:* 217–228 (1966).

11. Levey, R.H. and Medawar, P.B.: The mode of action of antilymphocyte serum. Ciba Foundation Symposium Study Group No. 29. Antilymphocyte Serum, pp. 72–80 (J. and A. Churchill Ltd., London 1967).

12. Levey, R.H. and Medawar, P.B.: Nature and mode of action of antilymphocyte antiserum. Proc. nat. Acad. Sci. *56:* 1130–1137 (1966).

13. Levey, R.H. and Medawar, P.B.: Some experiments on the action of antilymphoid antisera. Ann. N.Y. Acad. Sci. *129:* 164–177 (1966).

14. Martin, W.J. and Miller, J.F.A.P.: Site of action of antilymphocyte globulin. Lancet *ii:* 1285–1287 (1967).

15. Miller, J.F.A.P.:   Lancet *i:* 1299 (1967).

16. Miller, J.F.A.P.; Marshall, A.H.E. and White, R.G.: Role of the thymus in immunity. Adv. Immunol. *2:* 111–162 (1962).

17. Monaco, A.P.: (Unpublished observations.)

18. Monaco, A.P.; Wood, Mary L.; Gray, J.G. and Russell, P.S.: Studies on heterologous antilymphocyte serum in mice. II. Effect on the immune response. J. Immunol. *96:* 229–238 (1966).

19. Monaco, A.P.; Wood, Mary L. and Russell, P.S.: Adult thymectomy: Effect on recovery from immunologic depression in mice. Science *149:* 432–435 (1965).

20. Monaco, A.P.; Wood, Mary L. and Russell, P.S.: Studies on heterologous antilymphocyte serum in mice. III. Immunologic tolerance and chimerism produced across the H-2 locus with adult-thymectomy and antilymphocyte serum. Ann. N.Y. Acad. Sci. *129:* 190–209 (1966).

21. Monaco, A.P.; Wood, Mary L. and Russell, P.S.: Preparation of murine transplantation antigens: Ultracentrifugal analysis, physical properties, and biological activity. Transplantation *3:* 542–556 (1965).

22. Monaco, A.P.; Wood, Mary L.; Werf, B.A. van der and Russell, P.S.: Effects of antilymphocyte serum in mice, dogs, and man. Ciba Foundation Study Group, No. 29. Antilymphocyte serum p.p. 111–134 (J. and A. Churchill Ltd., London 1967).

23. Osoba, D. and Miller, J.F.A.P.: Evidence for a humoral thymus factor responsible for the maturation of immunological faculty J. exp. Med. *119:* 177–192 (1964).

24. Parrott, D.M.V.; Sousa, M.A.B. de and East, J.: Thymus-dependent areas in the lymphoid organs of neonatally thymectomized mice. J. exp. Med. *123:* 191–203 (1966).

25. Stimpfling, J.H.: The use of PVP as a developing agent in mouse hemagglutination tests. Transpl. Bull. *27:* 109–111 (1961).

26. Turk, J.L.: Action of lymphocytes in transplantation. Symp. Tiss. Org. Transpl., pp. 423–429, suppl. J. clin. Path. *20:* 430 (1967).

27. Turk, J.L. and Willoughby, D.A.: Central and peripheral effects of antilymphocyte sera. Lancet *i:* 249–251 (1967).

28. Werf, B.A. van der; Monaco, A.P.; Wood, Mary L. and Russell, P.S.: Immune competence of mouse lymph node cells after *in vivo* and *in vitro* contact with rabbit anti-mouse lymphocyte serum (RAMLS) in Advance in Transplantation, Proc. 1st Int. Congr. Transplant. Soc., pp. 133–140 (Munksgaard, Copenhagen, Denmark 1968).

Authors' address: Dr. A.P. Monaco, Dr. Dominique J. Franco and Dr. Mary L. Wood, Department of Surgery, Harvard Medical School and Transplantation Division, Sears Surgical Laboratory, Boston City Hospital, *Boston, Mass.* (USA).

Antibiotica et Chemotherapia, vol. 15, pp. 349–383 (Karger, Basel/New York 1969)

Perspectives in Organ Transplantation

T. E. STARZL, C. G. GROTH, L. BRETTSCHNEIDER, G. V. SMITH,
I. PENN and N. KASHIWAGI[1]

Department of Surgery, University of Colorado School of Medicine
and Veterans Administration Hospital, Denver, Col.

Human kidney homotransplantation was first attempted on a large
scale in 1962 and 1963. Even its most enthusiastic proponents could
not then predict that this procedure would within five years become
the preferred and the most effective way of treating patients with
renal failure. Almost all previous trials had ended in the early death
of the recipient [12] with the few notable exceptions recorded by
MERRILL [48], HAMBURGER [17, 19], KUSS [40], and SHACKMAN [67].
There are today only two patients still alive who were treated before
1962, one from Boston and the other from Paris; both received
kidneys from fraternal twins. Immunosuppression was with total body
radiation, a technique of host conditioning which has been replaced
in most centers by drug therapy. In contrast, successes in the suc-
ceeding years have been reported by many authors [6, 18, 27, 35, 36,
45, 55, 69, 101].

In this report, several issues will be reviewed on the basis of our
earlier experience with human renal transplantation. The questions
to be examined in distant retrospect concern the homograft rejection
seen after clinical renal transplantation and the measures necessary to
control and reverse this process; the life expectancy of patients
brought through early rejection episodes; the effect of prospective
histocompatibility matching upon survival; and the early and delayed
influence of thymectomy upon kidney transplant function. More
recent developments will also be mentioned including the use of
heterologous antilymphocyte globulin (ALG) in man, the role of the

[1] Supported by United States Public Health Service grants AM-06344, HE-07735,
AM-07772, AI-04152, FR-00051, FR-00069, AM-12148, and FO5-TW-1154.

Shwartzman reaction in "hyperacute rejection", the development of neoplasms after transplantation, attempts to alter graft antigenicity with ribonucleic acid (RNA) infusion, and the extension of transplantation techniques to human liver replacement.

Renal Homotransplantation

The Reversal of Rejection and Subsequent Adaptation or Tolerance

One of the most important contributions of clinicians was the demonstration that rejection is a highly reversible process. This concept had not emerged from the skin graft experiments upon which the foundations of transplantation biology were largely based, nor was it evident in the first trials of either canine or human renal homotransplantation.

It is probable in retrospect that the Boston and Paris fraternal twins mentioned earlier both passed through rejection crises. The events in HAMBURGER's case [17] were the most clear. For almost three weeks after operation, the transplanted kidney functioned perfectly. Fever, azotemia, and proteinuria then developed, but within a ten day period these findings receded without the institution of any specific therapy. HAMBURGER ascribed the changes to a spontaneously reversible immunologic crisis.

Evaluation of the course in MERRILL's case [48] was made difficult by complicating circumstances. Immediate good renal function was also obtained. Within a few weeks, fever and a rise in BUN were seen, but at the same time the patient's own kidneys had cortical and perinephric abscesses. After nephrectomies and drainage, the deterioration was reversed and MERRILL concluded that "the oliguria and nitrogen retention... were clearly associated with an episode of infection". Eight months later, a homograft biopsy revealed mononuclear cell invasion and other morphologic evidence of chronic rejection. Although function was stable and essentially normal, additional total body irradiation was given as well as a course of adrenal corticosteroids. Their opinion at the time these observations were reported was that a rejection had been thereby "aborted"; it is now well known as will be discussed later that kidney grafts, found with late biopsy to have such histologic changes, may function for years without intensification of therapy and without clinically evident rejection [61, 78]. In commenting on the significance and the earlier timing of events in HAMBURGER's case, MERRILL said [48] "it seems highly unlikely… that in a partially tolerant patient, rejection would begin at the time at which it might be expected for the non-tolerant person, only to abort spontaneously".

The first suggestion that rejection was a highly controllable and reversible phenomenon came from our institution [82]. That report began as follows:

"Because of the high failure rate after renal homotransplantation, there has been an air of pessimism concerning the possibility of long term function of the grafted kidney. The immunologic processes subserving rejection are generally thought to be so powerful and persevering that consistent success cannot be expected with the use of any of the currently available methods of antirejection therapy.

Recent personal experience in caring for patients with renal homografts has resulted in alterations in many of our preconceived notions concerning the management of such patients. It has led to the beliefs that the rejection process can almost never be entirely prevented, but that its effects can be reversed with a high degree of regularity and completeness. Furthermore, the subsequent behavior of patients who have been brought through a successfully treated rejection crisis suggests the early development of some degree of host-graft adaptation, since the phenomenon of vigorous secondary rejection has been encountered only once."

In that series there were ten patients treated in late 1962 and early 1963. In seven, clear cut rejection of variable intensity occurred from 4 to 34 days after operation (fig. 1), in one case actually leading to anuria. In each instance, the process was reversed by the addition of massive doses of prednisone to the pre-existing therapy with azathioprine (fig. 1). Three of these 7 patients are still alive five or more years later and are now amongst the longest living recipients of non-twin homografts in the world. After the remarkable effectiveness of steroid therapy in this situation had been established from our own experience, but before our findings were published, it was learned that the same kind of observation had been made by GOODWIN and his associates [11] in a young woman who ultimately died of sepsis 144 days after receipt of a maternal homograft. It was realized almost from the beginning that a reduction in homograft blood flow was an integral component of rejection crises and that the pharmacologically induced reversal was accompanied by relief of the organ ischemia [69, 77]; both conclusions have been corroborated in animal experiments [38, 39, 64, 65].

The reversibility of rejection in these patients was only one of the features which established the clinical feasibility of organ transplantation. The quantities of adrenal corticosteroids necessary to achieve reversal were often extremely large, too great for reasons of toxicity to be compatible with long survival of the recipient if continued indefinitely. Fortunately, another event of equal practical importance transpired coincidentally with the reversal of rejection or shortly afterwards. With the passage of time, the need for intensive therapy usually diminished both in patients who did and those who did not pass through a clinically evident rejection. Thus, the patient whose course is depicted in figure 1 had returned within five months after transplantation to treatment only with azathioprine, a drug which at the outset did not prevent the onset of a moderately severe rejection. An ultimate similar reduction in drug requirement is today seen in almost all new cases and it is probable that some patients could

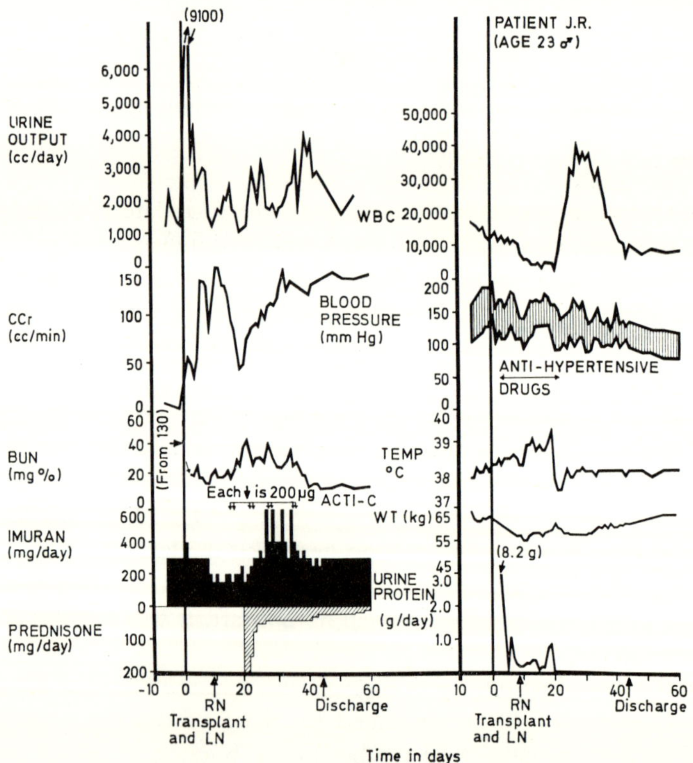

Fig. 1. Classical rejection crisis in patient (LD 6) treated with drugs alone. Deterioration of renal function began 19 days after transplantation. All stigmata of rejection were present except for acute hypertension and weight gain, which were successfully prevented by medical treatment. Acti-C---Actinomycin C; LN---Left nephrectomy at time of transplantation; RN---Right nephrectomy. Imuran is synonymous with azathioprine. (By permission of Surg. Gynec. Obstet. *117:* 385, 1963.)

eventually have all therapy stopped. In our laboratory, we have dogs
living for four to five years which were given treatment with immuno-
suppressants only for the first four months after receipt of life sustaining liver or renal homografts from non-related mongrel donors.

The foregoing phenomenon is so poorly understood that it is
still reasonable to refer to it by the originally used term [82] of
"a change in the graft-host relationship". Earlier animal experiments
of WOODRUFF and WOODRUFF suggested that a metamorphosis occurs
in transplants after long residence in a host [103], but, as MCGAVIC
and MURRAY of Boston showed [47, 54] by some other mechanism
than an alteration in intrinsic graft antigenicity. Both MERRILL [48]
and MCGAVIC [47] concluded that there was a host change (partial
tolerance) but on the basis of observations [47, 48, 54] that actually
tended to support WOODRUFF's point of view.

Whatever the explanation, there is no longer reason to doubt that
a homograft becomes more or less privileged if it can be kept alive
through the initial onslaught of rejection. This fact is detectable in
the shape of life survival curves after renal homotransplantation in
that the preponderant mortality is in the first few postoperative weeks
or months when stringent immunosuppression is required. It has
strongly influenced the way in which new therapeutic agents such as
heterologous antilymphocyte globulin (ALG) have been used clinically, and it has been a prime stimulus for the extension of transplantation
techniques to organs other than the kidney.

Chronically Tolerated Renal Homografts

Up-to-date reports about patients provided with renal homografts
several years ago are still of vital current interest since this is the only
data with which to obtain an idea of the long term prognosis of more
recently treated recipients. Consequently, the cases compiled in Denver
between the autumn of 1962 and March 1964 are particularly useful
since it is the first series in which a large number of patients were
successfully brought through the first few postoperative months.
There were 64 recipients who received their kidneys from healthy
volunteers; 30 (47%) of that original group are still alive.

The most encouraging results were where intrafamilial transplantation was the original procedure. There were 46 recipients of consanguineous kidneys. Of these, 15 died within the first year, but only
1, 1, and 1 were lost during the second, third, and fourth postoperative

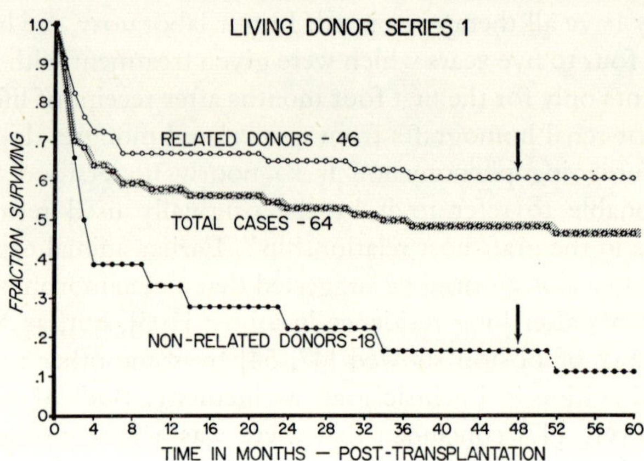

Fig. 2. Life survival curves of 64 patients treated in Denver with renal homotransplantation between November 1962 and March 1964. Preoperative histocompatibility testing was not done. The vertical arrows indicate the time of minimum followup.

years (fig. 2). The present survival after 4 to $5^1/_3$ years is 28 of 46 (60.9 %). None of the 28 patients have received late retransplantation and none have been returned to dialysis programs. The function of these chronically tolerated homografts has been shown by OGDEN [57] to be generally almost as good as the contralateral kidneys left in their donors.

With recipients of non-related homografts, the picture was by no means as good. There was a heavier early mortality inasmuch as 12 of the 18 patients entered into the series had died by the end of the first year (fig. 2). Furthermore, a steady attrition continued thereafter. Two more patients died in the second postoperative year, as well as another two who reached 33 and 51 months respectively. There are now only two of the original 18 recipients alive, one by virtue of a second homotransplantation 2 ½ years after the first. The other patient has had continuous excellent function from his non-related homograft for more than four years.

The foregoing observations in a large series of transplantations have made it clear that survival for several years can often be obtained, particularly if related donors can be found. However, it can hardly be expected that most of these homografts will function for a normal lifetime since the presence in them of more or less serious structural abnormalities is the rule rather than the exception. This conclusion was reached by Dr. K. A. PORTER of St. Mary's Hospital and Medical

School, London, on the basis of examination of 2-year renal biopsies obtained from all Denver patients who survived this long [60, 61].

An occasional homograft was completely normal. However, in the others there were pathologic changes which were not always reflected in impairment of renal function. There were vascular lesions; fibrous thickening of the intima of interlobular arteries often with rupture or duplication of the internal elastic lamina, deposition of a hyaline-like substance in the subintimal layer of afferent arterioles and deposition of the same PAS-positive hyaline material in the glomerular capillaries. The last finding has been shown by HARLAN et al. [20] to often be associated with a nephrotic syndrome.

The homografts with vascular lesions often had other secondary morphologic changes including fibrosis of the glomerular tufts, spotty periglomerular fibrosis, interstitial fibrosis, or tubular atrophy. The majority of the homografts also contained focal accumulations of mononuclear cells. Ten to 40 % of these cells consisted of the pyroninophilic variety which are found in acutely rejecting homografts. In the chronically functioning homografts, the presence of such cells was not incompatible with good or even normal long term function.

Further studies by PORTER and his associates with immunofluorescence techniques and with ferritin-conjugated antisera have shed additional light on some of the foregoing changes [60]. The deposits in the subendothelial layers of small vessels and glomerular capillaries were shown to consist at least in part of host antibodies, particularly in the IgM class but also often including complement, IgG, and fibrinogen. These were considered to represent the reaction of circulating host antibodies with antigens in the capillary basement membranes of the transplanted kidney.

In three exceptional grafts, the deposits were nodular and were along the subepithelial side of the glomerular capillary basement membranes. The authors suggested that these were caused by the transmission of active glomerulonephritis from the recipient to the homograft [60]. Morphologic evidence that this sequence of events was possible had previously been published by PORTER [62], O'BRIEN and HUME [56], and PETERSEN et al. [59]. More recently, LERNER et al. [43] have conclusively shown that anti-glomerular basement membrane (anti-GBM) antibodies present in the serum of a patient with active glomerulonephritis fixed to and adversely effected a subsequent transplanted homograft. Presumably, this complication could be avoided if patients with acute or subacute glomerulonephritis were subjected to preliminary nephrectomy and transplantation were then deferred until recipient serum levels of anti-GBM antibody disappeared.

The fact that many, or even most, renal homografts may gradually fail is not a serious argument against further clinical transplantation. The degree of social and vocational rehabilitation in the interval of satisfactory kidney function is usually relatively complete. Moreover, it is now known chiefly as the result of Hume's work [27], that retransplantation for the indication of a failing first homograft can be done with a reasonable expectation of success. This expedient was considered too late in some of the patients in our early series who died long after operation with diminishing renal function.

Histocompatibility Typing

During the time when the first Denver series was accumulated, there were no practical methods of predicting the vigor or tenacity of the anticipated rejection process. It was quickly recognized that red blood cell group incompatibilities between donors and recipients could lead to immediate loss of the transplanted kidneys, from which experience the now widely accepted rules were formulated [69, 75] concerning tissue transfer between people of different ABO types (table I). Since other preoperative analyses of donor-recipient compatibility were not available, the transplantation itself became a test system in which, presumably, the recipients of biologically unfavorable kidneys were ruthlessly weeded out in the early mortality. It was decided to retrieve the information derived from this unacceptable situation and use it to try to improve donor selection for future cases. The effort involved a collaboration with Dr. P. Terasaki of Los Angeles, and Dr. K. A. Porter of London, England. In the meanwhile, a six month moratorium on new cases was declared.

For some years, Terasaki, Dausset, Payne, van Rood, Ceppellini, Amos, and others [23] had been working on the characterization with a variety of serologic techniques of the antigens contained in leukocytes. These workers were convinced that most of the antigens contained in renal and other tissue were also to be found in the readily accessible peripheral lymphocytes. By studying the lymphocytes of prospective donors and recipients, it was hoped that an idea could be obtained of their general tissue compatibility. Unfortunately, there was at that time no proof that the antigen systems under investigation had any direct or indirect relationship to histocompatibility and it was to establish this point that the Denver patients were employed.

First, TERASAKI analyzed the antigenic constitution of a number of surviving recipients and their donors using his lymphocyte cytotoxicity test. The quality of the matches was graded and compared with clinical rankings accorded by those caring for the patients. The correlation was imperfect. It was evident that many patients had retained good homograft function for long periods in spite of what appeared to be poor matches with their donors. Nevertheless, most of the really superior clinical results were in patients who had received exceptionally well matched kidneys [78, 91]. Later, a far more striking correlation was found between the Terasaki results and the degree of histologic injury noted by PORTER in the two year biopsies mentioned in the preceding section [61].

Although much of the above-cited support for the validity of antigen typing was not yet available in 1964, there was even then enough favorable evidence to warrant a prospective clinical evaluation. When transplantation was resumed in October of that year, an effort was made by TERASAKI in every case to find the best possible donor amongst the volunteers available for each patient.

The selectivity was severely limited in most cases of intrafamilial transplantation. In most instances, only one or two blood relative were willing to donate or were acceptable on general medical or psychiatric grounds. Consequently, the matching was not improved to a statistically significant degree over that which could have been achieved with random intrafamilial pairing [88]. It was not, therefore, surprising to find that the ultimate survival in these related cases (fig. 3) was almost identical to that defined in the earlier Series I. Of 25 recipients, 16 (64%) were still alive at one year. Two more subsequently died after 26 and 30 months leaving a residual group of 14 (56%) with a follow-up of 23 months to 3 ½ years.

In the 17 non-related homotransplantations, the situation was different in that donors were picked from a pool which included as many as 80 volunteers. Perfect matches could not be found, but the quality of the pairing was improved over that which could have been expected by chance [88]. The recipients fared better than previously observed in Series I. Nine (52.9%) of the 17 recipients were still alive at the end of the first year (fig. 3). Three more patients were lost at 18, 27, and 35 months respectively but in two of these there was life sustaining renal function until death. Six of the 17 patients (35.3%)

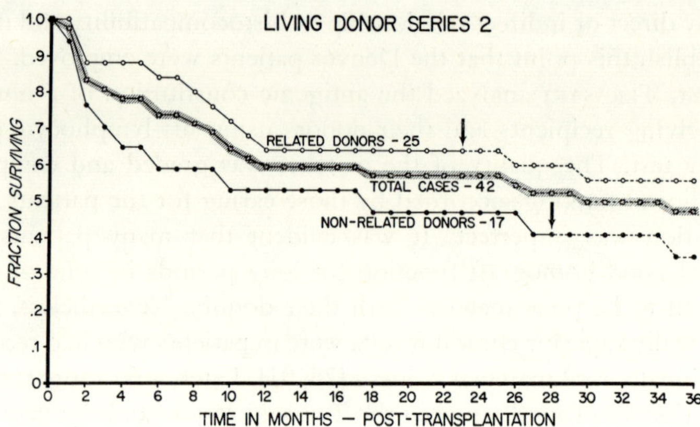

Fig. 3. Survival of 42 patients treated with renal homotransplantation between October 1964 and April 1966. An attempt was made by Terasaki to select the most compatible donor amongst available volunteers. See text for discussion of results.

are still living with good to excellent function of their original homografts from 28 to 40 months after transplantation. The mean creatinine clearance in the remaining group is 83.4 ± 26.2 (SD) ml/min.

In both the related and non-related cases, observations were made which were similar to those made retrospectively in Series I. Several recipients of poorly matched kidneys fared surprisingly well. A few patients with good matches experienced vigorous and prolonged rejection. However, the preponderance of the best results were in cases in which a close antigen match had been present.

The failure to improve survival at all in the related transplantations or to increase it more in the non-related cases was a keen disappointment since evidence from many investigators now suggested more strongly than ever that the tissue typing being used provided a measure of histocompatibility antigens [7, 41, 58, 63, 83, 90, 93, 98]. It seemed that safer methods of immunosuppression would be required before histocompatibility typing could receive a fair trial.

It had been recognized for several years that many and possibly even most of the deaths after clinical homotransplantation were due to drug toxicity. At the beginning, bone marrow depression from overdoses of azathioprine had been common, but with increased experience this complication was now rarely seen. Avoidance of the hazards of the steroid therapy which is usually combined with azathioprine was not so simple. In many cases, it had been found that continued function of a homograft was dependent upon continuation for long periods of unacceptably large quantities of prednisone. The complications which followed were exceedingly troublesome at best, and lethal at worst. These included cosmetic deformity, bone demineralization often with spontaneous fractures, muscle wasting, arrest of growth in infants, fatty infiltration of the liver, pancreatitis, and gastrointestinal ulceration and hemorrhage to name just a few. Most serious, however, was the consequent susceptibility to microorganisms of all types.

If the resultant infections were due to common pathogenic bacteria they could be treated effectively with properly chosen antibiotics. Very often, however, these were caused by fungi, protozoa, or viruses for which specific therapy was not available. The tragic consequences are illustrated in figure 4. This patient, who received a homograft from his brother, had an early rejection crisis followed by excellent renal function for the next nine months. After reduction of his prednisone to 10 mg/day, he had a delayed rejection which was controlled by increasing the prednisone dose to a level from which

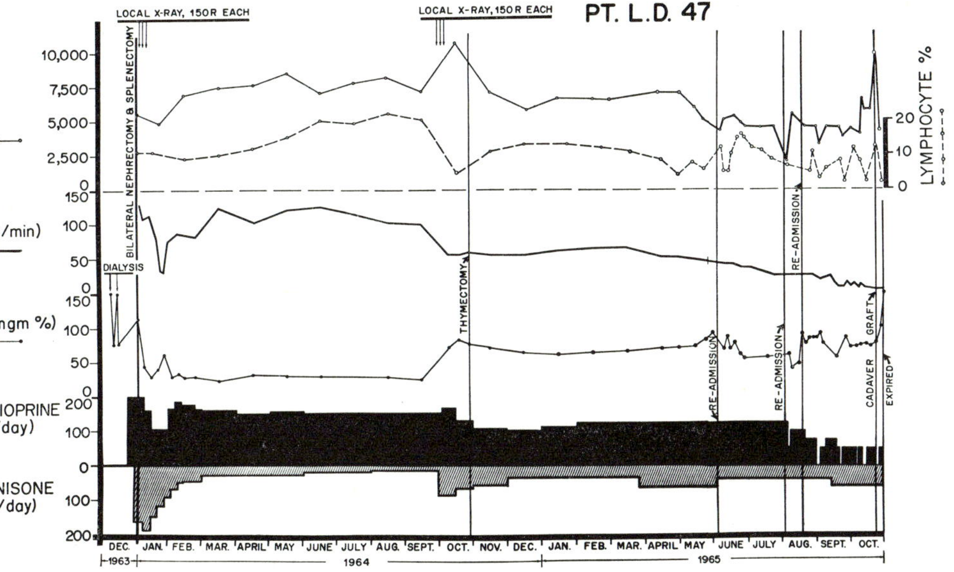

Fig. 4. Course of a 37-year-old man (LD 47) who received a kidney from his younger brother. Both were A+ blood type. Note the severe late rejection after nine months and the subsequent slow deterioration of renal function. The late thymectomy did not induce either lymphopenia or make the subsequent management easier; the post-thymectomy changes in lymphocyte counts were related to adjustments in steroid dosage. (By permission of Ann. N.Y. Acad. Sci. *129:* 605, 1966).

subsequent withdrawals were not possible without further deterioration of kidney function. He died 15 months later but not primarily from renal failure. He had fatty infiltration of the liver, a duodenal ulcer, and pancreatitis. There were cytomegalic inclusion viruses in the lungs and liver, and diffuse pneumonitis due to Pneumocystis carinii and Aspergillus fumigatum.

Improvements in Immunosuppression

For the aforementioned reasons, intensive efforts have been made in a number of laboratories to develop new and safer immunosuppressive agents. The most encouraging results have been with heterologous antilymphocyte serum (ALS) or its globulin derivative (ALG). These biologic agents were first evaluated in animals for their ability to prevent rejection by Waksman et al. [95] and Woodruff and Anderson [102]. Notable contributions have since been made by Monaco and Russell and their collaborators [13, 51, 52], Levey and Medawar [44], and many others [100].

In our laboratory, the horse has been used as the source of immune serum [28, 76]. After immunization with the lymphoid tissue of the species to be eventually treated, the horses are bled and the serum is separated. Undesirable anti-red cell and anti-plasma protein antibodies are absorbed with donor species red cells and plasma or serum. The antilymphocyte antibodies which are in the IgG fraction of the horse serum can then be removed with several techniques. Initially, we employed ammonium sulphate precipitation for crude globulin extraction (fig. 5) but more recently pure IgG has been removed in bulk quantities (fig. 6) by batch mixing with DEAE cellulose [33]. The ALG can then be given by intramuscular injection.

The guidelines for the clinical use of heterologous ALG were provided by extensive investigations in dogs. The ability of the anti-dog-lymphocyte globulin to mitigate homograft rejection was easily and unequivocally demonstrated [74, 76]. Nevertheless, the degree of protection was incomplete. In about a fourth of the animals rejection proceeded as might have been expected in untreated animals. Its onset was delayed or occasionally prevented altogether in the rest of the animals. However, survival of as long as 4, 8, or 12 months was observed in the minority of recipients of kidneys or livers. This spectrum of results was similar to that which can be obtained in dogs with other potent immunosuppressive agents such as azathioprine.

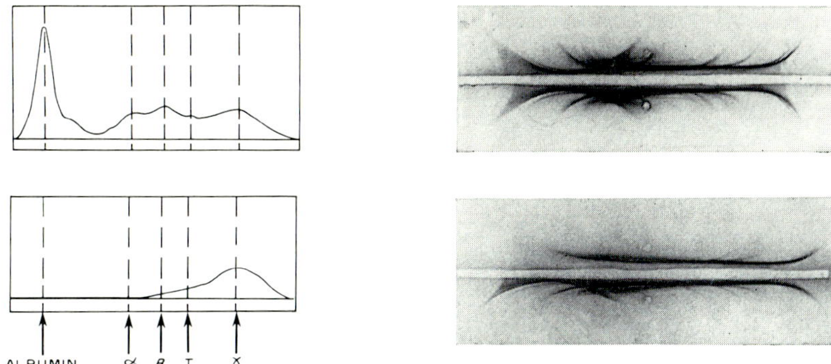

Fig. 5. Electrophoresis and immunoelectrophoresis of absorbed antihumanlymphoid serum and the protein obtained from it by two precipitations with 0.4 saturated ammonium sulphate, two dialyses, and lyophilization. The final product, which was used clinically, consisted mostly of gamma G globulin but it usually contained small quantities of alpha and beta globulins. (By permission of Surg. Gynec. Obstet. *124:* 1, 1967.)

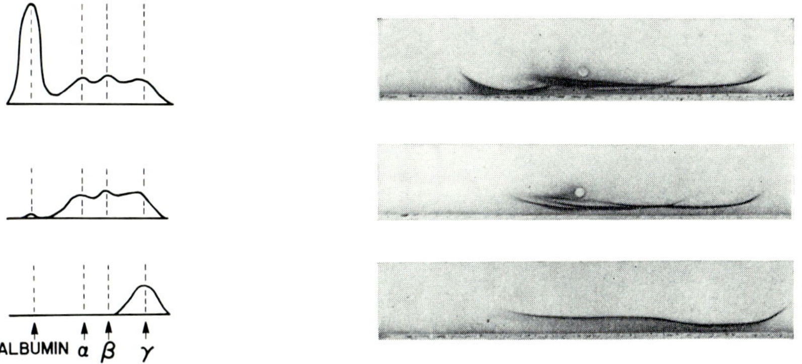

Fig. 6. Electrophoretic and immunoelectrophoretic patterns of unabsorbed antihuman ALS, the raw globulin obtained with a single ammonium sulphate precipitation of absorbed ALS, and the final product (pure gamma G globulin) after subsequent DEAE-cellulose batch extraction.

Other factors concerned with the toxicity of ALG influenced the therapeutic program finally adopted [28, 72, 76, 81]. After long term administration, the animals usually developed antibodies against the injected horse protein. Many of these dogs ultimately had microscopic renal lesions which consisted of deposits of horse protein, together with host gamma globulin and complement; the findings were characteristic of serum sickness nephritis [28].

For all these reasons it was decided to use ALG only as an adjuvant to the standard immunosuppressive agents azathioprine and prednisone. The regimen ordinarily followed is shown in figure 7. ALG was started a few days in advance of transplantation, continued daily for the first 10 to 14 postoperative days, then every other day for two weeks, twice a week for two months and once a week for a final month. The four month duration of the ALG course was selected since the greatest need for improvements in therapy was in this postoperative period of high risk. It was anticipated that an at least partial evolution of the state of "host-graft non-reactivity" discussed earlier would have occurred by the end of this time and that the need for maintenance treatment would be correspondingly reduced.

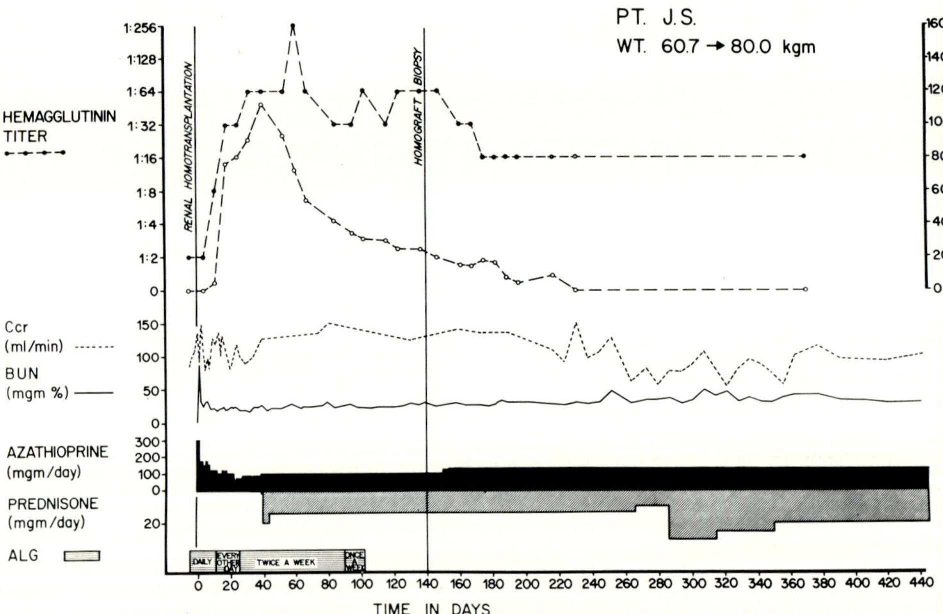

Fig. 7. The course of a patient who received antilymphocyte globulin (ALG) before and for the first four months after renal homotransplantation. The donor was an older brother. The Terasaki match was a good one. There was no early rejection. Prednisone therapy was started 40 days postoperatively because of the high rises in the serologic titers which indicated a host response against the injected foreign protein and which warned against a possible anaphylactic reaction. Note the insidious onset of late rejection after cessation of globulin therapy. This was treated by increasing the maintenance dose of steroids. This delayed complication was seen in only two of the original 20 patients whose survival is shown in figure 8. (By permission of Surg. Gynec. Obstet. *126:* May, 1968.)

The first patient was treated in this way in June 1966. From then until the following December, 19 more were added to the series One of the patients died during the second postoperative month as the direct consequence of a technical surgical accident. The others are alive with good renal function from their original homografts from 15 to 21 months later for a current survival of 95%. An additional 45 patients have since been treated with comparable results.

The ALG-treated recipients received kidneys from blood relatives. The results obtained in the first ALG series are shown graphically in figure 8 and compared with those obtained in previous intrafamilial transplantations in our institutions. For the latter purpose the consanguineous transplantations in the original Series I were divided into two consecutive groups, now termed Series 1A and 1B; this was done to evaluate the effect of increased experience upon results. The intrafamilial homotransplantations described in the above section on histocompatibility typing were Series 2. In each of the consecutive earlier series the mortality in comparable follow-up intervals had been from 28 to 31%.

The explanation for the improved results in the ALG-treated patients was not better histocompatibility matching as has been documented elsewhere in detail [72, 81]. The apparent reason is shown in figure 9. During the time when the sequential earlier series

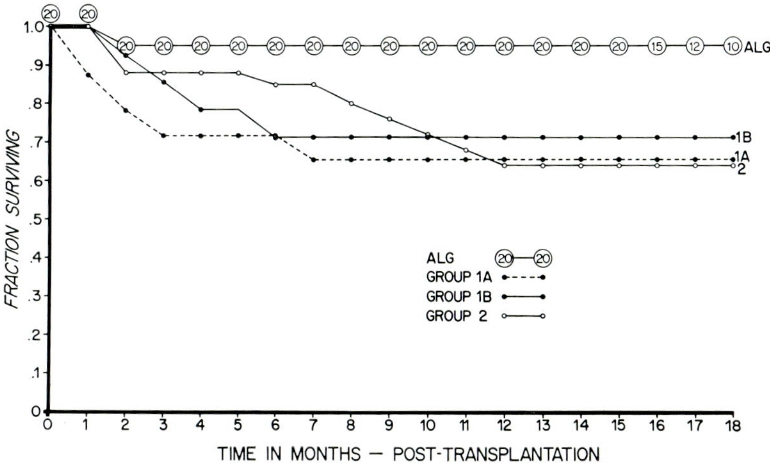

Fig. 8. Survival curve of the first 20 patients treated with antilymphocyte globulin (ALG) compared to that in three previous series of consanguineous transplantation at our institutions. Followups in the globulin-treated group are 15 to 21 months. The numbers in the upper curve indicate the patients at risk for each monthly interval.

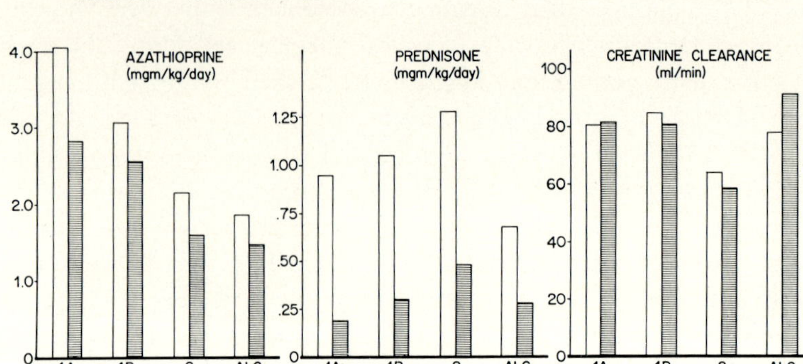

Fig. 9. The average azathioprine and prednisone doses per kg/day and the creatinine clearances for the first 16 postoperative weeks (shaded) and for the subsequent six months (solid). Shown are the retrospective control series (Groups 1A, 1B and 2) and the ALG series (Group 3). Inclusion in the analysis was contingent upon survival for 294 days, a condition which was met with the highest regularity in the ALG patients.

were being accumulated, there had been a progressive tendency to use smaller doses of azathioprine both during the first four and the subsequent six postoperative months. This trend continued into the ALG series.

However, as the average doses of azathioprine were cut, there had been compensatory increases in the quantities of prednisone which were necessary to maintain a somewhat poorer quality renal function (figure 9, middle and right). The result of the slowly evolving adjustments in policy was a change in the causes of death as described from our institutions by HILL *et al.* [22]. The early mortality from bone marrow depression and pyogenic infections was virtually eliminated. This was replaced by a delayed mortality which was usually due to untreatable infections caused by unusual opportunistic microorganisms.

The situation was drastically reversed in the ALG-treated patients in that the quantities of average daily prednisone could be sharply lowered during the first four postoperative months when ALG was being given. Furthermore, the steroid doses remained at acceptably low levels in the next six months after the ALG had been stopped. The ability to reduce the stringency of therapy with both azathioprine and prednisone was not paid for with a loss of renal function (fig. 9, right) since all measures of renal function in the ALG-treated patients were at least as adequate as in the earlier series.

The extremely favorable showing of the ALG as compared to earlier series was in spite of a sharp bias introduced by the method of analysis. Inclusion of any case in the studies shown in figure 9 was contingent upon survival for ten months. A substantial fraction of the worst patients in each of the retrospective series were thereby eliminated by their death. Inasmuch as only one of the 20 patients in the ALG group was similarly excluded, the latter series was much less selective.

This experience with ALG suggests that its use as an immuno-suppressive agent has improved the management of patients after transplantation. However, there have been a number of side effects, recently summarized by KASHIWAGI *et al.* [32]. Sensitization to the repeatedly injected horse protein has in time led to a number of skin rashes. Fever and pain at the injection sites were invariable. In nearly 20 % of cases an anaphylactic reaction occurred at some time during the course of therapy. The most serious of these adverse effects usually were observed when titers of host precipitating antibodies had reached high levels. Interestingly, the easily detectable antibodies were directed against the alpha and beta globulins which were present in small quantities in the ALG; only rarely were precipitins found against the equine gamma G globulin which is thought to be the biologically active part of ALG. Consequently, there is reason to hope that the pure gamma G globulin (IgG) which is now being produced in bulk as discussed earlier will eliminate some of the undesirable features of ALG.

One of the most disquieting possibilities with the clinical use of heterologous ALG was that the renal homografts would become the site of serum sickness or direct nephrotoxic Masugi-like nephritis. This fear has been largely dispelled. The first 8 patients treated with ALG received homograft biopsies at the end of their 4-month course of therapy. The specimens were studied with immunofluorescence and ferritin-labeled antibody techniques [81]. There was no trace of horse protein. Since then four more kidneys have been studied. In only one was there detectable horse protein, and in that patient there has been no clinical or biochemical evidence of serum sickness nephritis.

Thymectomy in Clinical Transplantation

In adult mice, rats, and hamsters the performance of complete thymec-tomy causes a slowly developing loss in immunologic reactivity in otherwise unaltered animals [49, 50, 68, 86]. The process can be accelerated in skin homotransplantation experiments if immunosuppressive therapy is given either with total body irradiation [9, 49] or with antilymphocyte serum [29, 51].

Shortly after the appearance of the first of the above reports, eight patients were subjected to thymectomy at our institutions 14 to 85 days before renal homotransplantation. Four of the patients died within a few weeks or months after receipt of their homografts. The other four are still alive more than five years later, all with excellent renal function. As has been previously stressed [78, 79], the role of thymectomy in the attainment of long term graft function in these cases was essentially unanalyzable.

In order to clarify this issue, a formal study of the effect of thymectomy was carried out in 46 more patients who were treated with renal homotransplantation from October 1964 until June 1966. All kidneys were provided by living donors of whom 37% were unrelated. A decision for or against thymectomy was made on the basis of random selection from appropriately marked cards. The spectrum of histocompatibility typing as well as a number of other variables proved to be almost identical in the 22 control cases as compared to the 24 cases in which transthoracic thymectomy was carried out before transplantation.

The duration of follow-up for these cases is now from 21 to 41 months. The results were assessed on the basis of early and late mortality (fig. 10), the dosages of immunosuppressive drugs necessary to retain stable homograft function, and the quality of both early and late renal function. There were no statistically significant differences between the thymectomized and non-thymectomized groups in any of these measures. In all 46 cases samples of the transplanted kidneys are now available for examination either as a result of autopsy or late biopsy. The histopathologic examination has not yet revealed clear differences between the test and control series of kidneys, although the specimens are currently being reviewed for the possibility that there may be subtle differentiating features.

At the moment, however, it can be concluded that an important benefit did not derive from thymectomy. This does not, of course, prove that the thymus has no immunologic function in adult man. At the least, however, it does indicate that other factors are so much more important in determining survival and homograft function that the loss of the thymus resulted in no detectable changes under the

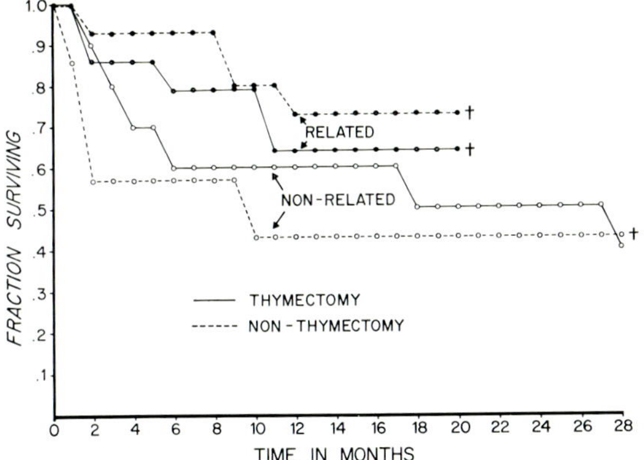

Fig. 10. Life survival curves of 24 patients who received pretransplantation thymectomy and 22 patients who did not. The minimum followup is 21 and 28 months in the related and non-related groups respectively. The crosses indicate that one additional patient in each of the three groups subsequently died after the period shown. Note that the thymectomy did not influence either the short- or long term survival.

experimental conditions which existed from 1964 to 1966. Conceivably future improvements in management might permit unmasking of a presently unrecognizable subtle effect of thymectomy but, at present, there seems to be no justification for the continued use of the procedure in clinical organ transplantation.

Post-Transplantation Neoplasia

In 1966, Schwartz *et al.* [66] described the development of malignant lymphomas after homotransplantation of lymphoid tissues in mice; the genesis of the neoplasm was thought to be related in some way to a subclinical graft-versus-host reaction. They stated: "The practical importance of these findings to those attempting the transplantation of allogenic bone marrow or lymphoid tissue remains to be determined. Nevertheless, it might be appropriate to consider them along with other possible hazards of tissue transplantation".

Two of our recipients of renal homografts have developed and died of reticulum cell or lymphosarcoma, and it is known that Dr. C. Hitchcock [24] of Minneapolis has had a similar patient. The close resemblance of the human tumors to some of those induced by Schwartz *et al.* in animals could conceivably be more than a coincidence. If so, these may be the first clinical examples of a new and serious complication of transplantation.

The three cases had in common the facts that consanguineous kidneys were transplanted (brother, father, and mother), that the donors have not subsequently had evidence of neoplasia with follow-ups of one to four years, and that the recipients were young (14 to 27 years) and all received immunosuppression with azathioprine and prednisone. One of the patients had thymectomy before transplantation. Another received heterologous antilymphocyte globulin (ALG) before and afterwards. The third received neither of these adjuvant measures. The malignancies led to death 6 months, 14 months and 2 ½ years after homotransplantation. It was not possible to determine where the tumors originated but the major sites of involvement were the brain in one patient, the liver in another, and the liver and lung in the third.

In connection with Schwartz's hypothesis of a graft-versus-host etiology of analogous neoplasms in mice, it is of interest that a small amount of lymphoid tissue is invariably transferred with renal homografts. This was well demonstrated by the studies of Wilson and Kirkpatrick [99] who showed that delayed hypersensitivity reactions present in donors were always transferred to previously negative recipients and there persisted for months.

Hyperacute Rejection

As mentioned earlier, it was soon learned that renal homografts had a significant risk of being immediately destroyed if the donors and recipients had different ABO red cell groups in the combinations shown in table I. A rational explanation was available since the iso-agglutinogens which allow red cells to be typed are also found in other tissues including the kidney [26, 85]. Thus if the kidney of an

Table I. Direction of acceptable mismatched tissue transfer[1]

0 to non-0	Safe
RH — to RH +	Safe
RH + to RH —	Relatively Safe
A to non-A	Dangerous
B to non-B	Dangerous
AB to non-AB	Dangerous

[1] 0 is universal donor; AB is universal recipient.

A or B donor were placed in a patient of 0 blood type, the naturally occurring anti-A and anti-B isoagglutinins respectively in the serum of the recipient could be expected to bind with the renal red cell antigens; serologic studies by WILSON and KIRKPATRICK provided strong evidence that this actually occurred [99].

In cases where the homografts were immediately lost, the sequence was typical. After opening the renal vessels, the kidney cortex was not well vascularized although the medulla, pelvis, and ureter apparently had a good blood supply. These soft and cyanotic kidneys which were removed within a few hours had histologic evidence of widespread small vessel thrombosis [69]. A frank red cell group mismatch did not always lead to this kind of accident. One of our patients has normal renal function more than five years after transplantation under such circumstances.

Recently, there have been reports of similar catastrophes where there was conformity of red cell types. The first case was described briefly by TERASAKI [87] and others were added by KISSMEYER-NIELSEN [37], WILLIAMS [96, 97], and TERASAKI [89]. In the serum of many but not all of these patients preformed antibodies were present preoperatively which reacted against donor white cells. This fact has resulted in speculation that such antibodies were directly responsible for the homograft destruction by virtue of a high grade nephrotoxicity [37, 96]. Our own studies on "hyperacute rejection" in the absence of red cell mismatching, carried out in collaboration with R. LERNER and F. DIXON of La Jolla, California, have led us to a different conclusion as recently reported in detail [73]. In five kidneys which sustained "rejection on the operating table", there was unequivocal evidence of a generalized Shwartzman reaction. With immunofluorescence techniques, LERNER and DIXON found massive fibrin deposition in the small vessels and glomerular capillaries and consequent cortical necrosis exactly as in an experimentally induced Shwartzman reaction. There was little or no immunoglobulin deposition detectable by immunofluorescence [73] although eluates of some of the kidneys were later shown by Dr. F. MILGROM of Buffalo, New York, to contain leukoagglutinins. In three of the five instances, the kidney donors had been shown by TERASAKI to have a good histocompatibility match with the recipients.

The generalized Shwartzman reaction was first described in 1934, but its significance as summarized by LEE and STETSON [42] and HJORT and RAPAPORT [25], was not understood until the last decade. Classically, it is produced in rabbits by two injections of endotoxin spaced at 24 h intervals. A generalized coagulapathy is produced. If the animal reticuloendothelial system (RES) can clear the breakdown products of fibrinogen rapidly enough, the kidney is spared from injury. If not, it becomes a primary target because the specific qualities of the renal microcirculation make it an exceptionally good fibrin filter. The result is cortical devascularization and necrosis.

A number of factors besides endotoxin can condition or precipitate a Shwartzman reaction, including antigen-antibody reactions; injection of thorotrast, carbon black, or steroids; or administration of an oxidized lipid diet. Their effects are incompletely understood but presumably they could be influential by either reinforcing the coagulapathy and/or by reducing the efficiency of RES function, or by suppressing counter-regulatory fibrinolysis.

In several ways, the recipient of a renal homograft could be expected to be a good candidate for a Shwartzman reaction. Before operation, he undergoes multiple hemodialyses with attendant risks from accidental exposure to endotoxin in the extracorporeal circuit [34], from an additional loss of RES efficiency caused by increased blood hemolysis [5] and other factors of extracorporeal circulation [84], and from the rapid changes in coagulation which occur with this procedure [94]. With multiple blood transfusions, there is an increased chance that he will develop antibodies against antigens in infused white blood cells or red cell subgroups, and that these will later react with the same antigens in the homograft. The operation itself introduces the latter possibility as well as that of a full spectrum of other potential triggering antigen-antibody reactions either within or outside the freshly transplanted kidney. Intra- and postoperatively steroids, which can potentiate a Shwartzman reaction by causing RES paralysis [92], are commonly used.

Recognition that many, and possibly even most, "rejections on the operating table" are due to Shwartzman reactions has practical implications. Prophylactic measures can be taken. Greater attention can be paid to the details of hemodialysis including asepsis and hemolysis rates. The value of white cell free blood for transfusion is obvious. Immunologic tests to detect presensitization are available; when such an examination is positive in a recipient, the hazards are predictably increased [89, 97]. Under these circumstances, it may be advisable to use total body heparinization at the time of transplantation. This was done in two of our patients whose previously placed kidney transplants had been immediately destroyed; the final homografts functioned well [73]. Once a Shwartzman reaction has started, a combination of heparin and fibrinolysin therapy might be worth a trial.

It is probable that most and perhaps even all Shwartzman reactions are ultimately triggered by antigen-antibody unions of one sort or other at the time of transplantation. If these are intrarenal, they may be inherently benign or even undetectable with immunofluorescence studies as in our cases and of significance only by virtue of the devastating secondary effects which they can initiate depending upon a variety of other conditions. If, as is now thought, the site of the immunologic reaction is not critical to the chain of events, it is conceivable that the Shwartzman reaction may lead to destruction of the kidneys after transplantation of other organs.

Cadaveric Transplantation

A cadaveric renal homograft was first transplanted in Denver in April 1963. This recipient, as well as the next two, died within 39 days. The kidneys either functioned poorly or not at all. No more cadaveric transplantations were performed for more than two years.

The program was reopened in November 1965. From then until July 1967, 12 patients received as their primary homograft the kidney of a blood group compatible cadaver. In each case, a minimum follow-up of eight months is available.

Six of these 12 recipients died after 13, 10, 8, 3 ½, 3 ½, and 3 months. The other six are still alive after 27, 24, 15, 10, 9, and 8 months. However, one of the latter patients required transplant nephrectomy and regrafting one year after receipt of his first kidney; another lost his homograft after a year and is presently anephric 15 months post-transplantation.

The last six patients in this series received ALG therapy for the first several postoperative months. In all cases, the donor-recipient histocompatibility matches as determined by TERASAKI were poor. Two of the recipients who had received their kidneys from a common cadaveric donor, died within a one day interval more than three months postoperatively. Death was caused by pulmonary emboli. The homografts had little or no evidence of rejection.

The other four patients including one with preformed lymphocytotoxic antibodies had good or excellent renal function during the four month period of ALG therapy. After its discontinuance, all have had evidence of slow but progressive rejection.

Other groups with much more extensive experience in cadaveric transplantation have repeatedly expressed optimism about the bright future of this approach [6, 27, 35, 36, 45]. It is a point of view with which few would disagree especially since the prospects of transplanting livers, lungs, and hearts will depend upon the use of cadaveric organs. Nevertheless, it is worth emphasizing that the costs in mortality, morbidity, and rehospitalization have been high in all centers. Furthermore, survival exceeding four years with continuous function of non-related renal homografts is rare. To our knowledge there are only four patients whose courses have been this long; one of Dr. W. GOODWIN who was treated at UCLA in June 1963, another who has been followed by Dr. D. HUME of Richmond since August of that year, and two more who were in our Series 1.

Ribonucleic Acid (RNA) Perfusion

Many of the problems of organ transplantation could be minimized if it were possible to mitigate graft rejection by modifying the transplanted tissue rather than the host immunologic response. Efforts to achieve this objective have been unsuccessful with occasional possible exceptions [2, 21, 30] of which the most intriguing was described by JOLLEY, HINSHAW, and PETERSON [30]. They reported that rabbit skin grafts which were first immersed in homologous ribonucleic acid (RNA) and then transplanted to recipient animals which were given intravenous RNA had a survival four times longer than controls. The role of the preliminary soaking was not analyzable in these experiments, but the authors also reported that human skin homografts subjected only to RNA soaking had unusually protracted viability when placed upon patients with burns [31].

In our laboratories similar attempts to "pre-treat" whole organ homografts have been made in dogs by perfusing kidneys for about 30 min with RNA prepared by phenol extraction from the spleens of the prospective recipients (autologous RNA) or other dogs (homologous RNA). After transplantation to unmodified recipients, about one fourth of these life sustaining organs had prolonged homograft viability [14]. Maximum survival of recipients, which were subjected to simultaneous removal of their own kidneys, was 123 days. The mean survival in a group of 40 recipients was more than 20 days as opposed to approximately 10 days in 30 control animals. Furthermore, there were seven homografts of the 40 which had no histologic evidence of rejection whereas all the control homografts had the typical findings of unmodified rejection. The protection afforded by recipient specific RNA was not significantly different from that obtained with homologous RNA.

The foregoing effect was not increased by the addition of a supposed RNase inhibitor, DEAE-dextran, but it was abolished by the addition of commercial RNase. The treatment of renal autografts with homologous RNA did not result in their rejection. The latter finding, and the fact that the results after homotransplantation were equivalent with either homologous or autologous RNA, suggest that the homograft protection was not due to RNA-induced changes in the genetic characteristics of the cells.

The significance of the foregoing findings is quite unclear since a logical explanation for the surprising results is not available, and because the degree of homograft protection was relatively limited. It will be of interest in laboratory experiments to determine whether or not such graft conditioning can be advantageously combined with effective host immunosuppression.

Liver Transplantation

Until last year, the kidney was the only vital organ which had been transplanted with resulting significant prolongation of life. There had been nine attempts at orthotopic liver transplantation; seven in Denver [70, 80], and one each in Boston [53] and Paris [10]. Two of these patients had succumbed within a few hours after operation, and none had lived for longer than 23 days.

This dismal picture has changed within the last nine months, inasmuch as six consecutive children treated with orthotopic liver transplantation from July 1967 to February 1968 all passed through this previously lethal operative and postoperative period. Two of the patients are still alive after 8 and 1 ½ months respectively; the others died after 2, 3 ½, 4 ½, and 6 ½ months. The better results were the product of several improvements in care as reported elsewhere [71].

First, a very efficient technique of preservation had been developed in dogs which permitted livers to be stored for 8 to 24 hours and then successfully transplanted as orthotopic homografts [3]. The method which combined hypothermia, low flow perfusion with diluted blood, and hyperbaric oxygenation, was used in the clinical cases for several hours after death of the donors and until the recipients could be prepared. Good immediate hepatic function was obtained in each case (fig. 11).

In each of these cases, the compatibility of the donor and recipient white cell antigens was studied by TERASAKI in advance of operation. A good match with compatibility in all six currently recognized components of the recently defined HLA system [90] was present only in one case. In three, there were breeches in one major antigen group and in the other two there were mismatches in two of the six groups.

A conservative attitude toward immunosuppression was taken during the early postoperative period, particularly in the dosages of

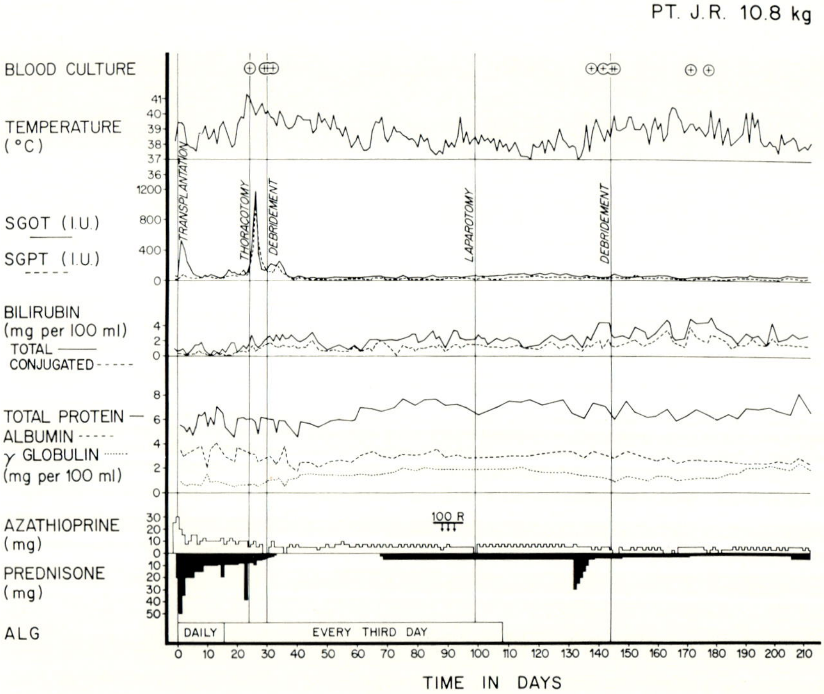

Fig. 11. Course of a 1 ½ year old girl who was treated with orthotopic hepatic homo-transplantation. The indication for the operation was a hepatoma. Note the essentially stable liver function except at the times of septic liver infarctions which were treated with debridement. The septicemia, indicated by encircled crosses, was with various gram negative rods or candida albicans. The thoractomy was for an unexpanded right upper lobe. The laparotomy was for excision of a tumor recurrence.

azathioprine (fig. 11). High initial doses of prednisone were given but rapidly reduced. Finally, heterologous antilymphocyte globulin (ALG) was administered in a course (fig. 11) similar to that described earlier after renal homotransplantation.

The six recipients were all infants. The indication for operation was a hepatoma in the first patient and extrahepatic biliary atresia in the other five. In all but one case, the early convalescence was remarkably rapid. Pre-existing jaundice was quickly cleared. Eating was begun on the second to fourth postoperative days.

A specific life threatening complication was encountered in five of the six patients. From two days to two months postoperatively, septicemia with gram negative microorganisms interrupted recovery. This was accompanied by high increases in SGOT and SGPT (fig. 11) and eventually septic infarctions within the liver were found. Liver scans showed filling defects which involved the right lobe (fig. 12).

In one case, the development of hepatic sepsis was not surprising inasmuch as a serious technical accident could be implicated. The homograft had been found to have a double arterial supply and the two vessels were anastomosed to the terminal right and left branches of the recipient hepatic artery. The artery to the right lobe thrombosed on the second postoperative day eventually necessitating a partial right lobectomy. In the four other children the complication occurred after a benign early postoperative course. Two of the latter patients who died from this complication were also found at autopsy to have thrombosed right hepatic arteries.

The unusual susceptibility of the transplanted liver to invasion by enteric organisms is not surprising in view of its perfusion by splanchnic venous blood, as well as the necessity for connecting its biliary drainage system to the intestinal tract. However, the precise pathogenetic events of the septic liver infarctions can only be speculated upon in the individual cases. In a recent analysis of the problem in dogs [4], any factor which caused liver necrosis, including the injury of rejection, was shown to predispose to liver abscess formation. It is possible that, in at least some of the clinical cases, the intensity of immunosuppression was inadequate, that the infarctions were a manifestation of the reduced blood flow known to accompany rejection [15], and that the bacterial invasion was a secondary event. In at least three of the patients, however, rejection did not seem to be severe when the right hepatic artery thrombosed. In these cases, the differentiation of mechanical from immunologic factors was not possible.

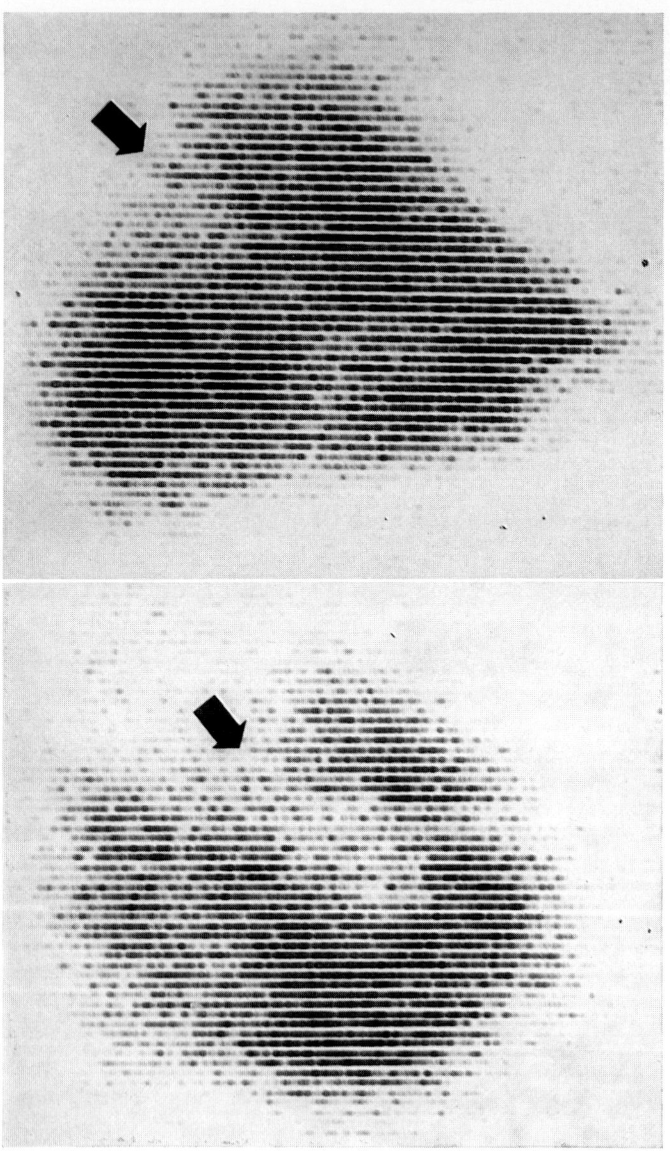

Fig. 12. Liver scan performed one month after hepatic homotransplantation in the 1 ½ year old patient whose course is depicted in figure 11. Anteroposterior (upper) as well as lateral views (lower) show large defect (arrows). Exploration revealed a septic infarct in the homograft.

Once established in the clinical cases, the infected liver infarcts required aggressive therapy. Debridement and drainage were carried out through lateral incisions in the right 10th intercostal space, taking care to enter neither the chest nor abdomen. These local measures plus therapy with properly chosen antibiotics tided three patients over the crisis but two of these eventually died. Two other recipients died within a few days after the onset of the complication.

An alternative to orthotopic liver transplantation has also been given a clinical trial, namely transplantation of an auxiliary organ. Only five cases have been reported [1, 8, 16] but it is known that many more have been attempted. The longest survival after auxiliary liver transplantation has been 34 days [16]. Analyses of the special physiologic and technical difficulties with this approach have been published [46], suggesting that it may be a less desirable procedure than the orthotopic operation.

Summary

Several separate issues in organ transplantation have been reviewed based upon our own experience with renal and liver transplantation. The topics surveyed include a reconsideration of rejection reversal and host-graft adaptation, projections of survival after renal homotransplantation in the past and today, the role of histocompatibility typing, improvements in immunosuppression, an evaluation of thymectomy, the development of neoplasms in post-transplantation patients, and the contribution of the Shwartzman reaction to "hyperacute rejection". In addition, a specific problem of hepatic sepsis after liver transplantation has been described.

References

1. ABSOLON, K. B.; HAGIHARA, P. F.; GRIFFEN, W. O. and LILLEHEI, R. C.: Experimental and clinical heterotopic liver homotransplantation. Rev. int. Hépat. *15:* 1481 (1965).
2. BONMASSAR, E.; FRANESCONI, G.; MANZONI, S. C. and PERELLI-ERCOLINI, M.: Chemical deletion of histocompatibility antigens. Homograft survival of rat skin treated with "Urethan" *in vitro*. Nature *209:* 1141 (1966).
3. BRETTSCHNEIDER, L.; DALOZE, P. M.; HUGUET, C.; PORTER, K. A.; GROTH, C. G.; KASHIWAGI, N.; HUTCHISON, D. E. and STARZL, T. E.: The use of combined preservation techniques for extended storage of orthotopic liver homografts. Surg. Gynec. Obstet. *126:* 263 (1968).
4. BRETTSCHNEIDER, L.; TONG, J. L.; BOOSE, D. S.; DALOZE, P. M.; SMITH, G. V.; HUGUET, C.; BLANCHARD, H.; GROTH, C. G. and STARZL, T. E.: Specific bacteriologic problems after orthotopic liver transplantation in dogs and pigs. Arch. Surg. *97:* 313 (1968).
5. BROWN, E.; SEIDEL, W. and KOLFF, W. J.: Hemolysis caused by pumps at flow rates of 2 liters. Trans. amer. soc. artif. Int. Organs *7:* 350 (1961).

6. Calne, R.Y.; Loughridge, L.; MacGillivray, J.B. and Swales, J.D.: Further observations on renal transplants in man from cadaveric donors. Brit. med. J. *2:* 1345 (1966).

7. Ceppellini, R.; Curtoni, E.S.; Mattiuz, P.L.; Leigheb, G.; Visetti, M. and Colombi, A.: Survival of test skin grafts in man: Effect of genetic relationship and of blood groups incompatibility. Ann. N.Y. Acad. Sci. *129:* 421 (1966).

8. Cree, I.C.: A liver transplant. Minn. Med. *50:* 1523 (1967).

9. Cross, A.M.; Leuchars, E. and Miller, J.F.A.P.: Studies on the recovery of the immune response in irradiated mice thymectomized in adult life. J. exp. Med. *119:* 837 (1964).

10. Demirleau; Nourreddine; Vignes; Prawerman; Reizicinar; Larraud and Louvier: Tentative d'homograffe hepatique. Mém. Acad. Chir. (Paris) *90:* 177 (1964).

11. Goodwin, W.E.; Kaufman, J.J.; Mims, M.M.; Turner, R.D.; Glassock, R.; Goldman, R. and Maxwell, M.M.: Human renal transplantation: Clinical experiences with 6 cases of renal homotransplantation. J. Urol. *89:* 13 (1963).

12. Goodwin, W.E. and Martin, D.C.: Transplantation of the kidney. Urol. Surv. *13:* 229 (1963).

13. Gray, J.G.; Monaco, A.P. and Russell, P.S.: Heterologous mouse anti-lymphocyte serum to prolong skin homografts. Surg. Forum *15:* 142 (1964).

14. Groth, C.G.; Porter, K.A.; Daloze, P.M.; Huguet, C.; Smith, G.V.; Brettschneider, L. and Starzl, T.E.: The effect of ribonucleic acid perfusion on canine kidney and liver homograft survival. Surgery *64:* 31 (1968).

15. Groth, C.G.; Porter, K.A.; Otte, J.B.; Daloze, P.M.; Marchioro, T.L.; Brettschneider, L. and Starzl, T.E.: Studies of blood flow and ultrastructural changes in rejecting and non-rejecting canine orthotopic liver homografts. Surgery *63:* 658 (1968).

16. Halgrimson, C.G.; Marchioro, T.L.; Faris, T.D.; Porter, K.A.; Peters, G.N. and Starzl, T.E.: Auxiliary liver transplantation. Effect of host portacaval shunt. Arch. Surg. *93:* 107 (1966).

17. Hamburger, J.; Vaysse, J.; Crosnier, J.; Tubiana, M.; Lalanne, C.M.; Antoine, B.; Auvert, J.; Soulier, J.A.; Dormont, J.; Salmon, C.; Maisonnet, M. and Amiel, J.L.: Transplantation d'un rein entre jumeaux non-monozygotes après irradiation du receveur: Bon fonctionnement au quatrième mois. Presse Méd. *67:* 1771 (1959).

18. Hamburger, J.; Crosnier, J.; Dormont, J.; Reveillaud, R.J.; Hors, J.H. and Alsina, J.: Homotransplantation renale humaine. Résultats personnels chez 52 malades. I. Téchniques et résultats d'ensemble. Presse Méd. *73:* 2793 (1965).

19. Hamburger, J.; Vaysse, J.; Crosnier, J.; Auvert, J.; Lalanne, C.M. and Hopper, J., Jr.: Renal homotransplantation in man after radiation of the recipient: Experience with six cases since 1959. Amer. J. Med. *32:* 854 (1962).

20. Harlan, W.R., Jr.; Holden, K.R.; Williams, G.M. and Hume, D.M.: Proteinuria and nephrotic syndrome in rejection of kidney transplants. New Engl. J. Med. *277:* 769 (1967).

21. Hellman, K.; Duke, D.I. and Tucker, D.F.: Prolongation of skin homograft survival by Thalidomide. Brit. med. J. *2:* 687 (1965).

22. Hill, R.B., Jr.; Dahrling, B.E.; Starzl, T.E. and Rifkind, D.: Death after transplantation: An analysis of 60 cases. Amer. J. Med. *42:* 327 (1967).

23. Histocompatibility Testing: National Academy of Sciences—National Research Council (Publ. 1229) Washington, D.C. (1965).

24. Hitchcock, C.: Personal Communication (March 10, 1968).

25. Hjort, P.F. and Rapaport, S.I.: The Shwartzman reaction: Pathogenetic mechanisms and clinical manifestations. Ann. Rev. Med. *16:* 135 (1965).

26. Hogman, C.F.: Blood group antigens A and B determined by means of mixed agglutination on cultured cells of human fetal kidney, liver, spleen, lung, heart and skin. Vox. Sang. *4:* 12 (1959).

27. Hume, D.M.; Lee, H.M.; Williams, G.M.; White, J.O.; Ferre, J.; Wolf, J.S.; Prout, G.R., Jr.; Slapak, M.; O'Brien, J.; Kilpatrick, S.J.; Kauffman, H.M., Jr. and Cleveland, R.J.: Comparative results of cadaver and related donor renal homografts in man, and immunologic implications of the outcome of second and paired transplants. Ann. Surg. *164:* 352 (1966).

28. Iwasaki, Y.; Porter, K.A.; Amend, J.; Marchioro, T.L.; Zuhlke, V. and Starzl, T.E.: The preparation and testing of horse antidog and antihuman antilymphoid plasma or serum and its protein fractions. Surg. Gynec. Obstet. *124:* 1 (1967).

29. Jeejeebhoy, H.F.: Effects of rabbit anti-rat lymphocyte plasma on immune response of rats thymectomized in adult life. Lancet *ii:* 106 (1965).

30. Jolley, W.B.; Hinshaw, D.B. and Peterson, M.: Effect of ribonucleic acid on homograft survival. Surg. Forum *12:* 99 (1961).

31. Jolley, W.B. and Hinshaw, D.B.: Basic studies on homograft acceptance including early clinical results. Amer. J. Surg. *112:* 308 (1966).

32. Kashiwagi, N.; Brantigan, C.O.; Brettschneider, L.; Groth, C.G. and Starzl, T.E.: Clinical reactions and serologic changes following the administration of heterologous antilymphocyte globulin to human recipients of renal homografts. Ann. int. Med. *68:* 275 (1968).

33. Kashiwagi, N.; Groth, C.G.; Amend, J.R.; Gecelter, L.; Blanchard, H. and Starzl, T.E.: Improvements in the preparation of heterologous antilymphocyte globulin with special reference to absorption and DEAE-cellulose batch production. Surgery (in press, 1968).

34. Kidd, E.E.: Bacterial contamination of dialyzing fluid of artificial kidney. Brit. med. J. *1:* 880 (1964).

35. Kincaid-Smith, P.; Marshall, V.S.; Methew, T.H.; Eremin, J.; Brown, R.B.; Johnson, N.; Lovell, R.R.H.; McLeish, D.G.; Fairley, K.F.; Allcock, E.A. and Ewing, M.R.: Cadaveric renal transplantation. Lancet *ii:* 59 (1967).

36. Kiser, W.S.; Straffon, R.A.; Hewitt, C.B.; Stewart, B.H.; Nakamoto, S. and Kolff, W.J.: Clinical experience with one hundred twenty-one human kidney transplants. Amer. Surg. *33:* 304 (1967).

37. Kissmeyer-Nielsen, F.; Olsen, S.; Petersen, V.P. and Fjeldborg, O.: Hyperacute rejection of kidney allografts associated with pre-existing humoral antibodies against donor cells. Lancet *ii:* 662 (1966).

38. Kountz, S.L.; Williams, M.A.; Williams, P.L.; Kapros, C. and Dempster, W.J.: Mechanism of rejection of homotransplanted kidneys. Nature (Lond.) *199:* 257 (1963).

39. Kountz, S.L.; Laub, D.R. and Cohn, R.: Detecting and treating early renal homotransplant rejection. J. amer. med. Ass. *191:* 997 (1965).

40. Kuss, R.; Legraine, M.; Mathé, G.; Nedy, R. and Camey, M.: Homologous human kidney transplantation. Experience with six patients. Postgrad. med. J. *38:* 528 (1962).

41. Lee, H.M.; Hume, D.M.; Vredevoe, D.L.; Mickey, M.R. and Terasaki, P.I.: Serotyping for homotransplantation. IX. Evaluation of leukocyte antigen matching with the clinical course and rejection types. Transplantation *5:* 1040 (1967).

42. Lee, L. and Stetson, C.A.: The local and generalized Shwartzman phenomena. In: The inflammatory process, pp. 791–817 (Eds.) L. Grant and R.T. McCluskey (Academic Press, New York 1965).

43. Lerner, R.A.; Glassock, R.J. and Dixon, F.J.: The role of antiglomerular basement membrane antibody in the pathogenesis of human glomerulonephritis. J. exp. Med. *126:* 989 (1967).

44. Levey, R.H. and Medawar, P.B.: Nature and mode of action of antilymphocyte antiserum. Proc. nat. Acad. Sci. (U.S.A.) *56:* 1130 (1966).

45. Martin, D.C.; Goodwin, W.E.; Kaufman, J.J.; Mims, M.M.; Goldman, R.; Rubini, M. and Gonick, H.: Ninety-two kidney transplants: Results, lessons learned, future prospects. J. Urol. (in press, 1968).

46. Marchioro, T.L.; Porter, K.A.; Dickinson, T.C.; Faris, T.D. and Starzl, T.E.: Physiologic requirements for auxiliary liver homotransplantation. Surg. Gynec. Obstet. *121:* 17 (1965).

47. McGavic, J.D.; Knight, P.R.; Tomkiewicz, Z.M.; Alexandre, G.P.J. and Murray, J.E.: Analysis of mechanisms of drug induced tolerance in canine renal homotransplants. Surg. Forum *14:* 210 (1963).

48. Merrill, J.P.; Murray, J.E.; Harrison, J.H.; Friedman, E.A.; Dealy, J.B. and Dammin, G.J.: Successful homotransplantation of the kidney between non-identical twins. New Engl. J. Med. *262:* 1251 (1960).

49. Miller, J.F.A.P.: Immunological significance of the thymus of the adult mouse. Nature (Lond.) *195:* 1318 (1962).

50. Miller, J.F.A.P.: Effect of thymectomy in adult mice on immunological responsiveness. Nature (Lond.) *208:* 1337 (1965).

51. Monaco, A.P.; Wood, M.L. and Russell, P.S.: Effect of adult thymectomy on the recovery from immunological depression induced by heterologous antilymphocyte serum. Science *149:* 432 (1965).

52. Monaco, A.P.; Wood, M.L.; van der Werf, B.A. and Russell, P.S.: Effect of antilymphocyte serum in mice, dogs and man. In: Antilymphocytic Serum, pp. 111–134. (Eds.) Wolstenholme, G.E.W. and O'Connor, M. (J. and A. Churchill Ltd., London 1967).

53. Moore, F.D.; Birtch, A.G.; Dagher, F.; Veith, F.; Krisher, J.A.; Order, S.E.; Shucart, W.A.; Dammin, G.J. and Couch, N.P.: Immunosuppression and vascular insufficiency in liver transplantation. Ann. N.Y. Acad. Sci. *120:* 729 (1964).

54. Murray, J.E.; Sheil, A.G.R.; Moseley, R.; Knight, P.R.; McGavic, J.D. and Dammin, G.J.: Analysis of mechanism of immunosuppressive drugs in renal homotransplantation. Ann. Surg. *160:* 449 (1964).

55. Murray, J.E.; Wilson, R.E. and O'Connor, N.E.: Evaluation of long functioning human kidney transplants. Surg. Gynec. Obstet. *124:* 509 (1967).

56. O'Brien, J.P. and Hume, D.M.: Membranous glomerulonephritis in two human renal homotransplants. Ann. int. Med. *65:* 504 (1966).

57. Ogden, D.A.: Donor and recipient function two to four years after renal homotransplantation. A paired study of 28 cases. Ann. int. Med. *67:* 998 (1967).

58. Ogden, D.A.; Porter, K.A.; Terasaki, P.I.; Marchioro, T.L.; Holmes, J.H. and Starzl, T.E.: Chronic renal homograft function: Correlation with histology and lymphocyte antigen matching. Amer. J. Med. *43:* 837 (1967).

59. Petersen, V.P.; Olsen, S.; Kissmeyer-Nielsen, F. and Fjeldborg, O.: Transmission of glomerulonephritis from host to human kidney allotransplant. New Engl. J. Med. *275:* 1269 (1966).

60. Porter, K.A.; Andres, G.A.; Calder, M.W.; Dosseter, J.B.; Hsu, K.C.; Rendall, J.M.; Seegal, B.C. and Starzl, T.E.: Human renal transplants. II. Immunofluorescent and immunoferritin studies. Lab. Invest. *18:* 159 (1968).

61. Porter, K.A.; Rendall, J.M.; Stolinski, C.; Terasaki, P.I.; Marchioro, T.L. and Starzl, T.E.: Light and electron micrographic study of biopsies from 33 human renal allografts and an isograft 1 ¾ to 2 ½ years after transplantation. Ann. N.Y. Acad. Sci. *129:* 615 (1966).

62. Porter, K.A.: Pathological changes in transplanted kidneys. In: Experience in renal transplantation, pp. 299–359 (Ed.) T.E. Starzl (W.B. Saunders Co., Philadelphia 1964).

63. RAPAPORT, F.T.; DAUSSET, J.; HAMBURGER, J.; HUME, D.M.; KANO, K.; WILLIAMS, G.M. and MILGROM, F.: Serologic factors in human transplantation. Ann. Surg. *166:* 596 (1967).

64. RETIK, A.B.; HOLLENBERG, N.K.; ROSEN, S.M.; MERRILL, J.P. and MURRAY, J.E.: Cortical ischemia in renal allograft rejection. Surg. Gynec. Obstet. *124:* 989 (1967).

65. ROSEN, S.M.; RETIK, A.B.; HOLLENBERG, N.K.; MERRILL, J.P. and MURRAY, J.E.: Effect of immunosuppressive therapy on the intrarenal distribution of blood flow in dog renal allograft rejection. Surg. Forum *17:* 233 (1966).

66. SCHWARTZ, R.; SCHWARTZ, J.A.; ARMSTRONG, M.Y.K. and BELDOTTI, L.: Neoplastic sequelae of allogenic disease. I. Theoretical considerations and experimental design. Ann. N.Y. Acad. Sci. *129:* 804 (1966).

67. SHACKMAN, R.; DEMPSTER, W.J. and WRONG, O.M.: Kidney transplantation in the human. Brit. J. Urol. *35:* 222 (1963).

68. SHERMAN, J.D.: Effect of thymectomy on the golden hamster, III. Studies on adult thymectomized hamsters. J. lab. clin. Med. *67:* 273 (1966).

69. STARZL, T.E.: Experience in renal transplantation (W. B. Saunders Co., Philadelphia 1964).

70. STARZL, T.E.; BRETTSCHNEIDER, L. and GROTH, C.G.: Recent developments in liver transplantation. In: Advance in transplantation (Eds.) DAUSSET, J., HAMBURGER, J. and MATHÉ, G, pp. 633–637 (Munksgaard Ltd., Copenhagen 1968).

71. STARZL, T.E.; GROTH, C.G.; BRETTSCHNEIDER, L.; MOON, J.B.; FULGINITI, V.A.; COTTON, E.K. and PORTER, K.A.: Extended survival in three cases of orthotopic homotransplantation of the human liver. Surgery *63:* 549 (1968).

72. STARZL, T.E.; GROTH, C.G.; TERASAKI, P.I.; PUTNAM, C.W.; BRETTSCHNEIDER, L. and MARCHIORO, T.L.: Heterologous antilymphocyte globulin, histocompatibility matching, and human renal homotransplantation. Surg. Gynec. Obstet. *126:* 1023 (1968).

73. STARZL, T.E.; LERNER, R.A.; DIXON, F.J.; GROTH, C.G.; BRETTSCHNEIDER, L. and TERASAKI, P.I.: The Shwartzman reaction after human renal transplantation. New Engl. J. Med. *278:* 642 (1968).

74. STARZL, T.E.; MARCHIORO, T.L.; FARIS, T.D.; McCARDLE, R.J. and IWASAKI, Y.: Avenues of future research in homotransplantation of the liver: With particular reference to hepatic supportive procedures, antilymphocyte serum and tissue typing. Amer. J. Surg. *112:* 391 (1966).

75. STARZL, T.E.; MARCHIORO, T.L.; HERMANN, G.; BRITTAIN, R.S. and WADDELL, W.R.: Renal homografts in patients with major donor-recipient blood group incompatibilities (Addendum). Surgery *55:* 195 (1964).

76. STARZL, T.E.; MARCHIORO, T.L.; PORTER, K.A.; IWASAKI, Y. and CERILLI, G.J.: The use of heterologous antilymphoid agents in canine renal and liver homotransplantation, and in human renal homotransplantation. Surg. Gynec. Obstet. *124:* 301 (1967).

77. STARZL, T.E.; MARCHIORO, T.L.; RIFKIND, D.; HOLMES, J.H.; ROWLANDS, D.T., Jr. and WADDELL, W.R.: Factors in successful renal transplantation. Surgery *56:* 296 (1964).

78. STARZL, T.E.; MARCHIORO, T.L.; TERASAKI, P.I.; PORTER, K.A.; FARIS, T.D.; HERRMANN, T.J.; VREDEVOE, D.L.; HUTT, M.P.; OGDEN, D.A. and WADDELL, W.R.: Chronic survival after human renal homotransplantation. Ann. Surg. *162:* 749 (1965).

79. STARZL, T.E.; MARCHIORO, T.L.; TALMAGE, D.W. and WADDELL, W.R.: Splenectomy and thymectomy in human renal homotransplantation. Proc. Soc. exp. biol. Med. *113:* 929 (1963).

80. STARZL, T.E.; MARCHIORO, T.L.; VON KAULLA, K.; HERMANN, G.; BRITTAIN, R.S. and WADDELL, W.R.: Homotransplantation of the liver in humans. Surg. Gynec. Obstet. *117:* 659 (1963).

81. STARZL, T.E.; PORTER, K.A.; IWASAKI, Y.; MARCHIORO, T.L. and KASHIWAGI, N.: The use of antilymphocyte globulin in human renal homotransplantation. In: Antilymphocytic serum, pp. 4–34. (Eds.) WOLSTENHOLME, G.E.W. and O'CONNOR, M. (J. and A. Churchill Ltd., London 1967).

82. STARZL, T.E.; MARCHIORO, T.L. and WADDELL, W.R.: The reversal of rejection in human renal homografts with subsequent development of homograft tolerance. Surg. Gynec. Obstet. *117:* 385 (1963).

83. STICKEL, D.L.; AMOS, D.B.; ZMIJEWSKI, C.M.; GLENN, J.F. and ROBINSON, R.R.: Human renal transplantation with donor selection by leucocyte typing. Transplantation *5:* 1024 (1967).

84. SUBRAMANIAN, V. and GANS, H.: Impaired reticuloendothelial function following extracorporeal circulation and its relationship to blood trauma. Arch. Surg. *97:* 330 (1968).

85. SZULMAN, A.E.: The histological distribution of the blood group substances A and B in man. J. exp. Med. *111:* 785 (1960).

86. TAYLOR, R.B.: Decay of immunological responsiveness after thymectomy in adult life. Nature (Lond.) *208:* 1334 (1965).

87. TERASAKI, P.I.; MARCHIORO, T.L. and STARZL, T.E.: Sero-typing of human lymphocyte antigens: Preliminary trials on long-term kidney homograft survivors. In: Histocompatibility testing, pp. 83–95 Nat. Acad. Sci. (National Research Council, Washington, D.C. 1965).

88. TERASAKI, P.I.; PORTER, K.A.; MARCHIORO, T.L.; MICKEY, M.R.; VREDEVOE, D.L.; FARIS, T.D. and STARZL, T.E.: Serotyping for homotransplantation. VII. Selection of kidney donors for 32 recipients. Ann. N.Y. Acad. Sci. *129:* 500 (1966).

89. TERASAKI, P.I.; TRASHER, D.L. and HAUBER, T.M.: Serotyping for homotransplantation. XIII. Immediate kidney transplant rejection and associated preformed antibodies. In: Advance in transplantation, pp. 225–229 (Munksgaard, Copenhagen 1968).

90. TERASAKI, P.I.; VREDEVOE, D.L. and MICKEY, M.R.: Serotyping for homotransplantation. X. Survival of 196 grafted kidneys subsequent to typing. Transplantation *5:* 1057 (1967).

91. TERASAKI, P.I.; VREDEVOE, D.L.; PORTER, K.A.; MICKEY, M.R.; MARCHIORO, T.L.; FARIS, T.D.; HERRMANN, T.J. and STARZL, T.E.: Serotyping for homotransplantation. V. Evaluation of a matching scheme. Transplantation *4:* 688 (1966).

92. THOMAS, L. and GOOD, R.A.: The effect of cortisone on the Shwartzman reaction. J. exp. Med. *95:* 409 (1952).

93. VAN ROOD, J.J., VAN LEEUWEN, A.; SCHIPPERS, A.; CEPPELLINI, R.; MATTIUZ, P.L. and CURTONI, S.: Leucocyte groups and their relation to homotransplantation. Ann. N.Y. Acad. Sci. *129:* 467 (1966).

94. VON KAULLA, K.N.; VON KAULLA, E.; WASANTAPRUCK, K.S.; MARCHIORO, T.L. and STARZL, T.E.: Blood coagulation in uremic patients before and after hemodialysis and transplantation of the kidney. Arch. Surg. *92:* 184 (1966).

95. WAKSMAN, B.H.; ARBOUYS, S. and ARNASON, B.G.: The use of specific "lymphocyte antisera" to inhibit hypersensitivity reactions of the delayed type. J. exp. Med. *114:* 997 (1961).

96. WILLIAMS, G.M.; LEE, H.M.; WEYMOUTH, R.F.; HARLAN, W.R.; Jr.; HOLDEN, K.R.; STANLEY, C.M.; MILLINGTON, G.A. and HUME, D.M.: Studies in hyperacute and chronic renal homograft rejection in man. Surgery *62:* 204 (1967).

97. WILLIAMS, G.M.; HUME, D.M.; KANO, K. and MILGROM, F.: Acute vasculitis in human renal transplants (Personal communication, January 6, 1968).

 98. WILLIAMS, G.M.; WHITE, H.J.O. and HUME, D.M.: Factors influencing the long-term functional success rate of human renal allografts. Transplantation *5:* 837 (1967).
 99. WILSON, W.E.C. and KIRKPATRICK, C.H.: Immunological aspects of renal homo-transplantation. In: Experience in renal transplantation, pp. 239–261 (Ed.) STARZL, T.E. (W.B. Saunders Co., Philadelphia 1964).
100. WOLSTENHOLME, G.E.W. and O'CONNOR, M. (Eds.): Antilymphocytic serum (J. and A. Churchill Ltd., London 1967).
101. WOODRUFF, M.F.: Experience with transplantation of the kidney in man. Ann. roy. Coll. Surg. Engl. *39:* 178 (1966).
102. WOODRUFF, M.F.A. and ANDERSON, N.F.: Effect of lymphocyte depletion by thoracic duct fistula and administration of antilymphocyte serum on the survival of skin homografts in rats. Nature (Lond.) *200:* 702 (1963).
103. WOODRUFF, M.F.A. and WOODRUFF, H.G.: The transplantation of tissue: with special reference to auto- and homotransplants of thyroid and spleen in the anterior chamber of the eye, and subcutaneously, in guinea pigs. Phil. Trans. B *234:* 559 (1950).

Authors' address: Prof. Dr. T.E. STARZL, Dr. C.G. GROTH, Dr. L. BRETTSCHNEIDER, Dr. G.V. SMITH, Dr. I. PENN and Dr. N. KASHIWAGI, Department of Surgery, University of Colorado School of Medicine and Veterans Administration Hospital, *Denver, Col.* (USA).

Antibiotica et Chemotherapia, vol. 15, pp. 384–392 (Karger, Basel/New York 1969)

Studies on the Mode of Action of Immunosuppressive Ribonucleases

J. F. Mowbray, A. W. Boylston, J. D. Milton and M. Weksler

Department of Experimental Pathology, St. Mary's Hospital Medical School,
London

Since the original description of a fraction of plasma protein from normal animals which had immunosuppressive properties [Mowbray, 1963] it has been found that this fraction contains a ribonuclease. This ribonuclease (RNase) is apparently distinct from other known RNases, of which the best studied, pancreatic ribonuclease A, does not have immunosuppressive activity. It has been possible to purify the enzyme and demonstrate that the immunosuppressive activity cannot be separated from the enzyme activity [Mowbray, 1967]. Mowbray and Scholand have shown that a series of immunosuppressive complexes of pancreatic RNase can be prepared, when the enzyme is covalently linked to a carrier protein [Mowbray and Scholand, 1966]. Of these complexes the one which has been most extensively studied is the polymer of pancreatic RNase (Poly-RNase). The trimer poly-RNase is the most immunosuppressive, and this paper describes the properties of trimer ribonuclease prepared by conjugation with difluorodintitrobenzene. The properties of all the immunosuppressive RNases are very similar, and this represents only an example of them. The finding by Mannick and his colleagues that the serum enzyme fraction inhibited phytohaemagglutinin transformation of lymphocytes *in vitro* suggested a method for investigating the immunosuppressive action of the RNases [Mannick, 1967].

Materials and Methods

Preparation of polyribonuclease. 100 mg of bovine pancreatic RNase (Koch Light 4X recryst.) were dissolved in 40 ml 0.1 M Na_2CO_3 at room temperature. To the solution 1.25 ml of a 1% solution of difluorodintitrobenzene in methanol was added rapidly. The mixture was left without stirring for 50 min and then 2.0 ml of 4M sodium acetate buffer pH 5 added. The mixture could then be left overnight for chromatography the next day. Just before application to the column the solution was adjusted to pH 10 by the addition of 1M NaOH. The sample was applied to a 3 × 40 cm column of Sephadex G100 in 0.05M glycine/0.04M NaOH buffer. The chromatographic peaks were identified by monitoring the column effluent at 280 mμ, and each peak concentrated by ultrafiltration. In some preparations, in order to produce high yields of monomer and high molecular weight fractions, the amount of coupling agent was varied. With the standard amount of coupling agent the yield of trimer ribonuclease was 70–85%.

Lymphocyte cultures. 2 ml cultures were used containing 2×10^6 lymphocytes, prepared by gelatin sedimentation of defibrinated human blood [Coulson and Chalmers, 1964]. The culture medium was composed of tris buffered Eagle's medium (3.2 ml 0.1M tris/HCl pH 7.2, 96.8 ml Eagle's medium) containing 20% autologous gelatin serum with added penicillin G and streptomycin. The cultures were maintained in tightly stoppered bijou bottles and phytohaemagglutinin (Burroughs Wellcome), mumps antigen [Eli Lilly] and purified protein derivative [Parke Davis] added as necessary. Incorporation of tritiated nucleic acid precursors was measured one hour after addition to the cultures. The cells were washed, and the nucleic acid precipitated with 10% trichloracetic acid. The precipitate, washed with methanol, was dissolved in formic acid/methanol prior to addition to a toluene/PPO/dimethyl POPOP scintillator. The radioactivity of the samples was measured in a Packard Tricarb liquid scintillation spectrometer.

Haemagglutinin assay. Mice were injected intravenously with 0.1 ml 10% washed sheep red cells, and bled six days later. The haemagglutinin titres were determined by the serial dilution technique previously described [Mowbray and Hargrave, 1966].

Anti-sheep red cell plaque assay. The spleens of the immunised mice were removed three days after injection of sheep cells, and the cells prepared from them by gentle teasing in 10 ml of Ringer's solution. 3 ml plates were poured in 9 cm petri dishes, each containing 1.0 ml of cell suspension, 0.5 ml 20% sheep cells and 1.5 ml 1.5% Difco agar. After 2 h incubation at 37°C, the plaques were developed by the addition of 0.5 ml fresh human serum and further incubation for 30 min. The counts were expressed as plaques per million nucleated cells from the spleen cell preparations.

Results

Inhibition of lymphocyte transformation in phytohaemagglutinin (PHA) cultures. It was found that addition of Poly-RNase to stimulated cultures at the start of the culture produced a decrease in ^{3}H-thymidine incorporation at three days which was arithmetically related to the dose of enzyme added to the culture (fig. 1). The same degree of inhibition was found when the enzyme was added up to 24 h after the PHA (table I). When the cells were incubated with Poly-RNase for 24 h, and then, after 24 h culture in medium without enzyme, cultured in

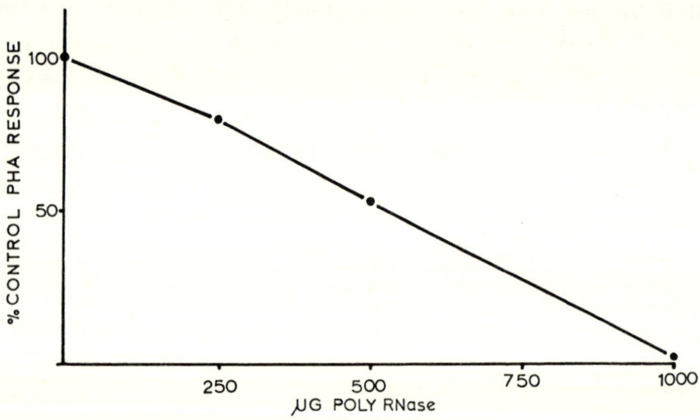

Fig. 1. Effect of increasing doses of trimer Poly-RNase on the uptake of tritiated thymidine in PHA stimulated human peripheral lymphocyte cultures.

Table I. Effect of addition of Poly-RNase to lymphocyte cultures at varying times after PHA.

Time of adding poly-RNase (h)	%inhibition of PHA response
0	98
3	97
6	96
13.5	95.5
24	85

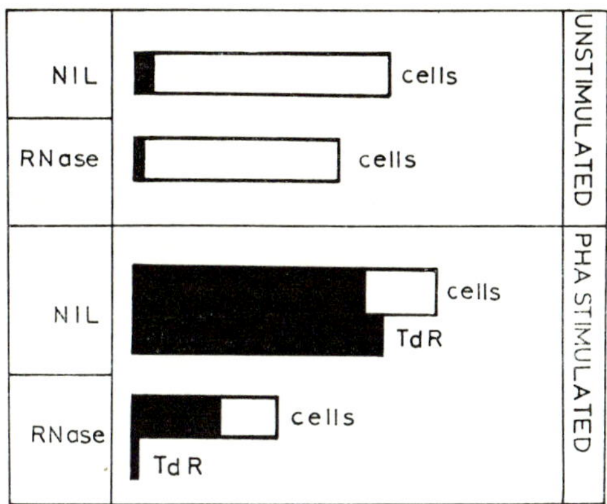

Fig. 2. Effect of addition of Poly-RNase on cell survival and thymidine incorporation in human lymphocyte cultures. Total cell count histograms have shaded areas to represent the fraction of large cells. Diminished total survival of cells in treated PHA cultures is by loss of large cell component. Surviving large cells incorporate practically no thymidine.

Table II. Morphological transformation, thymidine and uridine uptake of PHA cultures which had had 24 hours prior culture with Poly-RNase. The Poly-RNase was removed and the cultures incubated in medium alone for a further 24 h before addition of PHA.

	Preincubation	
	NO RNase	RNase
% Large cells	41 %	42 %
Thymidine incorporation (C.P.M./10^6 cells)	92	153
Uridine incorporation (C.P.M./10^6 cells)	175	320

the presence of PHA without Poly-RNase, normal transformation occurred (table II). However it will be seen from figure 2 that there was a considerable death of cells in the treated PHA cultures, whereas this was only seen to a limited degree in the unstimulated cultures treated by the addition of Poly-RNase. There was also an increase in the survival of small lymphocytes in treated PHA cultures in some experiments. Thus it seems that the addition of Poly-RNase results in the death of many cells after transformation, and some depression of transformation as well, as shown by the persistence of morphologically untransformed small lymphocytes. Attempts were made to measure the direct toxicity of Poly-RNase on cells which had been allowed to transform with PHA before addition of the enzyme. Figure 3 shows that the death of transformed and normal lymphocytes

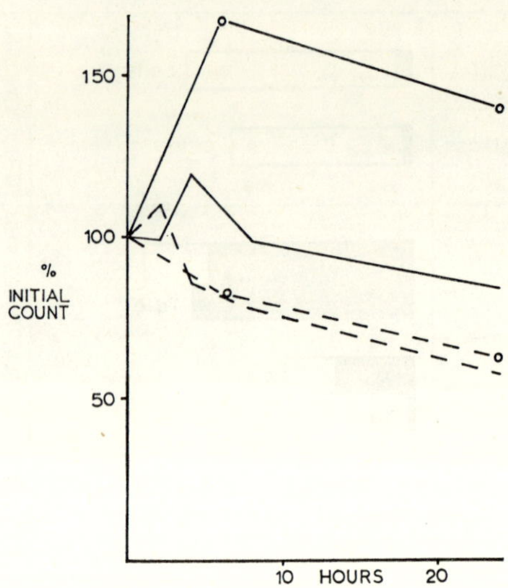

Fig. 3. Survival of PHA transformed cells (solid lines) and small lymphocytes (broken lines) with added Poly-RNase and without (open circles). There is no evidence for a differential toxicity of Poly-RNase on small or transformed lymphocytes. Multiplication of transformed cells is diminished by Poly-RNase.

is the same when Poly-RNase is added. Thus it appears that the death of transformed cells is associated with changes which occur close to the time of transformation, and not toxicity on the established transformed cell.

It has been found that poly-RNase also inhibits the stimulation of lymphocyte cultures with antigen. Figure 4 shows that the inhibition

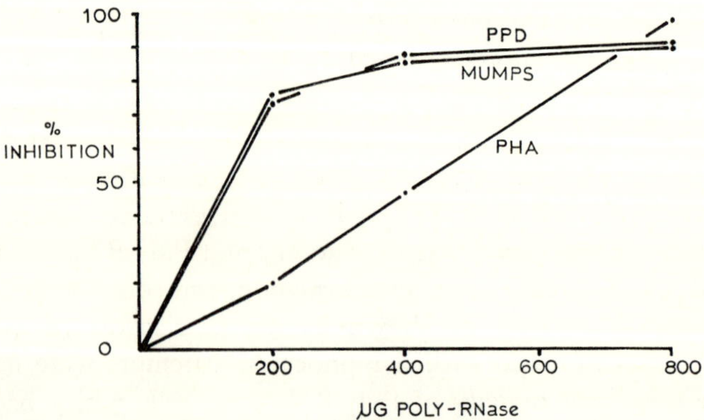

Fig. 4. Difference in dose/response for inhibition of thymidine incorporation in cultures stimulated by PHA or antigen.

of stimulation both by PPD and mumps antigens shows similar dose responses for both, and this is different from that found with PHA. A much greater sensitivity at low doses to poly-RNase is shown by the antigen cultures than the PHA cultures, and the response curve is not arithmetic in antigen cultures. Inhibition of mixed lymphocyte cultures has also been demonstrated in the presence of Poly-RNase, but to date dose response curves have not been obtained.

Figure 5 shows that there is a difference in efficacy of suppression with different sizes of polymer in different poly-RNase preparations. In addition it is shown that this difference occurs with both PHA cultures and the response to sheep red cells in the mouse. The finding that monomeric RNase is quite ineffective in either system has been a very consistent finding. The most effective size of polymer appears to be trimer, although some other polymers do show some activity. Recent studies have shown that trimer Poly-RNase is only effective

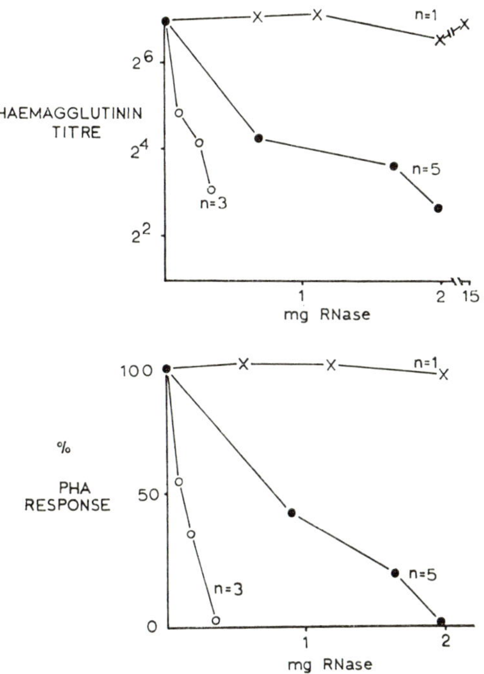

Fig. 5. Difference in efficacy of monomeric, trimeric and pentameric Poly-RNase on inhibition of immune response to sheep red cells in mice (top), and inhibition of thymidine incorporation in PHA stimulated human lymphocyte cultures (bottom). N=polymer number.

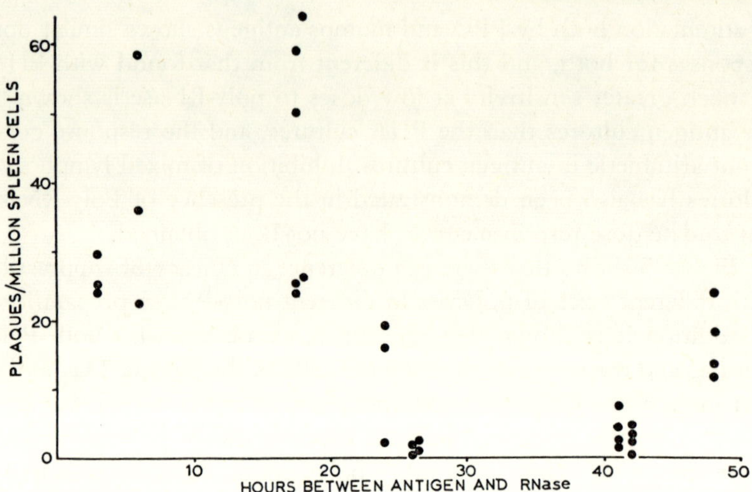

Fig. 6. Effect of Poly-RNase injection after the antigen on the number of plaque forming cells in spleens of mice three days after challenge with sheep red cells.

in suppressing the haemagglutinin response in the mouse if the preparation is soluble at neutrality, and it also seems that this is true in the lymphocyte cultures.

Previous experiments have shown that the optimal time of an injection of Poly-RNase or other forms of immunosuppressive RNase was either sixteen or one hundred hours before the antigen [Boylston, Mowbray and Ackermann, 1967]. The results presented above suggest that it should be possible to suppress the immune response in the intact animal by exposure to poly-RNase at the time when transformation occurs in response to the antigen. Figure 6 demonstrates that there is good suppression of plaque formation when the poly-RNase is given 26 to 42 h after the antigen. This timing of an immunosuppressive effect was not suspected until tested as a result of the culture findings.

Discussion

Our studies have shown that there appear to be three criteria for the immunosuppressive action of a ribonuclease preparation: (1) The size of the molecule must be greater than that of pancreatic ribonuclease A; (2) the preparation must be soluble at neutrality; (3) the enzyme activity of the preparation must be preserved.

The culture experiments show that the action of poly-RNase on lymphocytes seems to be on the cell at or near the time of transformation. The small lymphocyte is not apparently markedly affected, and pretreatment of small lymphocytes does not prevent their subsequent stimulation by PHA after the Poly-RNase has been removed. This should imply, if these results can be translated to the intact mouse, that the optimal time for exposure to the poly-RNase, in order to produce immunosuppression, should be after the injection of antigen, when transformation is occurring; we have shown that this time is an effective one. However the presence of two further periods of immunosuppression when the Poly-RNase is given before the antigen has been found previously [MOWBRAY, BOYLSTON and ACKERMANN, 1967]. These timings cannot be explained by the present study as an action on lymphocytes. This is because it has been shown that the cell will recover from culture in the presence of poly-RNase so that it can respond to stimulation, and injection simultaneously with the antigen does not produce immunosuppression. The difference in dose response curve for PHA and antigen stimulated cultures, presumably because of the participation of the phagocytic cells as well as lymphocytes, may suggest that there is an effect of poly-RNase on phagocytic cells. This effect, if present, might be responsible for different optimum timings of immunosuppression in the mouse. Alternatively the culture experiments in an artificial system with a PHA stimulus on human cells may not in all respects be comparable with antigenic stimulation of antigen sensitive cells in the intact mouse. Some of these problems may be resolved by studying the kinetics of antigen stimulated cultures suppressed with poly-RNase in the same way that has been done with PHA cultures.

The unusual findings of an arithmetic dose response for inhibition of PHA induced transformation suggests a stoichometric effect in which each cell should have only one binding site for enzyme, and that combination with this site would block the ability of the cell to respond to PHA. This seems unlikely because the same dose of poly-RNase blocks two million cells in culture and the response of a whole mouse. This suggests that the effect of a dose is dependent on concentration and not total amount, as the volumes of distribution in the culture and the mouse blood after an intravenous injection are comparable. This similarity of dose may be coincidental, but has occurred with several different types of immunosuppressive RNase. The difference in sensitivity between antigen and PHA stimulated cultures could also be related to enzyme concentration, as the poly-RNase may be carried in phagocytic cells so that when they interact with lymphocytes the local concentration may be higher than in the culture as a whole.

Summary

The study of the immunosuppressive action of RNase preparations in cell cultures has shown that the effect of lymphocytes appears to be one on the cell about the time of transformation. The unstimulated small lymphocyte is not irreversibly affected by RNases, but the recently transformed cell dies rapidly or fails to synthesise DNA.

Exposure of the mouse to polyribonuclease at the time of lymphocyte transformation after antigen injection produces immunosuppression. There is a good correlation between the dose of RNase which suppresses 2 ml human lymphocyte cultures and intact mice.

For immunosuppression ribonucleases must be soluble at neutrality, have the enzyme activity preserved, and have a size greater than that of pancreatic ribonuclease.

Acknowledgement

This work was supported in part by grants from the Medical Research Council and the Eleanor Countess Peel Trust.

References

BOYLSTON, A.W.; MOWBRAY, J.F. and ACKERMANN, J.R.W.: Immunosuppression by ribonucleases. Adv. Transplant., p. 189 (Munksgaard, Copenhagen 1967).

MANNICK, J.A.: Personal communication.

MOWBRAY, J.F.: Ability of an alpha$_2$ glycoprotein to inhibit antibody production. Immunology 7: 217 (1963).

MOWBRAY, J.F.: Immunosuppressive action of ribonucleases. Tissue and Organ Transplantation (Ed.) K.A. Porter Brit. med. Ass. (1967).

MOWBRAY, J.F. and SCHOLAND, J.: Inhibition of antibody production by ribonucleases. Immunology 11: 421 (1966).

Authors' address: Dr. J.F. MOWBRAY, Dr. A.W. BOYLSTON, Dr. J.D. MILTON and Dr. M. WEKSLER, Department of Experimental Pathology, St. Mary's Hospital Medical School, London (England).

Antibiotica et Chemotherapia, vol. 15, pp. 393–406 (Karger, Basel/New York 1969)

Immunodepression by Viruses

M. H. Salaman

Department of Pathology, Royal College of Surgeons, London

Introduction

In view of the vast labour expended on examination of immune reactions to viruses and their products, and of the cellular antigens they induce or uncover, it is surprising that so little attention had been given, until the last few years, to the possibility that some of them may affect the immune system itself.

Suppression of the tuberculin reaction during attacks of measles has been known for 60 years or more. Many other diseases, not certainly virus-induced, have long been known to be associated with defects of the immune system. A new interest in the specific effects of viruses on immunity is evident from recent work, which is growing rapidly in volume.

I shall first review what is known about immune depression by the non-oncogenic viruses.

Non-Oncogenic Viruses

Von Pirquet [47] noticed that tuberculin-positive children became negative a few days before a measles rash appeared and later reverted, and that tuberculosis became more active after measles. He also noticed disappearance of the symptoms of chronic nephritis during measles. Scarlet fever, epidemic meningitis, typhoid fever, and rubella did not affect the tuberculin response.

The effect of measles has been often confirmed, and further analysed with the help of the Mantoux test and the use of measles vaccine and immune γ-globulin [36, 13, 63]. Tuberculin insensitivity may appear one to three weeks before a measles rash and persist for an average of 18 days. In a recent series measles virus was added to peripheral lymphocytes of tuberculous children [60]: blast formation in the presence of tuberculin PPD was depressed in all of six cases. In one, the virus-treated lymphocytes were incubated with phyto-haemagglutinin (PHA) and were found to be fully responsive. In infants with congenital rubella, excretion of virus may persist for up to 18 months, and serum IgM levels are often elevated, while IgG levels are either depressed or normal [1, 3, 61]. There is no gross defect in antibody synthesis to rubella or to other antigens. The most striking change is failure of peripheral lymphocytes of these patients to respond to PHA *in vitro* [41, 44, 22]. Lymphocytes from patients with varicella, measles, pertussis, and undiagnosed fevers responded normally. Normal lymphocytes treated *in vitro* with rubella virus or Newcastle disease virus (NDV) did not respond to PHA. NDV has also been shown to reduce antibody production by sensitized rabbit spleen cells *in vitro* [35].

There is one old report [11] of suppression of tuberculin sensitivity during attacks of influenza, and recently it was shown [33] that treatment of sheep erythrocyte-sensitized mouse spleen cells *in vitro* with the PR8 strain of influenza virus reduced the number of haemolytic plaque-forming cells (PFC) among them, as estimated by the JERNE method [30], by about one half.

Oncogenic Viruses

In 1960 OLD *et al.* [43], in the course of a review of the behaviour of the reticuloendothelial system in neoplastic disease, made a passing reference to the fact, not previously reported, that FRIEND virus [26] depresses the haemolysin response to sheep erythrocytes (SE) and lowers properdin levels in mice.

The group of leukaemogenic viruses to which Friend virus (FV) belongs induce in mice of some strains a disease which has been compared to DI GUGLIELMO's erythroleukaemia in man (see [57] for clinical description).

My colleagues and I at the London Hospital had a twofold reason for interest in an immune depression by Friend virus. Firstly, as oncologists we were struck by the fact that an oncogenic virus has the property of immune depression in common with many chemical and physical oncogenic agents [10, 2]. As you know it is an assumption common to several theories of oncogenesis that a degree of inadequacy of the immune system is a necessary, though probably not a sufficient, cause of neoplastic growth [e.g. 48]. We need to know a lot more than we do about the mechanism of the immunodepressive action of oncogens, and the timing and persistence of this effect in relation to the appearance, persistence, and spread of neoplastic cells in the body.

Secondly, as virologists, and as immunologists perforce, we were interested in the site of attack of the virus: whether immune depression and malignant transformation were effects occurring in the same or in different cells, and at the same or at different times, and whether there was a connection between immune depression and the induction or uncovering of new cellular antigens. With regard to the last question, it now seems certain that viral-induced antigenic changes are not confined to neoplastic cells [29, 12, 64, 65].

Among oncogenic viruses, those that induce various neoplastic diseases of the blood-forming tissues of mice and rats have received most attention. Let us take first those that induce lymphoid leukaemia similar to the commonest type of spontaneous murine leukaemia. AK strain mice have an 80–90% spontaneous incidence of lymphoid leukaemia at 6 to 12 months, and are known to carry a virus, "Passage A", isolated by GROSS in 1951 [28], which induces a similar disease when injected into low-leukaemic mice or rats.

METCALF and MOULDS [38] have shown that proliferation of PFC in the spleens of AK mice after an injection of SE is delayed, slightly during the preleukaemic period and much more severely when they are overtly leukaemic.

GOOD *et al.* [45, 23] found that mice of a low-leukaemic strain injected with Passage A virus at three to four days of age, and tested about two months later (i.e. before overt leukaemia appeared), formed less antibody against T_2 phage than controls, and were unable to reject allogeneic skin grafts with a non-H_2 histocompatibility difference.

MOLONEY virus [40] is another lymphoid leukaemogen. It was isolated from the old, many-times-transplanted, murine Sarcoma 37. CREMER *et al.* [18, 19] found that this virus, injected into newborn rats, depressed haemagglutinin and haemolysin production to SE, and that IgA and IgG (but not IgM) production was reduced, from the fourth week after injection onwards. These changes began before leukaemia was detectable, though viraemia was already present.

In our hands Moloney virus (MLV) in mice has caused a variable immune depression during the later preleukaemic period, not appreciable till the sixth week or later. Overtly leukaemic animals, however, usually show a definite depression.

The class of murine viruses which includes Friend virus (FV) have a more rapid action. Infected mice develop splenomegaly, which may be detected at two weeks or less. In the spleen there is great proliferation of erythroblasts and stem cells, loss of lymphocytes, and multiple haemorrhages which often lead to death by rupture of the spleen. In survivors of the acute stage there is infiltration of other organs by erythroblasts and stem cells, and lymphoid or myeloid leukaemia may develop later. RAUSCHER [50], STANSLY [62], and KIRSTEN [31] viruses, and "UL" virus isolated in our laboratory from a urethane-induced leukaemia [53, 55], all belong to this class, though they show minor differences. Besides their rapid action they have the advantage over the lymphoid leukaemogenic viruses that adults are fully susceptible, so that the earliest effects of the virus can be looked for in immunologically mature animals.

During the past two years ODAKA et al. [42] and FRIEDMAN et al. [15, 16] have tested Friend virus, we have tested Friend, Rauscher, and UL viruses, and GELZER and DIETRICH [27] and SIEGEL and MORTON [58, 59] Rauscher virus, using SE or bovine albumen as antigens, and serum antibody titres and/or PFC formation in the spleen as test reactions.

In spite of differences of viruses and techniques used there is a fair measure of agreement. All report that these viruses, when injected into adult mice before a primary injection of antigen, significantly depress antibody titres; those who used the Jerne technique observed a similar reduction in PFC counts. Both IgM and IgG production were affected. Slight (barely significant) depression of peak responses was seen when the virus was injected on the same day as the antigen, little or none when it was injected one day after; but whatever the timing, mice in the terminal stage of the disease always showed immune depression. Though Friend virus injected after antigen had little or no effect on serum antibody level, virus injected four days before the 2nd of two injections of SE separated by five weeks depressed the secondary response even more than the primary, and here also IgM and IgG were both affected.

Analysis of the Immunodepressive Effects of Friend Virus

In recent years we have tried to define the characteristics of this immune depression. Much of this work, including all the Jerne tests, was done by Mrs. WEDDERBURN. Dr. BENDINELLI and I are responsible for part, and we collaborated in some experiments with Drs. G. L. ASHERSON and Dr. D. R. BAINBRIDGE [54, 66, 56, 68, 67].

Preliminary tests showed no qualitative differences in immune depressive effect between two different strains of FV, Rauscher virus, and UL virus.

As a control we chose a non-oncogenic virus with a rather similar proliferative behaviour in mice to the FV group: the plasma lactate dehydrogenase-elevating virus (LDV) of RILEY [51]. LDV was found to have no depressive effect on haemagglutinin titres to SE: in fact it enhanced them slightly when injected on Day –1 or Day –3, but not when injected on Day –7 or Day +1. This is of interest in itself, in view of a recent report [37] that LDV, when injected into mice one day before unaggregated human γ-globulin, acts as an adjuvant, converting the response from tolerance to antibody production, but when injected 10 days before or 11 days after the antigen it is ineffective.

As further controls we tested immune responses after injecting the following, four days before an injection of SE: (a) Formolized FV; (b) live FV into a resistant strain of mice (C_{57} Black); (c) live Moloney virus (MLV); (d) normal spleen extract.

No depression of serum titre and/or PFC count was observed. In the case of MLV, as mentioned above, though no depression is detectable at four days it develops later.

The two strains of Friend virus available to us induce slightly different diseases. In one, erythropoiesis outstrips red cell destruction, resulting in polycythaemia; in the other, the opposite happens, resulting in anaemia [39]. For further work we chose the anaemia-inducing variant, which is the one most workers have used.

Balb/c mice, two to three months old, were used. Injection of both virus and antigen was intravenous. Haemolysin and haemagglutinin production after injections of SE were measured by conventional methods. The numbers of PFC cells per spleen were measured by the JERNE technique [30].

Figure 1 shows seventh day titres of haemagglutinin to SE in mice inoculated with FV at intervals from four days before to four days after the antigen. Depression is definite if the virus is injected from –4 to –1 days, but not significant if injected later.

Figure 2 records a similar test in which numbers of PFC per spleen were counted. By this more sensitive method a depression, which is significant, is observed when virus is injected between Day –7 and Day 0. A slight depression by virus injected on Day +1 is probably not significant. Injecting the virus earlier than Day –7 did not increase the depression, but there was a further drop when it was injected so early that the antigen was given in the terminal stage of the disease.

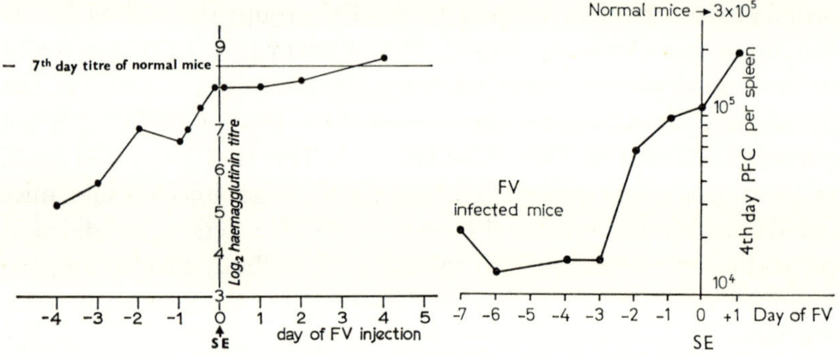

Fig. 1. 7th day—serum haemagglutinin titres against sheep erythrocytes (SE) related to interval between Friend virus (FV) and primary SE injection.

Fig. 2. 4th day—haemolytic plaque cell (PFC) (presumptive IgM) production related to interval between FV and primary SE injection.

Depression is inversely related to antigen dose, but is not abolished by a very large dose. Different doses of virus injected on the same day have effects directly dependent on dose, but a dose too small to produce a depression when injected at –4 days is active if injected earlier, though its effect does not equal that of a large dose injected at –4 days.

In order to trace the appearance of presumptive IgM and IgG antibody producing cells, respectively, we used a development of the Jerne method due to DRESSER and WORTIS [25]. By counting PFC on Jerne plates with and without the addition of an anti-mouse globulin serum (AMIgS) (for which we are grateful to Dr. DRESSER) the numbers of cells producing presumptive IgM and IgG is estimated [67].

Normal and infected mice produce IgM cells (fig. 3) in similar numbers for the first two days after antigen (at any rate no difference could be detected by this method), but then the counts diverge, and at the peak on Day +4 there is a 15 fold depression of the infected PFC count.

IgG cells, on the other hand, are not detectable till after Day +2 (fig. 4), and from their first appearance there is a depression of the count in infected spleens which reaches 15 fold at the peak and increases thereafter.

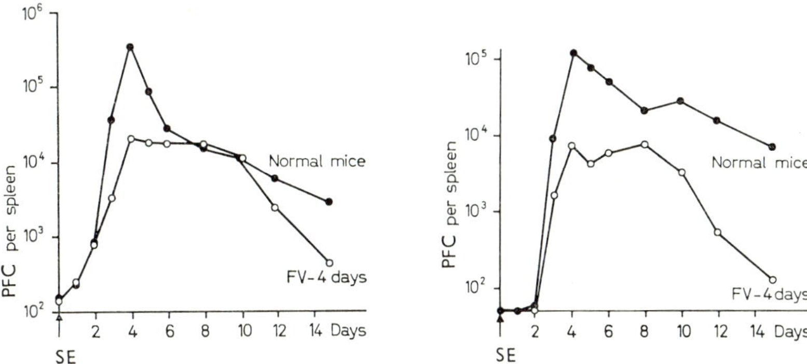

Fig. 3. PFC (presumptive IgM) counts after primary injection of SE in normal and FV-infected mice.

Fig. 4. PFC (presumptive IgG) counts after primary injection of SE in normal and FV-infected mice.

The delay in onset of depression of the IgM PFC count is not shortened by injecting the virus earlier than Day –4, though it can be lengthened somewhat by injecting the virus later than this. BENDINELLI has shown [4] that when a large dose of FV, such as was used in these tests, is injected intravenously into Balb/c mice, splenic virus content reaches a maximum four days later. The delay of immune depression cannot therefore be due to the virus not having reached a sufficient titre in the spleen when the antigen is injected.

The effect of FV on a secondary response was examined (figs. 5 and 6). Two injections of SE were separated by five weeks, and FV was injected four days before the second. IgM counts of both normal and infected spleens have risen by Day +1, the former more than the latter, and depression of the infected spleen cell count increases

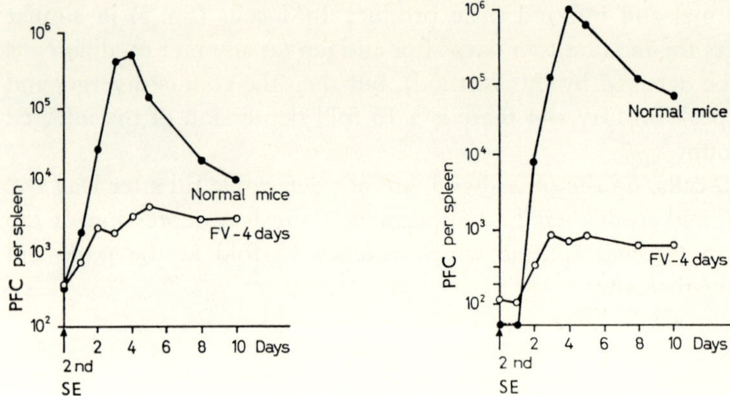

Fig. 5. PFC (presumptive IgM) counts after secondary (five weeks post primary) injection of SE in normal and FV-infected mice.

Fig. 6. PFC (presumptive IgG) counts after secondary (five weeks post primary) injection of SE in normal and FV-infected mice.

to 100 fold at the peak on Day 4. IgG counts have not risen by Day $+1$, but on Day $+2$ there is a large increase in the normal and a much smaller one in the infected spleens, and thereafter depression increases to 1000 fold at the peak at four days. Thus there is no detectable delay of depression of either IgM or IgG cell counts in the secondary response.

The delay in onset of depression of IgM cell production in the primary response is an intriguing phenomenon. In the next figure (fig. 7) the first five days of the primary response are recorded by more closely spaced observations. It clearly shows that IgM PFC

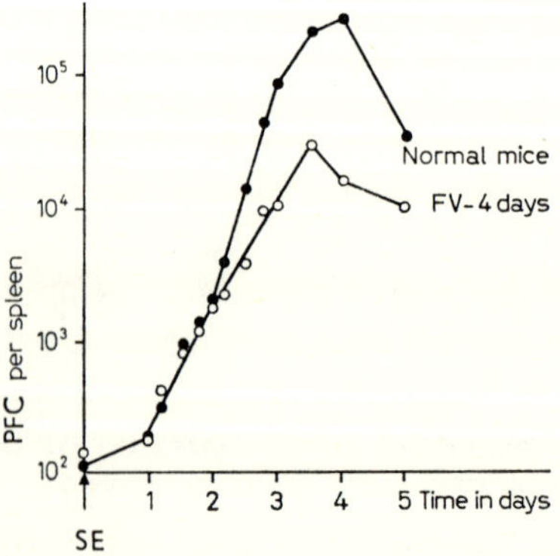

Fig. 7. As figure 3 but with more closely spaced observations.

Table I. Mean plaque-forming cells per spleen

2 days after SE			3 days after SE		
FV 4 days before SE	Uninfected	p of difference	FV 4 days before SE	Uninfected	p of difference
2,520	2,935	> 0.1	10,800	88,800	< 0.01

PFC (presumptive IgM) counts on 2nd and 3rd days after SE in normal and FV-infected mice.

counts in infected and normal spleens remain closely similar for the first 48 h, by which time there is already a 15 fold increase from background, and only then begin to diverge. Table I, which records representative results from a similar experiment, includes estimates of probability.

These observations on the timing of immune depression in primary and secondary responses have not yet been confirmed elsewhere. Taken at face value they suggest that an early stage of IgM response is resistant to FV, and that this stage does not occur, or is masked, in the secondary response.

We have made a few more relevant observations to which I will refer briefly.

Bendinelli and Wedderburn [9, 6] using a modification of the Bussard technique [14], measured PFC production by peritoneal cells from unimmunized mice in the presence of SE *in vitro,* and examined the effect of incorporating AMIgS in the medium. Their results support the view that it is the lymphocytes, not the macrophages, which actually produce Bussard plaques, and that the reaction has the character of a primary response. In further work Bendinelli [5] showed that peritoneal cells from a mouse infected 10 days before with FV produce as many PFC in Bussard cultures as normal cells do. However PFC formation is depressed 17 or more days after infection, but this may be accounted for by a fall in the lymphocyte/macrophage ratio.

Bendinelli and Asherson [7] studied the effect of FV on contact sensitivity in mouse skin. Picryl chloride was applied to the abdominal skin, and to the ear one week later. When FV was injected before the sensitizing dose reaction to challenge was significantly reduced, and antibody production to the picryl group was virtually abolished.

Bendinelli and Bainbridge [8] studied "homing" of intra-venously injected ^{51}Cr-labelled spleen cells from normal and FV-

injected mice to the spleens of normal and infected recipients. Fewer
infected than normal spleen cells were found in the recipients' spleens
24 h later. On the other hand FV infection of recipients did not
affect the result.

A recent development of great promise is the discovery by my
colleagues Drs. Rowson and Parr [52] of another virus in our FV
preparations. It produces a slight but definite splenomegaly, but no
overt signs of illness. Yet it has an immediate, though possibly
transient, immunodepressive effect of the same order as that of FV
itself. It is probably antigenically related to FV since it immunizes
against it. Mice infected with this "small" spleen virus do not die
of the infection, and we hope to be able to carry out long term
procedures such as tolerance induction, homograft rejection, and
perhaps chemical carcinogenesis, on them.

Little work has been done on immunodepressive effects of other
oncogenic viruses. A virus of the avian leucosis group, when injected into newly hatched chicks, depresses antibody titres to phage
T_2 and to bovine serum albumen at four weeks, but the depression
appears to be transient [46, 24, 20]. More definitive work on this
group of viruses is in press [17, 21, 49]. There is no convincing
evidence of depression of humoral antibody production by polyoma,
mammary tumour virus, or Shope fibroma virus, though defects in
cellular immunity have not been excluded. I have thought it best to
leave this rapidly expanding field to a future reviewer.

A great deal could be said about abnormal immunity in neoplastic
disease not yet proved to be of viral origin—too much to be included
in this review, even if it were judged germane to our subject.

The researches I have described must be regarded as a beginning
only. They have established that FV and other viruses affecting the
haemopoietic system interfere with immune reactions at some point.
To find out what point is the task of future work.

It is worth remembering that all these viruses are RNA, ether-
sensitive viruses, similar in many ways to the myxoviruses. Many
non-oncogenic members of this class have an effect on cell surfaces,
covering or stripping off some antigenic components and exposing
others. Their oncogenic analogues have been shown to form or expose immunologically foreign cellular antigens, to which an animal
who receives the virus in the perinatal period becomes tolerant, but
against which an adult can be immunized [e.g. 32, 34]. It is tempting,
but probably premature, to speculate on how an immunodepressive

virus might upset this balance, or affect the interplay of the many other local or systemic factors on which the issue of restraint versus release of neoplastic growth depends.

References

1. Alford, C.A.: Study on antibody in congenital rubella infections. Amer. J. Dis. Child. *110:* 455–463 (1965).
2. Ball, J.K.; Sinclair, N.R. and McCarter, J.A.: Prolonged immunosuppression and tumor induction by a chemical carcinogen injected at birth. Science *152:* 650–651 (1966).
3. Bellanti, J.A.; Artenstein, M.S.; Olson, L.C.; Buescher, E.L.; Luhrs, C.E. and Mitslead, K.L.: Congenital rubella. Amer. J. Dis. Child. *110:* 464–472 (1965).
4. Bendinelli, M.: Relation between Friend viraemia and immunodepression. Rep. Brit. Emp. Cancer Campgn. *44:* 110 (1966).
5. Bendinelli, M.: Haemolytic plaque formation by mouse peritoneal cells and the effect on it of Friend virus injection. Immunology (Lond.) *14:* 837–850 (1968).
6. Bendinelli, M.: The primary *in vitro* response of mouse peritoneal cells to sheep erythrocytes, and the effect on it of Friend virus. Rep. Brit. Emp. Cancer Campgn. *45:* 136 (1968).
7. Bendinelli, M. and Asherson, G.L.: Effect of Friend virus infection on contact sensitivity. Rep. Brit. Emp. Cancer Campgn. *45:* 137 (1968).
8. Bendinelli, M. and Bainbridge, D.R.: The effect of Friend virus infection on the distribution of infected lymphoid cells. Rep. Brit. Emp. Cancer Campgn. *45:* 137 (1968).
9. Bendinelli, M. and Wedderburn, N.: Haemolytic plaque formation by unimmunized mouse peritoneal lymphocytes. Nature (Lond.) *215:* 157–158 (1967).
10. Berenbaum, M.C.: Effects of carcinogens on immune processes. Brit. med. Bull. *20:* 159–164 (1964).
11. Bloomfield, A. and Mateer, J.: Changes in skin sensitiveness to tuberculin during epidemic influenza. Amer. Rev. Tuberc. *3:* 166–168 (1919).
12. Breyere, E.J. and Williams, L.B.: Antigens associated with a tumor virus: rejection of isogenic skin grafts from leukaemic mice. Science *146:* 1055–1056 (1964).
13. Brody, J.A. and McAlister, R.: Depression of tuberculin sensitivity following measles vaccination. Amer. Rev. resp. Dis. *90:* 607–611 (1964).
14. Bussard, A.E.: Antibody formation in non-immune mouse peritoneal cells after incubation in gum containing antigen. Science *153:* 887–890 (1966).
15. Ceglowski, W. and Friedman, H.: Suppression of the primary antibody plaque response of mice following injection with Friend virus. Proc. exp. Biol. N.Y. *126:* 662–666 (1967).
16. Chan, G.; Rancourt, M.W.; Ceglowski, W.S. and Friedman, H.: Leukaemia virus suppression of antibody forming cells: ultrastructure of infected spleens. Science *159:* 437–439 (1968).
17. Cooper, M.D.; Payne, L.N.; Dent, P.B.; Burmester, B.R. and Good, R.A.: Pathogenesis of avian leukosis. I Histogenesis. J. nat. Cancer Inst. (in press).
18. Cremer, N.E.: Selective immunoglobulin deficiencies in rats injected with Moloney virus. J. Immunol. *99:* 71–81 (1967).
19. Cremer, N.E.; Taylor, D.O.N. and Hagens, S.J.: Antibody formation, latency and leukaemia: infection with Moloney virus. J. Immunol. *96:* 495–508 (1966).

20. DENT, P.B.; COOPER, M.D.; PAYNE, L.N.; GOOD, R.A. and BURMESTER, B.R.: Characterization of avian lymphoid leukosis as a malignancy of the bursal lymphoid system. In: Perspectives in virology V. (Ed.) POLLARD, M., pp. 251–265 (Academic Press Inc., New York/London 1967).
21. DENT, P.B.; COOPER, M.D.; PAYNE, L.N.; SOLOMON, J.J.; BURMESTER, B.R. and GOOD, R.A.: Pathogenesis of avian leukosis. II. Immunological reactivity during lymphomagenesis. J. nat. Cancer Inst. (in press).
22. DENT, P.B.; OLSON, G.B.; GOOD, R.A.; RAWLS, W.E.; SOUTH, M.A. and MELNICK, J.L.: Rubella virus/leucocyte interaction and its role in the pathogenesis of the congenital rubella syndrome. Lancet *i:* 291–293 (1968).
23. DENT. P.B.; PETERSON, R.D.A. and GOOD, R.A.: A defect in cellular immunity during the incubation period of passage A leukaemia in C3H mice. Proc. exp. Biol. N.Y. *119:* 869–871 (1965).
24. DENT, P.B.; PETERSON, R.D.A. and GOOD, R.A.: The relationship of immunologic function and oncogenesis. In: Diseases of immunologic deficiency (Eds.) GOOD, R.A.; SMITH, R.T. and MIESCHER, P.B. (National Foundation Press 1967).
25. DRESSER, D.W. and WORTIS, H.H.: Use of antiglobulin serum to detect cells producing antibody with low haemolytic efficiency. Nature (Lond.) *208:* 859–861 (1965).
26. FRIEND, C.: Cell-free transmission in adult Swiss mice of a disease having the characteristics of a leukaemia. J. exp. Med. *105:* 307–318 (1957).
27. GELZER, J. and DIETRICH, F.M.: Haemagglutinin production in tumour-bearing and leukaemic mice. Int. J. Cancer *3:* 51–60 (1968).
28. GROSS, L.: "Spontaneous" leukaemia developing in C3H mice following inoculation, in infancy, with AK-leukemic extracts, or AK-embryos. Proc. Soc. exp. Biol. N.Y. *76:* 27–32 (1951).
29. ISACSON, E.P.: Myxoviruses and autoimmunity. Progr. Allergy, vol. 10, pp. 256–292 (Karger, Basel/New York 1967).
30. JERNE, N.K.; NORDIN, A.A. and HENRY, C.: The agar plaque technique for recognising antibody-producing cells. In: Cell-bound antibodies (Eds.) AMOS, B. and KOPROWSKI, H., pp. 109–122 (Wistar Inst. Press, 1963).
31. KIRSTEN, W.H.; MAYER, L.A.; WOLLMAN, R.L. and PIERCE, M.I.: Studies on a murine erythroblastosis virus. J. nat. Cancer. Inst. *38:* 117–139 (1967).
32. KLEIN, E. and KLEIN, G.: Immunological tolerance of neonatally infected mice to Moloney leukaemia virus. Nature (Lond.) *209:* 163–167 (1966).
33. MAZZUR, S.R. and PAUCKER, K.: Studies on the effect of interferon on the formation of antibody plaque formation and antibody production by transferred spleen cells. J. Immunol. *98:* 689–696 (1967).
34. McCOY, J.L.; FEFER, A. and GLYNN, J.P.: Comparative studies on the induction of transplantation resistance in Balb/c and $C_{57}Bl/6$ mice in three murine leukemia systems. Cancer Res. *27:* 1743–1748 (1967).
35. MEDZON, E.L. and VAS, S.I.: Studies on *in vitro* antibody production. II. The effect of Newcastle disease virus on antibody synthesis. Canad. J. Microbiol. *10:* 535–541 (1964).
36. MELLMAN, W.J. and WETTON, R.: Depression of the tuberculin reaction by attenuated measles virus vaccine. J. lab. clin. Med. *61:* 453–458 (1963).
37. MERGENHAGEN, S.E.; NOTKINS, A.L. and DOUGHERTY, S.F.: Adjuvanticity of lactic dehydrogenase virus: influence on the establishment of immunologic tolerance to a protein antigen in adult mice. J. Immunol. *99:* 576–581 (1967).
38. METCALF, D. and MOULDS, R.: Immune responses in preleukaemic and leukaemic AKR mice. Int. J. Cancer *2:* 53–58 (1967).
39. MIRAND, E.A. and GRACE, J.T., Jr.: Some current findings in Friend leukaemia. Proc. Int. Symp. Human and Murine Leukaemia, vol. 1 (Accad. Naz. dei Lincei, Rome 1964).

40. MOLONEY, J.B.: Biological studies on a lymphoid-leukaemia virus extracted from sarcoma 37. I. Origin and introductory investigation. J. nat. Cancer. Inst. *24:* 933–951 (1960).

41. MONTGOMERY, J.R.; SOUTH, M.A.; RAWLS, W.E.; MELNICK, J.L.; OLSON, G.B.; Dent, P.B. and GOOD, R.A.: Viral inhibition of lymphocyte response to phytohaemagglutinin. Science *157:* 1068–1070 (1967).

42. ODAKA, T.; ISHII, H.; YAMAURA, K. and YAMAMOTO, T.: Inhibitory effect of Friend leukemia virus infection on the antibody formation to sheep erythrocytes in mice. Jap. J. exp. Med. *36:* 277–290 (1966).

43. OLD, L.J.; CLARKE, D.A.; BENACERRAF, B. and GOLDSMITH, M.: The reticuloendothelial system and the neoplastic process. Ann. N.Y. Acad. Sci. *88:* 264–280 (1960).

44. OLSON, G.B.; SOUTH, M.A. and GOOD, R.A.: Phytohaemagglutinin unresponsiveness to lymphocytes from babies with congenital rubella. Nature (Lond.) *214:* 695–696 (1967).

45. PETERSON, R.D.A.; HENDRICKSON, R. and GOOD, R.A.: Reduced antibody forming capacity during the incubation period of Passage A leukaemia in C3H mice. Proc. Soc. exp. Biol. N.Y. *114:* 517–520 (1963).

46. PETERSON, R.D.A.; PURCHASE, H.G.; BURMESTER, B.R.; COOPER, M.D. and GOOD, R.A.: Relationships among visceral lymphomatosis, bursa of Fabricius, and bursa-dependent lymphoid tissue of the chicken. J. nat. Cancer Inst. *36:* 585–598 (1966).

47. PIRQUET, C. VON: Das Verhalten der kutanen Tuberculinreaktion während der Masern. Dtsch. med. Wschr. *34:* 1297–1300 (1908).

48. PREHN, R.T.: Function of depressed immunologic reactivity during carcinogenesis. J. nat. Cancer Inst. *31:* 791–805 (1963).

49. PURCHASE, H.G.; CHUBB, R.C. and BIGGS, P.M.: Effect of lymphoid leukosis and Marek's disease on the immunological responsiveness of the chicken. J. nat. Cancer Inst. *40:* 583–592 (1968).

50. RAUSCHER, F.J.: A virus-induced disease of mice characterized by erythrocytopoiesis and lymphoid leukaemia. J. nat. Cancer Inst. *29:* 515–532 (1962).

51. RILEY, V.; LILLY, F.; HUERTO, E. and BARDELL, D.: Transmissible agent associated with 26 types of experimental mouse neoplasms. Science *132:* 545–547 (1960).

52. ROWSON, K.E.K. and PARR, I.B.: Resistance inducing virus separated from Friend virus by end-point dilution. Biochem. J. *106:* 39P–40P (1968).

53. SALAMAN, M.H.: Attempt to isolate a leukaemogenic virus from urethane-induced leukaemia in mice. Rep. Brit. Emp. Cancer Campagn. *40:* 220–221 (1963).

54. SALAMAN, M.H.: Effect of viruses on haemagglutinin production in mice. Rep. Brit. Emp. Cancer Campgn. *42:* 193–194 (1964).

55. SALAMAN, M.H. and FLOCKS, J.: An attempt to isolate a leukaemogenic virus from urethane-induced leukaemia in mice. Rep. Brit. Emp. Cancer Campgn. *42:* 192–193 (1964).

56. SALAMAN, M.H. and WEDDERBURN, N.: The immuno-depressive effect of Friend virus. Immunology (Lond.) *10:* 445–458 (1966).

57. SCOTT, R.B.; ELLISON, R.R. and LEY, A.B.: A clinical study of 20 cases of erythroleukaemia (di Guglielmo's syndrome). Amer. J. Med. *37:* 162–171 (1964).

58. SIEGEL, B.V. and MORTON, J.I.: Depressed antibody response in the mouse infected with Rauscher leukaemia virus. Immunology (Lond.) *10:* 559–562 (1966).

59. SIEGEL, B.V. and MORTON, J.I.: Serum agglutinin levels to sheep red blood cells in mice infected with Rauscher virus. Proc. exp. Biol. N.Y. *123:* 467–470 (1966).

60. SMITHWICK, F.M. and BERKOVITCH, S.: *In vitro* suppression of the lymphocyte response to tuberculin by live measles virus. Proc. Soc. exp. Biol. N.Y. *123:* 276–278 (1966).

61. Soothill, J.F.; Hayes, K. and Dudgeon, J.A.: The immunoglobulins in congenital rubella. Lancet *i:* 1385–1388 (1966).
62. Stansly, P.G. and Soule, P.E.: Transplantation and cellfree transmission of a reticulum cell sarcoma in Balb/c mice. J. nat. Cancer Inst. *29:* 1083–1105 (1962).
63. Starr, S. and Berkovitch, S.: Effects of measles, gamma globulin-modified measles, and vaccine measles on the tuberculin test. New. Engl. J. Med. *270:* 386–391 (1964).
64. Svet-Moldavsky, G.J.; Mkheidze, D.M. and Liozner, A.L.: Two phenomena associated with skin grafting from tumor-bearing syngeneic donors. J. nat. Cancer Inst. *38:* 933–938 (1967).
65. Svet-Moldavsky, G.J.; Mkheidze, D.M.; Liozner, A.L. and Bykovsky, A.Ph.: Skin heterogenizing virus. Nature (Lond.) *217:* 102–104 (1968).
66. Wedderburn, N. and Salaman, M.H.: Effects of viruses on immune reactions in mice. Rep. Brit. Emp. Cancer Campgn. *43:* 171–172 (1965).
67. Wedderburn, N. and Salaman, M.H.: The immuno-depressive effect of Friend virus. II. Reduction of splenic haemolysin-producing cells in primary and secondary responses. Immunology (Lond.) *15:* 439–454 (1968).
68. Wedderburn, N.; Salaman, M.H. and Bendinelli, M.: Effects of viruses on immune reactions in mice. Rep. Brit. Emp. Cancer Campgn. *44:* 109–111 (1966).

Author's address: Dr. M.H. Salaman, Royal College of Surgeons of England, Lincoln's Inn Fields, *London, W.C. 2* (England).

Antibiotica et Chemotherapia, vol. 15, pp. 407–417 (Karger, Basel/New York 1969)

Suppression of Cellular Immunity by Gram-Negative Bacteria

G. L. FLOERSHEIM

National Institute for Medical Research, London, and
Pharmacological Institute, University of Basle, Basle

Vaccines or lipopolysaccharides of Gram-negative bacteria are known to modify the susceptibility of mice to infection with heterologous microorganisms. This effect has been demonstrated by several authors, including ROWLEY [1], FIELD *et al.* [2], LANDY [3], and DUBOS and SCHAEDLER [4]. The latter found that inoculation of mice with Pertussis vaccine or with *S. typhosa* lipopolysaccharide had a biphasic effect: a short phase, lasting a few hours, of increased susceptibility to infection with various bacteria, which was followed by a phase of heightened resistance lasting several weeks. Among the confirmations of these experiments were those of MICHAEL and MASSEL [5] who showed that endotoxin from *S. flexneri* protected mice from infection with *S. typhosa* if the interval between endotoxin and bacteria amounted to 24–48 h. Furthermore, resistance to mycotic infections could be enhanced in mice with *E. coli* endotoxins [6]. This latter resistance was transferable with serum obtained 24 h after the application of the endotoxin. The increase in resistance to infection is probably due to a non-specific release by endotoxins of natural antibody, followed by the replication of antibody-forming cells [7].

If we turn from the complex phenomenon of increased non-specific resistance against infectious agents towards the simpler situation where the antibody response to a given antigen is followed, then again the vast majority of studies demonstrate that endotoxins, administered before or together with the antigen, will increase serum antibody levels. As an illustration, we may consider the experiments of JOHNSON, GAINES and LANDY [8]. They observed in rabbits an enhancement of antibody formation to protein antigens if the latter were given simultaneously with *S. typhosa* lipopolysaccharide. Analogous increases in antibody titers have been demonstrated with a variety of antigens and the adjuvanticity of endotoxins is well established. Similarly, the efficiency of Freund's adjuvant is greatly increased by its *M. tuberculosis* component. Addition of endotoxin to tolerogenic antigens induces immunity. Moreover, Gram-negative bacterial materials administered prior to the transplantation of allogeneic or isogeneic tumours generally reduce tumour incidence, indicating a stimulation of the immune response against transplantation- or tumour-specific antigens [9, 10, 11, 12].

Despite this impressive body of evidence for the stimulating effects on immunity, some immune responses are less susceptible to enhancement by endotoxins. For instance, it seems that splenic antibody-forming cells appear earlier and persist longer, but the evidence for a genuine increase in their number after endotoxin administration is equivocal [13, 14]. Also, a suppression of antibody to actinophage in mice [15] and to bacterial antigen in rabbits has been reported [16]. In the latter experiment, endotoxin was only suppressive when injected as a mixture with the antigen and not when given separately. In one instance, suppression of antibody formation to a soluble antigen, bovine gamma globulin, by endotoxin has been reported in mice [17]. A study concerned with the influence of the time interval between endotoxin and antigen administration revealed that the hemolysin response to sheep erythrocytes in mice is suppressed if *S. typhosa* lipopolysaccharide is given before the antigen, while simultaneous application enhances antibody production [18]. Finally, the mechanism of the acute inhibition exerted by *Proteus* polysaccharides on systemic and local anaphylaxis in guinea-pigs and rabbits [19] remains to be clarified. A pertinent report deals with the effect of pretreatment with *Corynebacterium parvum* on the graft-versus-host reaction initiated by injection of parental strain spleen cells in adult *F. hybrid* mice [19a]. Mortality, phagocytic response and proliferation of donor cells in the spleen were all reduced.

It is interesting to note that the organisms displaying both immunostimulant and immunosuppressive properties belong almost uniquely to the class of Gram-negative bacteria. They are characterized by their endotoxins, which form a part of their cell walls. The endotoxins have been shown to be lipopolysaccharides, clearly different from the proteinic exotoxins synthesized by the microorganisms causing diphtheria, tetanus and botulism and also from the cytolytic toxins, comprising the streptolysins and staphylococcal toxins, which are also proteins.

The mechanisms by which bacterial products act as immuno-stimulants have not been elucidated. The same applies to the multi tude of other biological activities the endotoxins exert. Clearly, some of these are very likely to have some bearing on the modification of immune reactivity.

This would apply particularly to the effects of endotoxins on *macrophages*. They range from mild stimulation to frank destruction. Most important seems the effect on phagocytosis. Within a few hours after endotoxin, a decreased clearance of particulate material from the blood is observed, which is followed by the opposite effect. A similar biphasic change was observed in the number of spleen cells forming natural bactericidal antibody [7]. Incidentally, this coincides with the phases of enhanced and diminished susceptibility to infection. Other endotoxin effects which might possibly interfere with some step of the immune response include lymphocyte mobilization [20], thymic injury [21, 22], lysosomal damage, histamine sensitization, margination of neutrophils, chemotaxis and vascular changes. Moreover, it seems to be quite relevant that some endotoxin effects cannot be produced in germ-free animals.

The first hint that microorganisms might lead to a *decreased* immune reactivity came from two intriguing observations made in clinical medicine. One is the well known inhibition of the reactivity towards *M. tuberculosis* during an attack of measles [23], or during measles vaccination [24, 25]. The same applies—although less clear-cut than in measles—for pertussis infection [26]. Sensitivity to other infections and flare-up of latent ones during attacks of these diseases are notorious. Recently, a generalized depression of the delayed allergic inflammatory response was demonstrated also in patients with lepromatous leprosy [27]. The anergy occurring during pertussis infections prompted us to look into the effects of the pertussis agent on immune responses of the delayed or cell-mediated type.

As a first example, we investigated the tuberculin reaction [28]. Albino guinea pigs were immunized with BCG (a living lyophylized product) in Freund's complete adjuvant (Difco) in the foot pad. Four weeks later the guinea pigs were challenged intracutaneously with 750 I.U. tuberculin. The reaction intensity was assessed after 8 and 24 h by measuring the skin thickness at the reaction site and

Table I. Effect of *B. pertussis* on the tuberculin reaction.

Exp.	Group (No. of animals)	Treatment	Per cent increase in skin thickness		Relative difference to controls[1] (per cent)		Area of erythema (mm²)		Relative difference to controls[1] (per cent)	
			8 h	24 h	8 h	24 h	8 h	24 h	8 h	24 h
1	1 (8)	Controls, 1 ml aq.dest./kg	28 ± 16	48 ± 30			257 ± 62	222 ± 85		
	2 (6)	*B. pertussis*, 4×10^9 cells/kg[2]	8 ± 4	32 ± 16	—71[6]	—33	246 ± 48	178 ± 101	— 4	—20
	3 (8)	*B. pertussis*, 160×10^9 cells/kg	8 ± 11	19 ± 16	—71[5]	—60[6]	137 ± 92	134 ± 90	—47[6]	—40
2	4 (7)	Controls, 1 ml aq.dest./kg	34 ± 14	76 ± 25			204 ± 43	168 ± 68		
	5 (6)	Controls, 1 ml 0.01 % merthiolate/kg	47 ± 17	100 ± 24			219 ± 13	204 ± 46		
	6 (6)	*B. pertussis*, 40×10^9 cells/kg	20 ± 12	47 ± 17	—57[6]	—53[6]	121 ± 108	178 ± 56	—45	—13
	7 (6)	*B. pertussis*, 160×10^9 cells/kg	16 ± 15	37 ± 35	—66[6]	—63[6]	85 ± 98	158 ± 56	—61[6]	—23
	8 (6)	*B. pertussis*, 160×10^9 cells/kg[3]	40 ± 26	95 ± 31	—15	— 5	200 ± 45	176 ± 44	— 9	—14
3	9 (6)	Controls, 4 ml aq.dest./kg	32 ± 15	69 ± 16			283 ± 46	213 ± 89		
	10 (6)	*B. pertussis*, 160×10^9 cells/kg	10 ± 7	31 ± 14	—68[6]	—55[6]	126 ± 95	195 ± 75	—55[6]	— 8
	11 (6)	*B. pertussis*, 160×10^9 cells/kg[4]	30 ± 10	72 ± 26	— 6	+ 5	293 ± 50	272 ± 97	+ 4	+28

[1] Reaction of controls considered as 100 %.
[2] Single injection of pertussis vaccine 30 min prior to tuberculin.
[3] Single injection of pertussis vaccine 16 h prior to tuberculin.
± Standard deviation.

[4] Single injection of pertussis vaccine four days prior to tuberculin.
[5] p <0.05.
[6] p <0.01.

The average values for each group are presented. The animals in the experiments 1, 2 and 3 were sensitized respectively 6, 4 and 5 weeks prior to the tuberculin challenge. In experiment 2, the relative differences were correlated to the controls treated with 1 ml 0.01 % merthiolate/kg (group 5). 40×10^9 *B. pertussis* cells/kg were applied in 0.1 ml/100 g, 160×10^9 *B. pertussis* cells/kg in 0.4 ml/100 g [FLOERSHEIM, G. L.: Int. Arch. Allergy *26*: 340, 1965].

the area of the erythema. Pertussis vaccine was injected intraperitoneally 30 min before and 8 h after the tuberculin challenge. As can be seen from table I, a 60–70% decrease of the reaction intensity resulted. The effect was dose-dependent. Further investigations were directed towards the characterization of the active principle in the vaccine [29]. First, millipore filtration of the vaccine revealed that the filtrate retained the full activity. Treatment of the filtrate with enzymes including trypsin, papain, desoxyribo- and ribonuclease, lysozyme and hyaluronidase had no influence, nor had heating to 90°C for 30 min or dialysis. It was concluded that the active agent was not proteinic and probably a polysaccharide. A further purification of the active agent was performed by Hopff *et al.* [30]. As a source, the culture medium was used in which the organisms had been killed by heating to 56°C and by the addition of 0.5% phenol. The end product obtained after concentration, dialysis and drying of the supernatant had the chemical characteristics of a lipopolysaccharide. In addition, extracts obtained in a similar way from culture broths of *S. paratyphi A* and *B* were even more active than the lipopolysaccharide from *B. pertussis* (fig. 1). Other polysaccharides of non-bacterial origin, such as heparin or N-acetylneuraminic acid had no effect on the tuberculin reaction. It should be noted that the tuberculin reaction is very resistant to immunosuppressive drugs applied in the same way as the bacterial agents. Only occasionally inhibitions reaching 40–50% can be obtained [31]. It may be noted that prednisolone (3, 10 and 30 mg/kg) was only marginally effective, thus making it rather unlikely that the endotoxin-induced inhibition is mediated by corticosteroids. An even stronger argument against the stress theory are the immunostimulant effects displayed by endotoxins under different conditions. The possibility that the release of catecholamines is responsible for the inhibition should be dismissed on the basis that dibenamine, an α-adrenergic blocking agent, inhibits the reaction on its own [31].

As a second model to test the lipopolysaccharides, use was made of a normal lymphocyte transfer reaction in chickens [32, 33], in which lymphocytes obtained from the blood of Plymouth fowls are injected into the skin of three-week old Leghorn chickens. The resulting reaction consists of a circumscribed skin induration reaching its peak after four days and then declining during the following four days. The reaction has some characteristics of a graft-versus-host reaction. Histologically, massive granulomatous mononuclear infiltrates in the

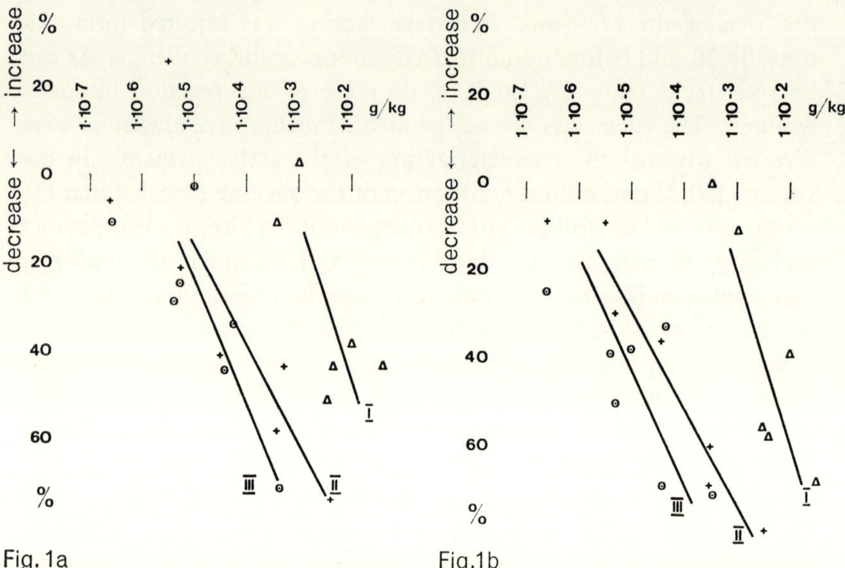

Fig. 1a and 1b. Effect of bacterial products in different dosages on the tuberculin reaction in guinea-pigs. The skin thickness over the reaction site at 8 (fig. 1a) and 24 h (fig. 1b) is expressed as percentage of the values in the saline-treated control group. I: *B. pertussis* crude product. II: *S. paratyphi B* crude product. III: Bacto lipopolysaccharide B, *S. typhosa* 0901. The entries represent mean values of groups of six guinea-pigs. Reproduced from HOPFF, W. L., FLOERSHEIM, G. L. and BUCHER, K.: Helv. Physiol. Acta *25:* 1 (1967). – [Ref. 30].

dermis with large pyroninophilic cells clustered around vessels are prominent. Administration of 3 mg/kg of the *S. paratyphi B* extract twice daily inhibited the reaction by about 30% (table II). The *B. pertussis* material had slightly less, but still significant depressing activity. This lesion, however, is more susceptible than the tuberculin reaction to inhibition by immunosuppressive or anti-inflammatory drugs. Nonetheless, only Methotrexate (3 mg/kg twice daily) and Actinomycin D (0.025 mg/kg twice daily) clearly exceeded the lipopolysaccharide effect.

Thirdly, the action of pertussis vaccine was tested on the growth of isogeneic YLI Moloney lymphomas in C571 mice [34]. Administration of pertussis vaccine simultaneously with the subcutaneous inoculation of graded doses of tumour cells led to an increased incidence of tumour takes at the threshold doses from 10^4 to 10^6 cells (table III). The assumption that the immune response to tumour-specific antigens has been decreased by the pertussis agent might explain these findings.

Table II. Effect of bacterial products on a cutaneous lymphocyte transfer reaction in chickens

Treatment	Dose (mg/kg twice daily)	Relative difference of skin thickness compared with controls (%)				Difference of % weight change against controls after 5 days
		48 h	72 h	96 h	120 h	
B. pertussis product	0.3	+ 7	+11	— 7	— 6	+ 9
	3	—15	—21[1]	— 6	+12	—27
S. paratyphi B product	0.3	—21[1]	—10	—13	+10	+ 6
	3	—21	—33[2]	—26[1]	—22	—12

3-week old Leghorn cockerels were injected at 0 h intradermally with 2.5×10^6 lymphocytes from the blood of Plymouth fowls. The ensuing reaction was evaluated daily by measuring the skin thickness over the reaction site and expressing it as percentage of the values in the saline-treated control group. The bacterial products (prepared according to Hopff, W.L., Floersheim, G.L. and Bucher, K.: Helv. Physiol. Acta *25:* 1, 1967) were injected intraperitoneally twice daily, except on day 0, when only one dose was given 15 min before the lymphocyte inoculation. The entries represent the mean values of groups of six chickens. Courtesy of Dr. K. Seiler.

[1] p <0.05, [2] p. <0.01.

A similar observation was made independently and simultaneously by Hirano *et al.* [35]. The intravenous injection of pertussis vaccine four days prior to the inoculation of a Rauscher lymphoma in mice was found to augment tumour growth. In addition, these authors observed that the vaccine prevented the proliferative effects brought about by phytohemagglutinin and Freund's adjuvant on spleen cells.

Interestingly, both in the tuberculin reaction as in the normal lymphocyte transfer reaction, the administration of pertussis vaccine two to four days *prior* to the antigen tends rather to increase the reaction [28, 33]. Moreover, prior administration of bacterial products to tumour iso- or allografts have been shown to lower the tumour incidence [9, 10, 11, 12], probably by increasing the immune response to the tumour inoculum. So although the immunosuppressive activity of the bacterial products has been documented in our studies with three types of cellular immune responses in three animal species, the hyporeactive phase is transient and depends on the time relationship between the administration of the antigen and the bacterial agent.

The suppressive effect was demonstrable both in presensitized animals (tuberculin reaction) and in primary responses (normal lymphocyte transfer reaction and tumour isograft rejection).

Table III. Effect of *B. pertussis* on the incidence of YLI lymphoma after the transplantation of various cell doses

No. of tumour cells transplanted	Treatment (No. of mice)	Tumour incidence (No. of takes, less No. of complete regressions) at the following intervals after transplantation (days)								Days on which death occured	Cumulative tumour incidence	No. of complete regressions
		12	15	19	24	33	41	50	60			
10^4	Controls (20)	0	0	7	4	4	4	4	4	68, 86, 94[1], 108[1]	8	4
	B. pertussis (20)	1	5[2]	12	8	8	8	8	8	55, 61, 70, 71, 74, 82, 82, 92[1]	17[2]	9
10^5	Controls (21)	1	2	5	6	6	7	7	7	44[1], 49, 44, 68, 75[1], 76, 76	10	3
	B. pertussis (21)	4	12[3]	16[3]	10	10	10	11	11	40, 48, 49, 53[1], 55[1], 56, 56, 58, 61, 68, 86	19[2]	8
10^6	Controls (14)	4	1	0	0	0	0	0	0		4	4
	B. pertussis (15)	7	5	8[3]	8[3]	7[2]	7[2]	8[3]	8[3]	43, 49, 50, 59, 61, 71[1], 86[1], 86[1]	13[3]	5
10^7	Controls (10)	8	6	6	5	5	5	5	5	35, 48[1], 57, 65, 70[1]	9	4
	B. pertussis (9)	7	7	8	8	7	7	7	7	35, 37, 43, 50[1], 75[1], 82, 90	9	2

[1] Mice dead with generalized leukaemia after regression of the solid tumour (counted as takes throughout the observation period).
[2] p <0.05   [3] p <0.01
[FLOERSHEIM, G. L.: Nature *216:* 1235, 1967].

As to the mechanism of the effect, several hypotheses may be put forward. Besides antigenic competition or preoccupation of immunologically active cells, the effects of endotoxins on macrophage activity deserve mention. Furthermore, the hypothesis that endotoxin interferes with the feedback inhibition by antibody should be considered. The most attractive possibility seems to me that the suppression of delayed-type hypersensitivity is due to an acute release of antibody from cells as recently described [36]. Antibody then could either combine with the eliciting dose of antigen and thereby prevent its interaction with antibody attached to cells or, more likely, the released antibody might suppress the formation of other antibody participating in the delayed-type immune response. At any rate, the clear dissociation the bacterial products display with regard to their effects on humoral and cellular immunity may provide an opportunity for the analysis of the respective mechanisms.

It is not established if the immunosuppressive properties of bacteria are limited to Gram-negative organisms. A recent report shows that cytoplasmic components of group A streptococci, which also have some other endotoxin-like properties, suppress both 7S and 19S antibody responses of mice to sheep erythrocytes [37].

In summary, products of Gram-negative bacteria cause both increased non-specific resistance to infection and enhanced humoral antibody titers to a variety of antigens. Occasionally, inhibition of humoral antibody formation has been reported. The evidence presented discloses a further property of bacterial lipopolysaccharides, the depression of cell-mediated immune reactions.

References

1. Rowley, D.: Stimulation of natural immunity to *Escherichia coli* infections. Lancet *i:* 232 (1955).
2. Field, T.E.; Howard, J.G. and Whitby, J.L.: Studies on the non-specific immunity to *Salmonella typhi* infection in mice. J. roy. Army med. Corps. *101:* 324 (1955).
3. Landy, M.: Increased resistance to infection developed rapidly after administration of bacterial lipopolysaccharides. Fed. Proc. *15:* 598 (1956).
4. Dubos, R.J. and Schaedler, R.W.: Reversible changes in the susceptibility of mice to bacterial infections. I. Changes brought about by injection of pertussis vaccine or of bacterial endotoxins. J. exp. Med. *104:* 53 (1956).
5. Michael, J.G. and Massell, B.F.: Factors involved in the induction of non-specific resistance to streptococcal infection in mice by endotoxin. J. exp. Med. *116:* 101 (1962).
6. Kimball, H.R.; Williams, T.W. and Wolff, S.M.: Effect of bacterial endotoxin on experimental fungal infections. J. Immunol. *100:* 24 (1968).

7. Michael, J.G.: The release of specific bactericidal antibodies by endotoxin. J. exp. Med. *123:* 205 (1966).

8. Johnson, A.G.; Gaines, S. and Landy, M.: Studies on the O-antigen of *Salmonella typhosa*. V. Enhancement of antibody response to protein antigens by the purified lipopolysaccharide. J. exp. Med. *103:* 225 (1956).

9. Old, L.J.; Clarke, D.A. and Benacerraf, B.: Effect of *Bacillus* Calmette-Guérin infection on transplanted tumours in the mouse. Nature *184:* 291 (1959).

10. Old, L.J.; Benacerraf, B.; Clarke, D.A.; Carswell, E.A. and Stockert, E.: The role of the reticuloendothelial system in the host reaction to neoplasia. Cancer Res. *21:* 1281 (1961).

11. Weiss, D.W.; Bonhag, R.S. and DeOme, K.B.: Protective activity of fractions of tubercle bacilli against isologous tumours in mice. Nature *190:* 889 (1961).

12. Woodruff, M.F.A. and Boak, J.L.: Inhibitory effect of injection of *Corynebacterium parvum* on the growth of tumour transplants in isogeneic hosts. Brit. J. Cancer *20:* 345 (1966).

13. Freedman, H.H.; Nakano, M. and Braun, W.: Antibody formation in endotoxin-tolerant mice. Proc. Soc. exp. Biol., N.Y. *121:* 1228 (1967).

14. Finger, H.; Emmerling, P. and Schmidt, H.: The influence of bacterial endotoxins on the formation of antibody-forming spleen cells in mice immunized with sheep red blood cells. Experientia *23:* 849 (1967).

15. Bradley, S.G. and Watson, D.W.: Suppression by endotoxin of the immune response to actinophage in the mouse. Proc. Soc. exp. Biol., N.Y. *117:* 570 (1964)

16. Whang, H.Y. and Neter, E.: Immunosuppression by endotoxin and its lipoid A component. Proc. Soc. exp. Biol., N.Y. *124:* 919 (1967).

17. Johnson, A.G.; Jacobs, A.; Abrams, G. and Merritt, K.: Comparative changes in the mouse spleen during immuno-stimulation or immuno-suppression. *In* Germinal Centers in Immune Responses. (Eds.) H. Cottier, N. Odortchenko, R. Schindler and C.C. Congdon (Springer-Verlag, New York 1967).

18. Franzl, R.E. and McMaster, P.D.: The primary immune response in mice. I. The enhancement and suppression of hemolysin production by a bacterial endotoxin. J. exp. Med. *127:* 1087 (1968).

19. Meier, R.; Bein, H.J. and Jaques, R.: The action of bacterial polyssacharides on allergic phenomena. Int. arch. Allergy *11:* 101 (1957).

19a. Howard, J.G.; Biozzi, G.; Stiffel, C.; Mouton, D. and Liacopoulos, P.: An analysis of the inhibitory effect of *Corynebacterium parvum* on graft-versus-host disease. Transplantation *5:* 1510 (1967).

20. Morse, S.I.: Studies on the lymphocytosis induced in mice by *Bordetella pertussis*. J. exp. Med. *121:* 49 (1965).

21. Rowlands, D.T.; Claman, H.N. and Kind, P.D.: The effect of endotoxin on the thymus of young mice. Amer. J. Pathol. *46:* 165 (1965).

22. Landy, M.; Sanderson, R.P.; Bernstein, M.T. and Lerner, E.M.T.: Involvement of thymus in immune response of rabbits to somatic polysaccharides of Gram-negative bacteria. Science *147:* 1591 (1965).

23. von Pirquet, C.E.: Das Verhalten der kutanen Tuberkulinreaktion während der Masern. Dtsch. med. Wschr. *34:* 1297 (1908).

24. Mellman, W.J. and Wetton, R.: Depression of the tuberculin reaction by attenuated measles virus vaccine. J. Lab. clin. Med. *61:* 453 (1963).

25. Starr, S. and Berkovich, S.: Effect of measles, gamma-globulin-modified measles and vaccine measles on the tuberculin test. New Engl. J. Med. *270:* 386 (1964).

26. Fanconi, G. and Wallgren, A.: Lehrbuch der Pädiatrie (Benno Schwabe, Basel 1954).

27. Bullock, W.E.: Studies of immune mechanisms in leprosy. I. Depression of delayed allergic response to skin test antigens. New Engl. J. Med. *278:* 298 (1968).

28. FLOERSHEIM, G. L.: Effect of Pertussis vaccine on the tuberculin reaction. Int. Arch. Allergy *26:* 340 (1965).
29. FLOERSHEIM, G. L.: Further studies pertaining to a *B. pertussis* factor inhibiting the tuberculin reaction. Experientia *22:* 219 (1966).
30. HOPFF, W. L.; FLOERSHEIM, G. L. and BUCHER, K.: Alteration der Tuberkulinreaktion durch mikrobielle Polysaccharide. Helv. Physiol. Acta *25:* 1 (1967).
31. FLOERSHEIM, G. L.: Pharmakologische Beeinflussbarkeit cellulärer Immunität. Z. naturwiss.-med. Grundlagenforsch. *2:* 307 (1965).
32. FLOERSHEIM, G. L. and SEILER, K.: Differential effects of immunosuppressive drugs on a cutaneous graft-versus-host reaction in chickens. Transplantation *5:* 1355 (1967).
33. SEILER, K.: Prüfung von Antiphlogistica an einer immunologischen Entzündung des Hühnchens. Arch. int. Pharmacodyn. *169:* 452 (1967).
34. FLOERSHEIM, G. L.: Facilitation of tumour growth by *Bacillus pertussis*. Nature *216:* 1235 (1967).
35. HIRANO, M.; SINKOVICS, J. G.; SHULLENBERGER, C. C. and HOWE, C. D.: Murine lymphoma: augmented growth in mice with pertussis vaccine-induced lymphocytosis. Science *158:* 1061 (1967).
36. HILL, W. C. and ROWLEY, D.: The origin of the antibody released into serum following injection of bacterial lipopolysaccharide. Austr. J. exp. Biol. med. Sci. *45:* 693 (1967).
37. MALAKIAN, A. and SCHWAB, J. H.: Immunosuppressant from group A streptococci. Science *159:* 880 (1968).

Author's address: PD. Dr. G. L. FLOERSHEIM, Pharmacological Institute, University of Basle, Spitalstrasse 21, *4000 Basle* (Switzerland).

Subject – Index

From the contents of

Antibiotica et Chemotherapia, Vol. 16

Experimental and Clinical Evaluation of the Tuberculostatics Capreomycin /
Isoxyl / Myambutol / Rifampicin

Edited by
E. FREERKSEN, J. THUMIN and E.-H. ORLOWSKI

S. KARGER · BASEL (Switzerland) · NEW YORK